Pressure Ulcers

Guidelines for Prevention and Management

Third Edition

Pressure Ulcers

Guidelines for Prevention and Management

Third Edition

JoAnn Maklebust, MSN, RN, CS, CNP

Clinical Nurse Specialist/Nurse Practitioner
Harper Hospital/Detroit Medical Center
Detroit, Michigan

Mary Y. Sieggreen, MSN, RN, CS, CNP, CVN

Clinical Nurse Specialist/Nurse Practitioner
Harper Hospital/Detroit Medical Center
Detroit, Michigan

Springhouse Corporation / Springhouse, Pennsylvania

To the patients and caregivers we know personally
and to those we touch with our writings, we dedicate this book.
—J.M. and M.Y.S.

Senior Publisher
Donna O. Carpenter

Clinical Director
Ann Barrow, RN, MSN, CCRN

Creative Director
Jake Smith

Design Director
John Hubbard

Executive Editor
H. Nancy Holmes

Clinical Project Manager
Beverly Ann Tscheschlog, RN

Editors
Audrey Selena Hughes, Peter H. Johnson, Jennifer P. Kowalak, Elizabeth Jacqueline Mills

Copy Editors
Dolores P. Matthews, Celia McCoy

Designers
Arlene Putterman (associate design director), Debra Moloshok (designer and project manager), Joseph John Clark, Jean Gardner (illustrator), Jeffrey Sklarow

Cover Illustration
Stage III pressure ulcer/Anatomical Chart Company

Electronic Production Services
Diane Paluba (manager), Joyce Rossi Biletz

Manufacturing
Deborah C. Meiris (director), Pat Dorshaw (manager), Otto Mezei (book production manager)

Editorial Assistants
Carol Caputo, Arlene Claffee, Tom Hasenmayer, Elfriede Young

Indexer
Ellen Brennan

The clinical procedures described and recommended in this publication are based on currently accepted clinical theory and practice and on consultation with medical and legal authorities. Nevertheless, they cannot be considered absolute and universal recommendations. For individual application, all recommendations must be considered in light of the patient's clinical condition and, before administration of new or infrequently used drugs, in light of the latest package-insert information. The authors and the publisher disclaim responsibility for any adverse effects resulting directly or indirectly from the suggested procedures, from any undetected errors, or from the reader's misunderstanding of the text.

For information, write Springhouse Corporation, 1111 Bethlehem Pike, P.O. Box 908, Springhouse, PA 19477-0908.

Printed in the United States of America.

PU3-D N O S

03   10 9 8 7 6 5 4 3 2

Library of Congress Cataloging-in-Publication Data
Maklebust, JoAnn.
  Pressure ulcers: guidelines for prevention and
  management / JoAnn Maklebust, Mary Sieggreen.—
  3rd ed.
    p. ; cm.
  Includes bibliographical references and index.
  ISBN 1-58255-035-2
  1. Bedsores—Prevention. 2. Bedsores—Nursing. I.
Sieggreen, Mary. II. Title.
    [DNLM: 1. Decubitus Ulcer—prevention & control.
2. Decubitus Ulcer—nursing. 3. Wound Healing.
WR 598 M235p 2000]
RL675.M35 2000
616.5'45—dc21   00-044625

Contents

Advisory Board

David Hoffman, JD
Assistant District Attorney
Philadelphia, Pa.

Mary Ellen Posthauer, RD, CD
MEP Healthcare and Dietary Services, Inc.
Evansville, Ind.

Steven Reger, PhD, CP
Director of Rehabilitation Technology
The Cleveland Clinic Foundation
Cleveland, Ohio

Marlys Staley, MS, PT
Independent Wound Care Consultant
Pleasant Plain, Ohio

David R. Thomas, MD, FACP
Saint Louis University
Division of Geriatrics
Saint Louis, Mo.

Foreword

This new edition of *Pressure Ulcers: Guidelines for Prevention and Management* continues to serve as an invaluable resource for the practicing wound care professional. JoAnn Maklebust and Mary Sieggreen, the book's authors, are recognized experts in the field and have contributed to the national guidelines on pressure ulcer prevention and management that were originally published in 1992 and 1994 by the Agency for Health Care Policy and Research, now the Agency for Healthcare Research and Quality.

The pressure ulcer problem continues to be a very significant one, in terms of numbers of cases and the costs entailed in managing these wounds. The true size of the pressure ulcer problem in the United States is unknown because pressure ulcers aren't a reportable condition for which national records are kept. Data from a variety of studies reveal pressure ulcer prevalence ranging from 2% to more than 15% among general hospital populations. Among spinal cord injury patients, a high-risk population, a 1998 study by Salzberg et al. estimated a 17% prevalence.* The same researchers postulated that treating pressure ulcers in all types of patients in the U.S. cost more than $1.3 billion dollars in 1998.

Maklebust and Sieggreen have addressed the pressure ulcer problem by taking a large volume of literature and distilling it to its essence. They have explained characteristics of the normal skin and how those characteristics interact with prolonged pressure that is in excess of normal soft tissue resistance to injury. For example, 32 mm Hg represents the generally accepted value for normal capillary closing pressure, a value used by many manufacturers of therapeutic support surfaces to show that their products are capable of reducing pressure to levels that will not cause damage. However, this value is unlikely to be accurate because it's a figure derived from studies done on normal, healthy, medical students in their twenties and thirties. The patient with a spinal cord injury and the elderly patient almost certainly have significantly lower capillary closing pressures. This means that effective support surfaces for these two types of patients would need to maintain supporting pressures at the tissue interface considerably lower than 32 mm Hg in order to prevent or delay skin breakdown.

The authors discuss the size and cost of the pressure ulcer problem based on their experiences and the findings of other researchers. An official data-

---

*Salzberg, C.A., Byrne, D.W., Cayten, C.G., Kabir, R., van Niewerburgh, M.A., Viehbeck, M., Long, H., Jones, E.C. (1998) "Predicting and preventing pressure ulcers in adults with paralysis," *Advances in Wound Care* 11(5), 237-246.

base on pressure ulcers is lacking — a situation that should be remedied by the federal government. Pressure ulcers should become a reportable condition so that centralized factual data would exist upon which to base the efficacy of prevention and treatment regimens such as those proposed in this book.

The section on wound healing and the types of products available will aid practicing professionals in making decisions about which products should or should not be used in a wound. The damage to wounds that is done by well-intentioned efforts on the part of caregivers is much greater than has been appreciated. For example, wet-to-dry dressings disrupt not only necrotic tissue in the wound bed, but also normal cells growing there. Utilizing the principles discussed by the authors will help minimize the use of inappropriate dressings, support surfaces, and systemic treatments and maximize the use of those products that will yield the best results in a given wound.

Maklebust and Sieggreen go beyond the individual patient to discuss the way in which a successful wound care program can be established, monitored, evaluated, and improved. Their work at Harper Hospital serves as a basis for the recommendations.

Readers of *Pressure Ulcers: Guidelines for Prevention and Management*, Third Edition, will find essential information that has been tried and proven by two of the most experienced and best-informed experts in the field of wound care. Those who read and master the content contained herein will be able to use their resulting knowledge base to bring about improvement in agency wound care programs throughout the country.

Mary L. Shannon, EdD, RN
Founding Member, National Pressure Ulcer Advisory Panel
Professor and Chair, Adult Health Nursing
School of Nursing
University of Texas at Galveston

Preface

Pressure ulcer management consumes a large percentage of healthcare time and resources and is financially and emotionally costly to the patient. There is little to guide the bedside practitioner in providing safe, economic, and effective care for patients with pressure ulcers. Scientific rationales for pressure ulcer management are often lacking in the health care literature. Consumers are confused by conflicting manufacturers' claims for products and equipment.

The Agency for Healthcare Research and Quality (formerly the Agency for Health Care Policy and Research) recognizes pressure ulcers as a continuing major health care problem in the United States. This book is an attempt to address this problem.

Our original interest in pressure ulcers was stimulated by the lack of standards for pressure ulcer care and by a seemingly disorganized attempt to educate the staff about pressure ulcer management. As clinical nurse specialists, we were consultants to the nursing staff providing care for patients with multiple complex problems. We received many requests to assist in planning care for chronic wound management, and we found that each patient care unit had a different favorite remedy for pressure ulcers. In our attempt to study the etiology of pressure ulcers and the scientific basis for treatment, we carefully researched the problem and then assumed accountability for investigating the management of pressure ulcers. This investigation led us to formal research on the topic, and we have published many reports to share our findings. However, these reports are scattered among several journals and are often inaccessible to staff nurses. Thus we decided to combine our findings with the findings of others who were studying pressure ulcers, and our original book evolved.

This third edition of *Pressure Ulcers: Guidelines for Prevention and Management* includes care maps, and policies and procedures have been updated to include the latest developments in caring for patients with pressure ulcers. The expanded content enhances the book's usefulness to caregivers in extended care facilities as well as in home care settings.

We hope that our work will be used by bedside caregivers to improve the quality of care for patients who are at risk for pressure ulcers and for patients who already have pressure ulceration.

Pressure ulcers are more than physical wounds. In our quest for scientific understanding, compassion and empathy must not be lost. Nothing stirs one to action more than seeing a part of oneself reflected in the suffering of others. The story on page 15 helps to place in perspective the true significance of pressure ulcers — a human condition.

JoAnn Maklebust
Mary Sieggreen

We gratefully acknowledge the ongoing work of the Pressure Ulcer Committee of Harper Hospital.

Chapter 1

Skin anatomy and physiology

The skin is the largest organ of the body and provides the interface between the body and the rest of the world. Actual or potential impairment of skin integrity has important implications for a person's well-being because loss of tissue integrity compromises skin function. A basic clinical knowledge of skin structure and function is the basis of good pressure-ulcer management. Through a thorough understanding of skin function, careful skin assessment, selection of appropriate interventions, and development of public education programs and materials, health care professionals can promote the maintenance of healthy skin and decrease the risk of pressure ulcers.

Human skin, also known as the cutis or integument, is a large organ that covers the entire external surface of the body. It's composed of tissue that constantly grows and renews itself. Skin appearance and texture reflect regional variations in blood flow, distribution of glandular structures, and hairiness. Healthy skin must adapt to all body contours and conform to all body movements.

The skin is a sensitive and readily accessible indicator of both physical and emotional status. Unscarred, disease-free, flexible skin has functional benefits as well as cosmetic appeal. Functionally, it provides the first line of host defense mechanisms and protects the integrity and functioning of internal organ systems. The psychosocial aspect of skin appearance is extremely important to a person's well-being. In our beauty-conscious society, cosmetic factors, such as scarring, can trigger social discrimination.

Characteristics and functions

The skin of an average-sized adult weighs 6 to 8 pounds and covers more than 20 square feet. Skin thickness ranges from $\frac{1}{50}$ of an inch over the eyelids to $\frac{1}{3}$ of an inch on the palms of the hands and the soles of the feet. Specialized skin cells harden to form nails and elongate to form hair. The pH of skin normally ranges from 4.5 to 5.5, thus providing the so-called pro-

Skin assessment

Assessment should address the skin's functional integrity. Findings indicate whether the skin is functioning properly or malfunctioning.

Function	Action	Findings
Temperature regulation	Palpate surface, including extremities; observe color.	• A warm flesh tone is normal. • Hot, red or purplish skin color suggests increased blood flow as a result of the body's response to inflammation or infection. • Cool or cold, pale skin suggests decreased blood flow to the surface as a result of impaired circulation from internal or external factors.
Sensory communication	Check temperature, tactile, and two-point discrimination on various parts of the body.	• Patient should be able to distinguish variations of temperature, sharpness, dullness, and pressure sensations against skin surface. • Diminished sensation may be generalized or may affect only a part of the body, such as lower extremities.
Storage of water and fat	Observe tone (turgor and tension) and body build.	• Smooth and resilient skin is normal. • Very wrinkled, withered, or dry skin may signal dehydration. • Taut, shiny skin may indicate underlying edema. • Pronounced bony prominences reflect low-body-weight persons. • Obesity may cause extra folds and consequent friction and irritation to approximating skin surfaces.
Absorption and excretion	Observe texture and moisture.	• Dry or oily skin texture depends on the quantity of body secretions. • Skin usually becomes drier with advancing age; excessive perspiration may reflect environmental factors or elevated body temperature.
Protection	Observe for loss of structural integrity.	• Skin surface should be free of eruptions or wounds.
Physical beauty	Observe texture, color, and general appearance.	• Blemishes, rashes, lesions, and discolored areas on the skin surface reflect inflammation, irritation, or trauma.

Adapted with permission from Gosnell, D.J. "Assessment and evaluation of pressure sores," *Nursing Clinics of North America* 22(2):401, February 1987.

tective acid mantle of the skin, which serves to maintain the skin's normal flora.

Assessment of the skin should consider the integrity of each of the skin's several vital functions, such as:

■ regulating body temperature
■ transmitting such sensations as touch, pressure, and pain
■ preventing excessive loss of body fluids
■ acting as an excretory organ
■ providing an interface between the body and its environment
■ protecting the inner tissues from invasion.
(See *Skin assessment.*)

Skin layers

Anatomically, the skin consists of epidermal, dermal, and subcutaneous layers of tissue, each of which has distinctive structures and cell types. (See *Layers of the skin,* page 4.) Each layer has its own function, which is interrelated with the functions of the other two.

Epidermis

The epidermis, or cuticle, is a thin, avascular structure that is further divided into five structurally and functionally distinct layers, or strata. (See *Layers of the epidermis,* page 5.)

Stratum corneum, or horny layer. This tough, outer layer of the epidermis provides the major chemical and mechanical defenses of the body. Its surface includes several layers of anucleated, flattened, desiccated cells, which are dead keratinocytes. Keratinocytes contain keratin, a protective protein that is the principal constituent of the epidermis and makes the skin waterproof. New keratinocytes are constantly being formed in the stratum germinativum, and dead (keratinized) cells are constantly shed; a new epidermis is formed about every 4 to 6 weeks. This normal shedding of the keratin layer of skin is a defense mechanism against infection.

Stratum lucidum. This densely packed, translucent line of flat cells is found only on the palms and soles. Thin skin has no stratum lucidum.

Stratum granulosum. This metabolically active layer contains active, differentiated keratinocytes and Langerhans' cells. Langerhans' cells originate in the bone marrow and migrate to all regions of the body, including the skin. They play a primary role in immune reactions and affect the inflammatory phase of allergic contact dermatitis. They participate in immunologic responses by functioning in antigen recognition and processing. They act as macrophages that ingest potential antigenic compounds to prevent allergic reaction. Langerhans' cells are particularly susceptible to destruction by ultraviolet irradiation, which may be important in the pathogenesis of sunlight-induced skin malignancy.

Layers of the skin

The skin consists of three functional and anatomic layers: epidermis, dermis, and subcutaneous tissue. Between the dermis and the epidermis lies the dermal-epidermal junction, consisting of contact points between the papillary dermis and the rete pegs of the epidermis.

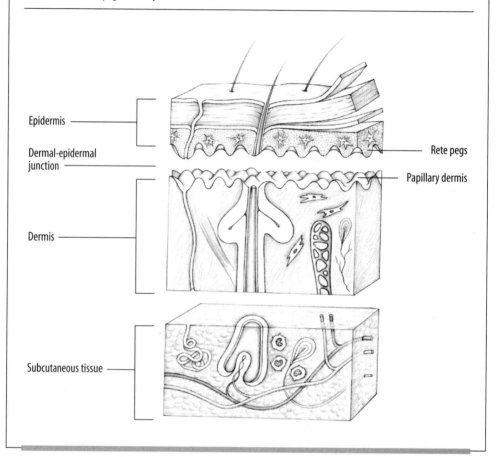

Stratum spinosum. Several layers of spinelike extensions of the basal layer constitute the spinosum. It may be considered part of the underlying basal layer, but it cannot regenerate. The stratum spinosum also contains large numbers of immunologically active Langerhans' cells.

Stratum germinativum, or basal layer. This single layer of cells is the only layer that can regenerate or undergo mitosis to form new cells. Cells that do not regenerate are repaired by scar formation.

Melanocytes migrate into this layer during embryologic development. Melanocytes release melanosomes — granules of melanin, a pigment that

Layers of the epidermis

The five layers, or strata, of the epidermis are, from the outermost inward, the corneum, lucidum, granulosum, spinosum, and germinativum.

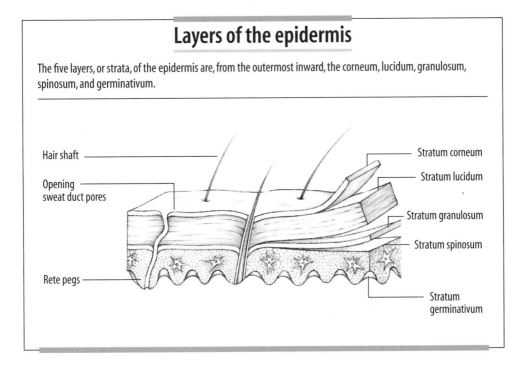

provides yellow, brown, and black skin tones. Everyone has approximately the same number of melanocytes, although melanosomes may be larger and more heterogeneous in aging skin. Darkly pigmented skin results from both increased size and enhanced function of the melanocyte. Normal melanocytes produce melanin at a steady rate to provide continual protection from damage to cellular DNA by solar radiation. Ultraviolet light increases skin pigmentation through two pathways: photo-oxidation of existing melanin and delay of new melanin production through the process of tanning.

Melanosomes migrate into keratinocytes in the basal layer and are degraded by intracellular lysosomal enzymes as the keratinocytes migrate upward to the stratum corneum.

Dermal-epidermal junction

Between the epidermis and dermis is the *basement membrane,* an undulating junction that both separates and attaches the epidermis and the dermis. The configuration of the dermal-epidermal junction provides structural support and allows exchange of fluids and cells between the skin layers.

The epidermis has an irregular surface, with downward fingerlike projections known as rete ridges or pegs. These pegs of epidermis interface with upward projections of the papillary dermis. The two opposing surface projections anchor the epidermis to the dermis and help prevent the epidermis

Layers of the dermis

The dermis consists of two layers, the papillary dermis and the reticular dermis.

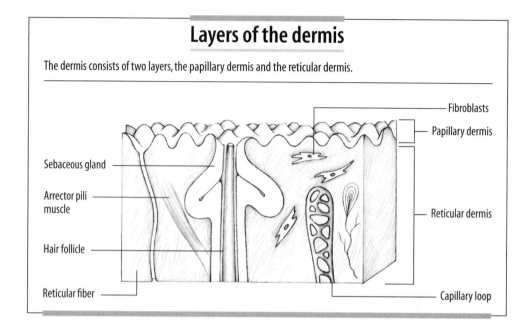

from sliding back and forth on the dermis. As the skin ages, this dermal-epidermal junction tends to flatten, as the contacting surfaces of epidermis and dermis decrease by one-third. This loss increases the potential for dermal-epidermal separation and places older people at risk for skin tears.

Dermis

The dermis, or corium, lies directly beneath the epidermis. It supports and supplies nutrition to the epidermis. The dermis consists primarily of fibroblasts and a strong extracellular matrix of collagen and elastic fibers that provide the skin with mechanical strength. It contains blood vessels, nerves, and integumentary appendages: hair, nails, and skin glands.

Fibroblasts are the most important cells of the dermis. Fibroblasts are connective tissue cells that perform the following functions:

■ produce collagen, a protein that gives the skin strength
■ synthesize the elastic fibers that help the skin stretch and recoil
■ produce ground substance that serves as a cushion and lubricant.

The dermis has two layers characterized by structural and functional differences. (See *Layers of the dermis.*) The outer layer, the *papillary dermis,* is formed of collagen and reticular fibers that are important for healing. Also present are capillaries that supply nourishment to support the metabolic activity of the epidermis and appendages. The inner layer, the *reticular dermis,* consists of thick networks of collagen bundles that enhance elasticity and anchor the skin to the subcutaneous tissue.

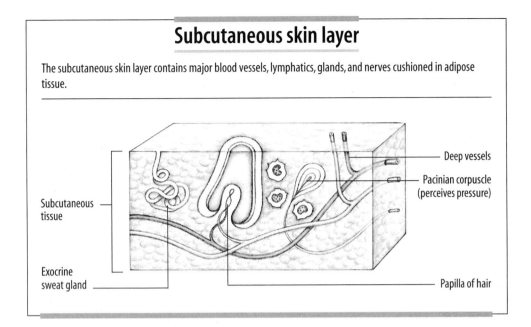

Subcutaneous skin layer

The subcutaneous skin layer contains major blood vessels, lymphatics, glands, and nerves cushioned in adipose tissue.

Deep vessels

Pacinian corpuscle (perceives pressure)

Subcutaneous tissue

Exocrine sweat gland

Papilla of hair

Subcutaneous tissue

The hypodermis, also called the subcutis or subcutaneous tissue, is made up of dense connective and adipose tissue. (See *Subcutaneous skin layer.*) It houses major blood vessels, lymphatics, and nerves; acts as a heat insulator; and provides a nutritional depot that is used during illness or starvation. The subcutaneous fat also acts as a mechanical shock absorber and helps the skin move easily over the underlying structures. The distribution of the subcutaneous fat tissue depends on age, heredity, and gender.

Fascia

Below the subcutaneous layer is a layer of superficial fascia, a type of dense, firm, membranous connective tissue that covers muscles, nerves, and blood vessels. Fascia varies in function, thickness, and strength depending on its location. The superficial fascia connects the skin to subjacent parts, facilitating movement. The deep fascia, which is less elastic, forms sheath or envelope-like coverings for muscles, blood vessels, and nerves.

Blood supply

The skin's blood supply comes from cutaneous branches of arteries in the subcutaneous muscles. With the exception of the perforating muscular vessels, most of the cutaneous circulation is microcirculation (arterioles, capillaries, and venules), which supplies oxygen and nutrients directly to sur-

Cutaneous blood supply

The illustration depicts the microcirculation in the dermis and subcutaneous tissue.

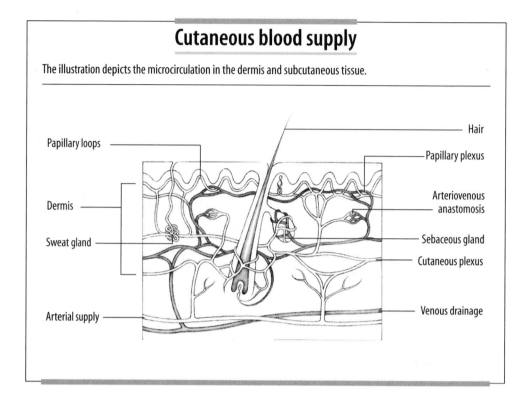

rounding fibroblasts and to basal keratinocytes by diffusion across the basement membrane of the vessel.

The blood supply to the skin originates in the underlying muscles. (See *Cutaneous blood supply*.) The cutaneous vasculature consists of arteries that supply the blood to the skin, capillary beds that permit blood flow from arteries to veins, and veins that drain the blood from the skin.

Blood pressure in the cutaneous capillary beds is far lower than in the larger arteries. It drops from approximately 32 mm Hg at the arteriolar end of the capillary bed to approximately 12 mm Hg at the venous end, averaging about 20 mm Hg.

The vasculature of the dermis is the most expansive of any organ system. The main purpose of this vast blood supply to the skin is to regulate body temperature. Unlike muscle and subcutaneous fat, the skin does not use all of its blood supply to nourish the tissue and, in fact, is oversupplied with blood when compared with its metabolic needs. Muscle and fatty tissue do not tolerate ischemia or hypoxia, and they are more susceptible to the effects of pressure than are the dermis and epidermis.

Pressure ulcers form when the relationship between anatomy and physiology of the cutaneous blood supply is compromised. They usually result from a prolonged failure of capillary blood supply as a consequence of externally applied pressure.

Clinical implication of skin color

Human skin comes in a continuum of colors from white to yellow, tan, red, dark brown, and black. In general, color has no effect on structure and function, but subtle variations can lead to different skin care needs and require different assessment skills. Most of the published studies deal with black or dark brown skin.

The variation in melanin pigmentation is the most obvious difference between light and dark skin. As mentioned earlier, in the section on skin layers, the number of melanocytes does not differ with skin color. In darker skin, the melanocytes are more active and melanosomes, or melanin granules, are larger. Electron microscopy of melanosomes shows that melanosomes involved in the synthesis of different-colored pigments (black or brown, red or yellow) have distinctive shapes and internal structures.

Another difference between very dark and very pale skin is the structure of the stratum corneum, the outer layer of the epidermis. Its thickness is the same, but in dark skin it's denser and has more cell layers. For this reason, dark skin resists chemical irritation and offers a more effective barrier against external stimuli.

Dark skin is generally smooth and dry. As the stratum corneum flakes off, it gives the underlying skin an "ashy" look. Application of petroleum jelly or lotion helps to eliminate flaking. Soap should be used sparingly on dry skin of any color. Use of lanolin-based lotion is preferable to either water-based or perfumed lotions, which dry the skin.

Changes in skin color, such as those characterizing erythema, are not easily recognizable in patients whose normal skin color is dark. Good lighting is particularly essential to an accurate assessment of pressure-related skin changes. Bennett has studied the problem of assessing darkly pigmented skin and has developed criteria to facilitate accurate assessment. The best way to assess erythema is to use the sensitive dorsal surface of the fingers to palpate the area for increased warmth, a feeling of tightness, and areas of hardness under the skin.

Hypopigmentation frequently accompanies healing of superficial injuries to dark skin. When the outer layer heals, the melanin commonly requires time to reach the stratum corneum. Postinjury hypopigmentation may cause a patient more anxiety than the primary cutaneous lesion.

The etiology of postinflammatory hypopigmentation is unknown, but it's thought to be familial and may be associated with diabetes mellitus, pernicious anemia, hypothyroidism, and hyperthyroidism. Vitiligo, or partial loss of pigmentation, can occur in all races, but dark-skinned persons are more frequently affected. The most commonly affected sites are the face and

Age-related skin changes

The illustration at left schematizes youthful skin. Thinning and other changes that occur with aging are shown at right.

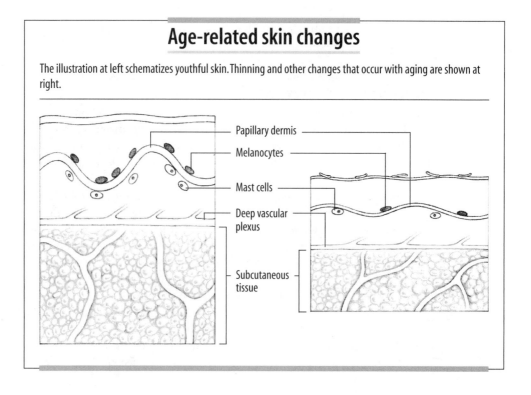

around the eyes, the chest, the axilla, the groin, and the dorsal aspects of the hands. The pale patches are sensitive to ultraviolet rays and burn easily if exposed to sunlight. Few skin changes other than the absence of melanocytes in the affected area accompany vitiligo.

Posttraumatic keloid formation is more common in dark-skinned than in light-skinned people. Males and females are equally affected. These dense collagenous growths are easily distinguished by clawlike projections but may be confused with hypertrophic scarring. Keloid tissue tends to be pruritic and may be very painful or tender. Treatment is difficult because keloids recur and may even enlarge after surgical attempts at correction. Intralesional injection of corticosteroid solution has demonstrated varied degrees of success. Recently, the carbon dioxide laser has been used with good results. Keloid formation can occur without injury and also may be familial.

Age-related changes

Dramatic changes in the skin occur with aging. (See *Age-related skin changes*.) Sweat glands diminish in number. The epithelial and fatty layers of tissue atrophy and become thin. The thickness of subcutaneous fat on the legs or forearms diminishes, even if abdominal or hip fat remains abundant. One result of the general loss of fat from the subcutaneous tissue is the relative prominence of the bony protuberances of the thorax, scapula, trochanters, and knees. The loss of this valuable padding contributes to the development of pressure ulcers.

The appearance of skin changes with progressive destruction of the delicate architecture of the dermal connective tissue. Dermal fibroblasts, which are among the few body cells that possess a finite replicative capacity (50 to 100 doublings), cease replicating. Collagen and elastin shrink and degenerate. Collagen content of the skin decreases by approximately 1% per year throughout adult life. The net effect of all these changes is thin, dry, and inelastic skin that is increasingly susceptible to separation of dermis and epidermis as minor friction or shearing forces cause an injury known as skin tear.

Aging people may begin to complain of dryness and itchiness of the skin. They also complain of being cold. Most likely, both are due to loss of insulating subcutaneous fat. Graying of the hair and pallor or loss of ruddiness of light-colored skin may result as melanin production diminishes and cutaneous blood vessels become smaller.

In general, aging people tend to lose their body hair and to develop wrinkles, which are permanent infoldings of the skin and subcutaneous structures. Repeated stress on the skin during changes in facial expression is a partial reason that wrinkles are most noticeable on the face. The single most important factor that causes wrinkles and other age-related changes is exposure to sun; heredity and hormonal fluctuations also contribute.

The thin, fragile skin of the elderly needs special care. Intermittent gentle cleansing with warm water alone is generally sufficient for daily skin hygiene. During the cleansing and drying processes, care should be taken to minimize friction against the skin. Use of a soft cloth to pat the skin dry is better than rubbing with a towel. Forceful scrubbing and use of caustic agents and harsh cleansers should be avoided.

Selected references

Bennett, M.A. "Spotting pressure ulcers in patients with dark skins," *Nursing96* 26(6):24q-24r, June 1996.

Brown-Etris, M. "Measuring healing in wounds," *Advances in Wound Care* 8(4):53-58, 1995.

Grous, C.A., et al. "Skin integrity in patients undergoing prolonged operations," *Journal of Wound Ostomy Continence Nursing* 24(2):86-91, 1997.

Lewicki, L.J., et al. "Patient risk factors for pressure ulcers during cardiac surgery," *AORN Journal* 65(5):933-942, 1997.

Maklebust, J. "Pressure ulcer assessment," *Clinics in Geriatric Medicine* 13(3):455-481, August 1997.

Maklebust, J. "Pressure ulcer staging systems: Intent, limitations, expectations," *Advances in Wound Care* 8(4):11-14, 1995.

Margolis, D. "Definition of pressure ulcer," *Advances in Wound Care* 8(4):8-10, 1995.

McGuckin, M. "The case for evidence-based practice standards," *Advances in Wound Care* 11:46, 1998.

Robson, M.C. "Wound infection: A failure of wound healing caused by an imbalance of bacteria," *Surgical Clinics of North America* 77(3):637-650, 1997.

Steed, D.L. "The role of growth factor in wound healing," *Surgical Clinics of North America* 77(3):575-586, 1997.

Stotts, N.A. "Evidence-based practice: What is it and how is it used in wound care," *Nursing Clinics of North America* 34(4):955-963, 1999.

Stotts, N.A., and Cavanaugh, C.E. "Assessing the patient with a wound," *Home Healthcare Nurse* 17(1):27-36, 1999.

Stotts, N.A., et al. "Underutilization of pressure ulcer risk assessment in hip fracture patients," *Advances in Wound Care* 11(1):32-38, 1998.

Stotts, N.A., and Hunt, T.R. "Pressure ulcers, managing bacterial colonization and infection," *Clinics in Geriatric Medicine* 13:565-573, 1997.

Straus, S.E. "Evidence-based medicine as a tool," *Hospital Medicine* 59:762-765, 1998.

Quigley, S.M., and Curley, M.A.Q. "Skin integrity in the pediatric population: Preventing and managing pressure ulcers," *JSPN* 1(1):7-18April-June 1996.

Van Rijswijk, L., and Braden, B. "Pressure ulcer patient and wound assessment: An AHCPR clinical practice guideline update," *Ostomy/Wound Management* 45(1A suppl):56s-67s, 1999.

Chapter 2
The challenge

Common terms used for tissue destruction resulting from prolonged pressure are "bedsore," "decubitus ulcer," "pressure sore," and "pressure ulcer." "Decubitus ulcer" and "bedsore" originated from the observation that ulcers frequently occur in persons who are bedridden. However, patients need not be lying down or bedridden to develop tissue ulcerations related to pressure. Ulcers can form when a patient constantly maintains any position. Because the primary cause is pressure, "pressure ulcer" most accurately describes both the lesion and the etiology.

The size of the problem

The incidence and prevalence of pressure ulcers vary among populations. The variability reflects methodologic inconsistency in interpreting the data. In 1989, the National Pressure Ulcer Advisory Panel sponsored a pressure ulcer consensus development conference. Participants defined the following problems in calculating accurate incidence and prevalence rates:

■ Studies often confused incidence (onset of new cases over time) and prevalence (number of patients with pressure ulcers in a facility on a given day).

■ Study populations varied.

■ Sources of information ranged from direct observation of patients to chart reviews of discharged patients.

■ Investigators used different definitions to stage pressure ulcers.

The question of stage definitions has been central. Prevalence rates reported in the literature vary, depending on whether stage I ulcers are defined as superficial breaks in the epidermis or reddened areas of unbroken skin.

Despite the problem of inaccurate statistics identified over a decade ago, pressure ulcers remain a national health concern. Although incidence is difficult to determine, published estimates have ranged as high as 30% among elderly bedridden and chairbound patients at an acute care hospital. The risk of pressure ulcers persists as long as a patient resides in a long-term care facility. The incidence of pressure ulcers is highest during the first few weeks after admission to a long-term care facility, but this may be because a clinician examining a new patient may be the first to diagnose a previously unrecognized pressure ulcer.

Patients in long-term care facilities may be more "at risk," yet the reported prevalence of pressure ulcers is no higher in such facilities than in acute care hospitals. About 20% of patients with pressure ulcers develop them at home, and these figures represent pressure ulcer patients being cared for by health care professionals. The total number of homebound patients who have pressure ulcers remains unknown.

The cost of pressure ulcers

It is impossible to predict the total national cost of pressure ulcers because no one knows the precise incidence and prevalence. However, in 1994, Miller and Delozier estimated that the total national cost of pressure ulcer treatment exceeded $1.335 billion. Published estimates of treatment costs vary widely, perhaps because data collection is all too often inconsistent or inaccurate. Nosocomial infections and other hospital complications add to consumption of health resources among patients at risk for pressure ulcers. The estimated cost of healing one pressure ulcer including long-term care and hospital costs was $2,731. A single pressure ulcer can lengthen a patient's hospital stay by a factor of 3.5 to 5. Xakellis and colleagues studied the actual cost of preventing pressure ulcers. Not surprisingly, the cost increased in parallel with the patient's level of risk. Turning patients was the most expensive component of prevention.

Of course, in addition to financial costs, there are a number of "intangible" costs, as stated by Alterescu:

" . . .the nurse who is emotionally drained because the pressure ulcer patient requires frequent, difficult dressing changes contributes to the nonfinancial cost of pressure ulcers. Other patients in the facility pay the penalty of receiving less nursing care, or waiting longer for certain services, when a person with a pressure ulcer requires treatment. If a facility is operating at capacity, there may be increased waiting times for ancillary services or admission because patients with pressure ulcers require services. Most importantly, irrespective of the financial costs to treat pressure ulcers, they are a source of anxiety and pain for the patient, the family, and the staff."

Nurses and other health care professionals must not allow such "intangible" costs to be underestimated because pressure ulcers are indeed more than physical wounds. (See *Case history: On deeper reflection*.)

Case history: On deeper reflection

Mrs. Smith had been transferred to our geriatrics and chronic disease ward. Her lengthy record looked painfully similar to so many others I had read during the first five months of my geriatrics fellowship. She was 87 years old. The chart listed her diagnoses as dementia, pressure sores, incontinence, diabetes, anemia, malnutrition, and multiple fractures. The history did not describe the fractures.

She was bedridden and responsive only to painful stimuli. An indwelling urinary catheter and a gastrostomy feeding tube were in place. Her albumin level was 1.5. She had been in this state for at least three months, as she had been in the transferring hospital for that long after being admitted there in a hypoglycemic coma. The head nurse informed me that Mrs. Smith was hypothermic.

"The temperature is 94.8 rectally," the nurse said as I entered Mrs. Smith's room. She cried out, seemingly in pain, as the nurse turned her on her left side. The rest of her vital signs were surprisingly normal. She had many pressure sores, including large ones on both heels that were still covered by thick, black eschar.

"I'm Dr. Sachs, Mrs. Smith," I introduced myself. I placed a hopefully reassuring hand on the patient's shoulder. Her skin was cool and clammy. She cried out as I touched her. "I'm one of the doctors here on the floor," I said. "I'm going to examine you to see what we can do to help you feel better." I began to examine an open wound over her right trochanter. The hip sore was 2 by 3 centimeters on the surface but was extensively undermined.

Wound infestation?

As I moved forward to look deeper into the sore, I thought I saw movement within the wound. I immediately felt repulsed and feared that there might be maggots in this poor woman's hip. I saw no organisms, the wound looked clean, and there was a strange clearness in the center of the crater. I took a deep breath and looked again at the ulcer. Once more, I noted movement within the sore. This time the move-

ment paralleled my own motions. I moved closer and peered deeper into the cavity. Right in the center, in the deepest portion of the wound, I saw my own reflection staring back at me.

Again I looked to convince myself that I was indeed seeing my own reflection, moving in the wound as I moved outside of it. I moved the opening in the skin back and forth to see more of the tissues below. As more was revealed, it dawned on me that I was seeing myself in Mrs. Smith's hip prosthesis, the shiny artificial head of her femur mirroring the image of my face. I took one more look at myself and then left the room.

Sad realization

Seeing oneself in a pressure sore is a stark and frightening vision, disturbing on many levels. In addition to the grotesque wound and personal reflection, it seemed to mirror the topsy-turvy medical care given to many such patients. Mrs. Smith came from a hospital where she received mechanical ventilation for a respiratory arrest suffered when she was hypoglycemic. She had pleural effusions tapped and analyzed and innumerable laboratory tests performed. Yet she lay long enough without being turned for all the tissue between her skin and bones to necrotize.

It is sad that somewhere in the course of a dementing process, Mrs. Smith lost many of the characteristics that most of us associate with meaningful adult life. It is sadder still that she received medical treatment that forgot about her as a human being.

Debilitated and dependent patients need us most to reach out and care for them when we are starting to push them away. It is our distancing of ourselves from these people that is the true dehumanizing act.

Frequently, I have caught myself praying that I would not contract any of the horrible diseases I saw during residency. Now, mostly, I pray, "Please, dear Lord, do not let me die with pressure sores."

Greg A. Sachs, MD
Chicago

Adapted with permission from JAMA, vol. 259, p. 2145, April 8, 1988. ©.1988, American Medical Association.

Separating fact from fiction

Health care practices must be grounded in science. All too often, "old wives' tales" and "lore" permeate teachings of care of the ill. Pressure ulcer care is no exception. Common misconceptions about pressure ulcers may prevent caregivers from providing appropriate care. The following are a few common misconceptions:

■ All pressure ulcers develop because of poor nursing care.
■ All pressure ulcers are preventable.
■ All pressure ulcers result from pressure only.
■ Massaging reddened tissue helps prevent pressure ulcers.
■ The use of specialty equipment, such as air-fluidized beds, prevents pressure ulcers independently and indefinitely.

Poor nursing care is not the only cause of pressure ulcers. Most pressure ulcers are preventable, but even the most conscientious care cannot prevent some ulcers. A patient who falls at home and remains in the same position until help arrives will have soft-tissue ischemia over bony prominences that were subjected to pressure. The tissue breakdown may not become evident until the patient is hospitalized, but the original damage occurred at home. Another example is the patient who is in a catabolic state. Poor nutrition or chronic disease commonly causes loss of pressure-absorbing soft-tissue padding over the bone and consequent pressure ulcers, even in the face of careful preventive measures. LaPuma, in discussing the ethics of pressure ulcers, questioned why pressure ulcers are considered a sign of inadequate care. He pointed out that failure of the heart, lungs, or kidneys is not considered a sign of inadequate care. So why, he asked, should failure of the skin be treated as inadequate health care when it may be only a sign of physical decline and mortality?

Pressure is seldom the only cause of a pressure ulcer. More often, two causes (for example, pressure and shear) or frequently three (such as pressure, shear, and friction) coexist. At a sufficiently high level of shear, vascular occlusion occurs at half the pressure that causes occlusion in the absence of shear. Isolated shear and isolated pressure are equally rare.

Historically, nurses were taught to massage reddened tissue over bony prominences. In recent years, massage has gone out of favor. Massaging reddened, hyperemic tissue may cause maceration in the already ischemic tissue. Massaging the hyperemic area may rupture capillaries that already are maximally dilated to compensate for temporary ischemia.

The use of specialty beds to relieve pressure may help prevent pressure ulcerations. However, the use of such equipment does not eliminate the need for vigilance and regular patient assessment. High-tech equipment may give a caregiver a false sense of security. Remember that no piece of equipment ever substitutes for good nursing care.

Experience-based practice

A substantial amount of literature offers suggestions for health care professionals who are attempting to reduce or prevent pressure ulcers. The information in many articles is derived from experience, intuition, and common sense. Few reports are the result of systematic study. In the current and future health care environment of monetary limits and nursing shortages, hard data support decisions about where to direct energy and dollars.

In an attempt to enhance the quality and decrease the cost of health care, in 1989 the U.S. government established the Agency for Health Care Policy and Research (AHCPR), now renamed the Agency for Healthcare Research and Quality (AHRQ). One of its missions is to establish clinical practice guidelines to assist practitioners in the prevention and treatment of various clinical conditions. In May 1992 and December 1994, the agency released guidelines for preventing and treating pressure ulcers, providing practitioners with current practice parameters based on a synthesis of research findings and expert opinion. Each guideline was developed by an interdisciplinary panel convened by the agency. To support their recommendations, panel members evaluated hundreds of abstracts from the National Library of Medicine and then developed scientific evidence tables and methodology ratings.

The release of clinical practice guidelines placed pressure ulcers in the limelight and had a significant impact on patient care. The Joint Commission for Accreditation of Healthcare Organizations (JCAHO) recommends use of the clinical practice guidelines; the Health Care Financing Administration (HCFA) used these guidelines to create medical policy and reimbursement criteria; and auditors of long-term care facilities use the guidelines as quality criteria. The guidelines for prevention and treatment of pressure ulcers are meant to be living documents — that is, interested individuals and organizations must make them keep pace with science, research, and technology. There is much work to be done to fill scientific gaps noted by the AHRQ Pressure Ulcer Guideline Panels.

Goals of care

"Pressure ulcers" may be an admitting medical diagnosis or a nursing diagnosis for a patient with other medical problems. To help determine goals of care, one must take into account the whole person. Nursing goals must be consistent with both patient and medical goals. For example, if there is no hope for recovery and a patient will receive only palliative care, the goal of care related to the pressure ulcer would be to provide comfort. A frequent, painful dressing change to debride a pressure ulcer would not be consistent with goals for a patient who is not expected to live long. However, for another patient who has developed a pressure ulcer, or for one whose medical treatment places him at risk for developing a pressure ulcer, the goal may include measures to reduce the risk or heal the ulcer. Decisions relating to treatment, therefore, reflect the goals of care.

Summary

When evaluating pressure ulcer management, health care professionals must consider all of the following:

■ goals of patient care
■ physiological principles
■ science-based interventions
■ judicious use of products.

The real key to the pressure ulcer problem is to focus on prevention. The authors hope that this text will heighten interest in interventions aimed at preventing pressure ulcers and will provide a guide to the effective management of those patients who already have developed pressure ulcers.

Selected references

Allman, R.M. "Pressure ulcer prevalence, incidence, risk factors, and impact," *Clinics in Geriatric Medicine* 13(3):421-436, August 1997.

Alterescu, V. "The financial costs of inpatient pressure ulcers to an acute care facility," *Decubitus* 2(3):14-23, 1989.

Barezak, C.A. "Fourth national pressure ulcer prevalence survey," *Advances in Wound Care* 10(4):18-26, 1997.

Bergstrom, N., et al. "Multi-site study of incidence of pressure ulcers and the relationship between risk level, demographic characteristics, diagnoses and prescription of preventive interventions," *Journal of the American Geriatric Society* 44(1):22-30, 1996.

Capobianco, M.L., and McDonald, D.D. "Factors affecting the predictive validity of the Braden Scale," *Advances in Wound Care* 9(6):32-6, 1996.

Frantz, R.A. "Measuring prevalence and incidence of pressure ulcers," *Advances in Wound Care* 10(1):21-24, 1997.

LaPuma, J. "The ethics of pressure ulcers," *Decubitus* 4(2):43-44, 1991.

Lewicki, L.J., et al. "Patient risk factors for pressure ulcers during cardiac surgery," *AORN Journal* 65:933-42, 1997.

Miller, H., and Delozier, J. *Cost Implications of the Pressure Ulcer Treatment Guideline.* Columbia, Md.: Center for Health Policy Studies. Contract No. 28-91-0070. 17 p. Sponsored by the Agency for Health Care Policy and Research, 1994.

National Association for Home Care. *Home care basic statistics.* Washington, DC: National Association for Home Care, 1997.

Norton, D. "Calculating the risk: Reflections on the Norton Scale," *Advances in Wound Care* 9(6):38-43, 1996.

Thomas, S. "The cost of wound care in the community," *Journal of Wound Care* 4:395-398, 1995.

Tourtual, D.M., et al. "Predictors of hospital-acquired heel pressure ulcers," *Ostomy/Wound Management* 43:24-8, 1997.

Xakellis, G.C., et al. "Cost of pressure ulcer prevention in long-term care," *Journal of the American Geriatric Society* 43(5):496-501, 1995.

Welch, H.G., et al. "The use of the medicare home health care services," *New England Journal of Medicine* 335:324-329, 1998.

Chapter 3
Etiology and pathophysiology

Pressure ulcers are the clinical manifestation of local tissue death. Cellular metabolism depends on blood vessels to carry nutrients to the tissues and to remove waste products. When the soft tissues are subjected to prolonged pressure and insufficient nutrients, cells die. Pressure ulcers usually occur in soft tissue over bony prominences that remain in contact with compressing surfaces. Unrelieved pressure applied to the skin surface exerts its greatest force near the bone, so that much damage may occur between skin and bone before it becomes apparent when the skin is broken. Many other factors — primarily shear, friction, excessive moisture, and possibly infection — interact to mechanically damage soft tissue.

Pressure

Pressure, the amount of force exerted on a given area, is measured in millimeters of mercury (mm Hg). External pressure greater than capillary perfusion pressure compresses the vessels and causes ischemia. Normal capillary filling pressure is approximately 32 mm Hg at the arteriolar end and 12 mm Hg at the venous end. External pressure greater than 32 mm Hg may cause tissue damage by restricting blood flow to the area. Continued pressure on soft tissue causes capillaries to collapse and form thrombi. Oxygen and nutrients can no longer reach the involved tissues, toxic metabolic by-products accumulate, and cells die.

Body tissues have different tolerances for pressure and ischemia. Muscle is more sensitive to compression than skin. The deeper muscle tissue may be necrotic before damage to the overlying skin is apparent. Thus, the ulcers of many bedridden patients may reflect pressure-induced muscle ischemia, which can develop in as little as 2 days.

The force of pressure increases as the affected body surface area decreases. For instance, the pressure on a ballerina's toe is 2,600 mm Hg, and the

Pressure points in various body positions

Arrows show important pressure points on patients in supine, prone, side-lying, and sitting positions.

Supine

Prone

Side

Sitting

pressure against the skin of a person floating in water is 20 mm Hg. Clinical studies have shown that pressures on the buttocks and ischial tuberosities of a healthy person who is supine or sitting are high enough to cause tissue ischemia. (See *Pressure points in various body positions.*) Pressure over bony prominences intensifies the response of soft tissue and blood vessels. If the external pressure exceeds venous capillary pressure, leakage from the vessels causes edema, which further impedes circulation and again increases the pressure. Eventually, when the interstitial pressure equals or exceeds the arterial pressure, blood flows through the vessel walls into the tissue (nonblanchable erythema). The continued capillary occlusion, lack of oxygen and nutrients, and buildup of toxic wastes lead to necrosis of muscle, subcutaneous tissue and, ultimately, the dermis and epidermis. This irreversible ischemic response has been referred to as the "no reflow" phenomenon.

The normal response to prolonged pressure is a change in body position before tissue ischemia occurs. In pressure ulceration, this time-pressure relationship is critical. Low pressure endured for long periods of time is believed to be more significant in producing pressure ulcers than higher pressure of short duration. For example, constant pressure of 70 mm Hg for longer than 2 hours can cause irreversible tissue damage, and a short interval at 240 mm Hg may cause only minimal changes. If the time-pressure threshold is reached or exceeded, tissue damage continues even after pressure is released.

Not surprisingly, free radicals play a significant role in pressure ulceration. In animal studies, damage to the vascular system and parenchyma has been consistent with an ischemia/reperfusion insult initiated through a free radical mechanism. Neutrophils, which accumulate at the border between viable and nonviable tissue, presumably generate free radicals and contribute to proteolytic digestion of the connective tissue. Production of free radicals may initiate a cascade of events that significantly contribute to pressure ulceration.

Repetition of pressure on vulnerable bony areas of the body is important and needs to be considered by clinicians. Although pressure ulceration can result from one period of sustained pressure, most pressure ulcers probably occur secondary to repeated ischemic events without adequate time for recovery.

Pressure ulcers can form over any bony prominence or any area of soft tissue that is subjected to prolonged pressure — over the sacrum, coccyx, ischial tuberosities, greater trochanters, elbows, heels, scapulae, occipital bone, sternum, ribs, iliac crests, patellae, lateral malleoli, and medial malleoli. Because most body weight, as well as the major bony prominences, is in the lower half of the body, that is where most pressure ulcers occur. Two-thirds of all pressure ulcers occur in the area of the pelvic girdle. (See *Common sites of pressure ulcers,* page 22.)

Untreated contractures may cause pressure ulceration. At the very least, caregivers must consider any contractures as a possible cause of pressure necrosis. Assessment for pressure ulcer risk must include the pressure exerted by dysfunctional alignment of the body and its extremities. Contract-

Common sites of pressure ulcers

The illustration depicts the most common locations where pressure ulcers develop.

Scapula

Iliac crest

Sacrum

Trochanter

Ischium

Lateral edge of foot

Lateral malleolus

Heel

ed limbs may exert pressure on adjacent areas other than bony prominences. A contracted limb may exert more pressure on the mattress than does a non-contracted limb. Contracture of a leg or foot may cause pressure ulcers of the lower extremity. Remember to consider the contracture, as well as the ulcer, when assessing the patient for tissue breakdown.

One of the most commonly overlooked factors in the development of pressure ulcers is sitting posture. Preventive measures include limited use of

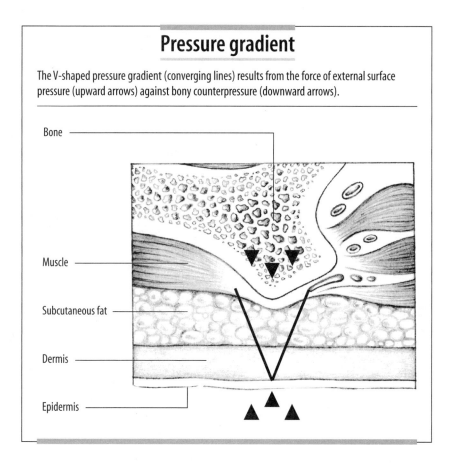

Pressure gradient

The V-shaped pressure gradient (converging lines) results from the force of external surface pressure (upward arrows) against bony counterpressure (downward arrows).

Bone

Muscle

Subcutaneous fat

Dermis

Epidermis

the geriatric chair and proper lumbar support to prevent the kyphotic or slumping position. If a footstool is used, it must not position the feet so high that body weight shifts from the posterior thighs to the ischial tuberosities.

Pressure gradient

When blood vessels, muscle, subcutaneous fat, and skin are compressed between bone and the surface where a patient is lying or sitting, pressure is transmitted from the body surface toward the bone, and the bone exerts counterpressure. These opposing forces result in a cone-shaped pressure gradient. (See *Pressure gradient.*) Pressure affects all of the tissue between the external surface and the skeletal anatomy, but the greatest tissue destruction is at the bony interface. Because fat and muscle have little tolerance for decreased blood flow, they are less resistant than skin to pressure. Therefore, destruction in the subcutaneous tissues and muscle may be far worse than the surface damage indicates. Assessment of pressure ulcer size must take into consideration the presence of unseen necrosis in the area of the pressure gradient.

Pressure ulcer formation

There are two schools of thought regarding where and how pressure ulcers begin. The top-to-bottom view is that tissue destruction occurs first in the epidermis and later in the deeper tissue layers. The earliest discernible clinical sign of damage in that model is blanchable erythema. Another school of thought uses a bottom-to-top model, in which injury to skeletal muscle precedes evident damage to the skin surface. Both models of pressure necrosis may be correct, and superficial and deep pressure ulcers may have different etiologies. Only continued research on the basic science of pressure ulceration will determine the true etiologic model.

Shear

Shear is a mechanical force that is parallel rather than perpendicular to an area. The main effect of shear occurs in deep tissues. Elevating the head of the bed increases shear and pressure in the sacral and coccygeal areas. Body weight pulls the deep tissues attached to the bone in one direction while the surface (skin) or tissue sticks to the sheets and remains stationary. The body skeleton actually slides downward inside the skin. (See *Shearing force over the sacrum.*) The skin in the sacral area may pucker. The mechanical forces can obstruct or tear and stretch blood vessels. Shear is greatest when a caregiver drags a patient along the surface of the sheets during repositioning or allows the patient to slide down from high-Fowler's position. Minimizing shearing forces involves raising the head of the bed to no more than a 30-degree angle, except for short periods while the patient is eating or if medically contraindicated.

The presence of shearing forces decreases the time that tissue can remain under pressure before ischemia or destruction occurs. In the presence of shear, vascular occlusion may occur at half the usual amount of pressure. Shearing forces may cause triangular-shaped sacral ulcers with tunneling or deep sinus tracts.

Friction

The force of two surfaces moving across one another causes friction and may create a wound that resembles an abrasion. Friction is a common cause of skin damage in patients who are unable to reposition themselves. Pulling a patient across the bed linen may rub away the protective outer layer of skin.

Shearing force over the sacrum

Shearing force develops over the sacrum as gravity exerts downward pull on the skeleton while skin adherence to the underlying surface tends to hold the body stationary.

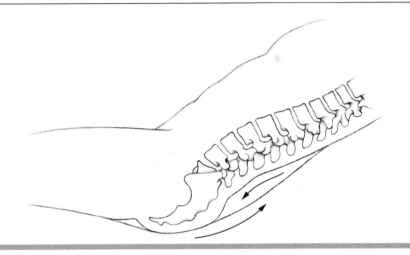

This mechanical erosion of surface tissue increases the potential for deeper tissue damage because friction is the precursor of shear. When transcutaneous water loss becomes abnormally high, moisture can accumulate on the surface of the body. When the interface between body and bedding is moist, the coefficient of friction rises sharply and, if it becomes great enough, actually causes the skin to stick to the sheets. If the head of the bed is high, gravity pulls the skeleton downward, and the friction and shearing forces cause necrosis in the sacral area.

Patients who have uncontrollable movements or spastic conditions, patients who wear braces or appliances that rub against the skin, and the elderly are at high risk for tissue damage by friction. Dry lubricants, such as cornstarch, and adherent dressings with slippery backings can help keep friction at a minimum.

Excessive moisture

Moist skin is five times as likely to become ulcerated as dry skin. Constant exposure to wetness can waterlog or macerate the skin. Maceration becomes a contributing factor in the etiology of pressure when the excessive moisture softens the connective tissue. Macerated epidermis is easily eroded. Eventually, degenerative changes take place, and the tissue sloughs. As mentioned earlier, the adherence of wet skin surfaces to bed linen increases the risk of friction as the patient is moved across the surface of the bed linen.

Excessive moisture may be the result of perspiration, wound drainage, soaking during bathing, and fecal or urinary incontinence. Fecal incontinence exposes the skin to bacteria in the stool and adds the risk of infection. When a patient is incontinent of both urine and stool, the urea from the urine reacts chemically with the stool and causes further damage.

Infection

The role of infection in pressure ulceration isn't fully understood. In animal studies, compression alone allowed local increases in bacterial concentration after intravenous injection of bacteria. The bacteria localized at the site of compression and caused necrosis at pressures lower than those needed to cause necrosis in animals who weren't given a bacterial load. Several investigators have concluded that compression makes local skin less resistant to bacterial infection and that compression-induced ischemia inhibits the first line of defense against bacterial invasion. Other investigators, who studied the role of denervation in soft tissue infection in animals, have shown that local neurologic impairment increases susceptibility to infection and pressure ulceration.

Summary

The unquestionable cause of pressure ulcers is irreversible ischemia due to compression. Other significant contributors are shear, friction, moisture, and possibly infection. Tissues vary in their resistance to the effects of pressure. Although clinical awareness of impending necrosis occurs only when skin becomes inflamed, deep necrosis most likely has already occurred in areas not apparent on visual inspection. We believe we know the etiology of pressure ulcers, but we don't know exactly how they develop. High-risk patients, whether in an institution or at home, should be assessed regularly for the presence of pressure ulcers. Understanding the etiology of pressure ulcer development is the foundation for planning prevention and treatment.

Selected references

Bergquist, S. *Risk for Pressure Ulcers in Community-based Older Adults Receiving Home Health Care.* Doctoral dissertation. Iowa City: The University of Iowa; 1998.

Cherry, G.W., and Wilson J. "The treatment of ambulatory venous ulcer patients with warming therapy," *Ostomy/ Wound Management* 45(9):65-70, 1999.

Parish, L.C., et al. *The Decubitus Ulcer in Clinical Practice.* New York: Springer-Verlag, 1997.

Santilli, S.M., et al. "Use of a non-contact radiant heat bandage for the treatment of chronic venous stasis ulcers," *Advances in Wound Care* 12(2):189-193, 1999.

Chapter 4

Wound healing

Understanding the nature of wound healing is fundamental to caring for patients who have pressure ulcers. As in many other areas of study, several disciplines have claimed the territory of wounds and wound healing. Communication among these disciplines will facilitate progress toward understanding the problem and devising solutions.

In an effort to provide a universal language for research, clinical practice, regulatory agencies, and payers, the Wound Healing Society in Richmond, Virginia, proposed common terminology for defining a wound and the process of wound healing. (See *Glossary of wound healing*, page 28.)

Wound closure is classified according to the amount of tissue loss, which determines the time required for healing, and the amount of granulation tissue and contraction necessary to close the defect.

■ *First*, or *primary*, *intention healing* occurs when a wound with little or no tissue loss, such as a surgical wound, is sutured and it heals by direct union.

■ *Delayed primary intention healing* occurs when significant tissue loss can be repaired surgically with a skin or muscle graft.

■ *Indirect union* or *secondary intention healing* occurs when tissue loss is significant, such as with burns or pressure ulcers, and the wound can't be corrected surgically.

Wounds into the epidermis or dermis can heal by *tissue regeneration*. Wounds through the dermis heal by *scar formation* because deeper structures, such as subcutaneous tissue, glands, and hair follicles, can't regenerate. *Contraction* is the main mechanism that closes large defects during secondary intention healing.

The process of wound healing begins at the moment of injury and may continue for years. Careful assessment and continuous monitoring of wound healing are essential to wound care.

Glossary of wound healing

- *Wound* describes the disruption of the normal anatomic structure and function of a tissue.

- *Acute* wounds proceed through an *orderly* and *timely* repair process that results in sustained restoration of anatomic and functional integrity.

- *Chronic* wounds either fail to proceed through an *orderly* and *timely* process to produce anatomic and functional integrity, or they proceed through the repair process without establishing a sustained anatomic and functional result.

- *Healing* is a complex dynamic process that results in the restoration of anatomic continuity and function.

- *Orderly* healing is a sequence of inflammation, angiogenesis, tissue matrix regeneration, contraction, epithelialization, and remodeling.

- *Timely* healing is determined by the nature of the pathologic process; it varies with the uniqueness of each wound as it interacts with the patient's internal and external environment.

- An *ideally* healed wound has returned to normal anatomic structure, function, and appearance.

- An *acceptably* healed wound has sustained functional and anatomic continuity.

- A *minimally* healed wound has anatomic continuity without a sustained functional result and is therefore subject to recurrence.

Phases of healing

The body responds to wounding by an ongoing process often called the tissue repair cascade. (See *Wound-healing cascade.*) No matter how trivial or extensive the wound, healing always includes three overlapping phases: inflammation, proliferation, and differentiation. Each phase is regulated by growth factors that are created and secreted by cells present during that phase. Activity differs according to the type of growth factor that is secreted; effects include increased protein synthesis, cellular proliferation, and alterations in cellular activity. Growth factors attract other cells needed to promote subsequent phases. They have the unique capability of acting on distant or adjacent cells or on the cells they came from.

Inflammatory phase

The inflammatory phase of the healing process activates the tissue repair cascade. A chemical action during this phase stimulates the healing process. The first response to wounding is local vasoconstriction that lasts about 5 to 10 minutes. During this time, several cell types arrive at the wounded area to defend and revitalize traumatized tissue. First, platelets aggregate and deposit granules that affect clotting and stimulate growth factors. The granules promote fibrin deposition to form a thrombus or clot to seal the wound.

Wound-healing cascade

This algorithm depicts the tissue repair cascade from injury through the healing process.

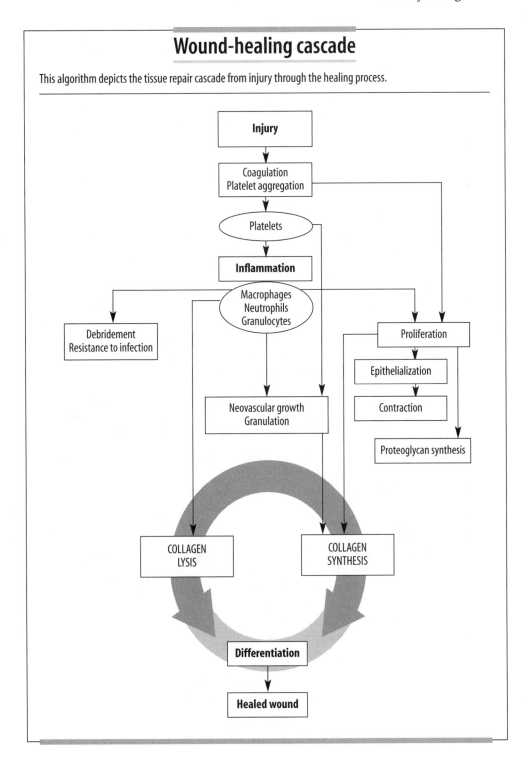

Factors that inhibit collagen synthesis

Many factors, including the following ones, contribute to a decrease in collagen synthesis.

Advanced age	Infection	Traumatic injuries
Diabetes mellitus	Malnutrition	Uremia
Emotional stress	Radiation injuries	
Hypoxemia	Steroids	

The surrounding tissues become ischemic, and vasodilation occurs. Vascular permeability increases, and neutrophils migrate from the vessels into the wound space, along with enzymes, fluid, and protein. These cells and substances are trapped in the extracellular space, where they cause inflammation.

The neutrophils start to recede after about 24 hours as monocytes enter the wound. Monocytes are soon converted to macrophages, which are key cells in the wound-healing process. Macrophages not only debride the wound, they also regulate the development of fibrous tissue (fibroplasia) and degrade collagen during the wound-healing process. They release an angiogenic factor, which stimulates formation of both new blood vessels to feed the growing new tissue, and a growth factor, which stimulates fibroblast production and promotes collagen synthesis during the second phase of wound healing.

The main function of the inflammatory phase of healing is to initiate the wound-healing cascade, remove the debris, and prepare the wound for the regeneration of new tissue. Clinically, the inflammatory phase is characterized by local erythema, edema, and tenderness of the affected tissue.

Proliferative phase

The proliferative phase of wound healing overlaps the inflammatory phase. It begins 3 to 4 days after wounding and lasts for approximately 15 or 16 days. The main events during this phase are deposition of connective tissue and collagen cross-linking. During this time, epithelial cells migrate across the wound surface, guided by the wound matrix and anatomic tissue planes.

Fibroblasts, the key cell type in this phase, multiply and actively synthesize collagen, the principal component of connective tissue. Collagen fills the wound and provides strength. Several factors can inhibit collagen synthesis. (See *Factors that inhibit collagen synthesis*.)

Granulation

During collagen production, new capillaries are forming as budlike structures on nearby vessels. Stimulated by a relatively hypoxic environment, capillaries penetrate the wound, grow into loops, and carry nutrients to the newly generating tissue. These bright red loops of blood vessels impart a granular appearance to the wound surface. For this reason, the new tissue is often
called *granulation tissue*. Granulation tissue, when kept moist, provides good
tissue for advancing epithelial cells, but when dried out, as in a scab, it provides a different terrain. Occasionally, excessive amounts of granulation tissue, or "proud flesh," form over a wound, rising above the skin level; epithelial
cells cannot "climb the hill." Nonocclusive dressings dehydrate the granulation buds and reduce inflammation; the hypergranulation tissue then re-
cedes and reepithelialization can occur.

As the wound matures and the synthesis of collagen decreases, the new
vascular channels regress, and the wound undergoes a transformation from
capillary-rich, highly cellular tissue to comparatively avascular, cell-free scar
tissue composed of dense collagen bundles.

Epithelialization

The replacement of dead or damaged surface tissue by new and healthy cells
begins by a process called *epithelialization*. Epithelial cells migrate from the
wound margins across the wound surface to create a watertight seal over the
wound. Cells have an insatiable drive to contact cells of their own type. A
network of fibrin strands functions as a scaffolding over which the cells creep.
Sheets of new epithelial cells continue to grow until they come into contact
with others moving across the wound from other directions.

In primary healing, fibrin closes the wound within a few hours and epithelialization begins in 1 to 2 days. Epithelial cells may arise from the hair
follicles in a partial-thickness wound if the shaft of the follicle still is intact.
In secondary healing, migration of cells is rapid at first but gradually slows,
so that days or weeks may elapse before epithelialization is complete. If a
scab is covering the wound surface, the epithelial cells must migrate under-
neath the scab.

A wound covered by epithelial cells stops weeping body fluid and elec-
trolytes. The new epithelium protects the wound against direct bacterial invasion only as long as it remains intact. And, because the new epithelium is
hardly more than a gelatinous film, the slightest trauma will destroy it.

Contraction

The scar in a wound that has healed by secondary intention shrinks by a
process called *wound contraction*. Contraction of scar tissue occurs as surrounding tissue moves toward the center of the wound. Contraction overlaps the proliferation and differentiation phases. It begins on about the fifth

day, when collagen-synthesizing contractile cells called *myofibroblasts* appear in the wound. Myofibroblasts do not appear in sutured wounds but are common in granulating wounds.

Surgeons use the skin's inherent tendency to contract to help them place incisions. Skin contracts in the plane perpendicular to lines of tension in the skin called Langer's lines. Incisions made along Langer's lines place little tension on the skin. Reducing the tension produces a less noticeable scar.

Contraction ceases when the counteracting force of the surrounding skin begins to exceed the force of the contracting wound. Secondary intention healing continues for months or even years, as is described in the next section. Over time, the diameter of collagen fibrils increases, and the fibrils become more compact.

Differentiation phase

In the differentiation, or remodeling, phase of wound healing, a wound matures and the collagen in the scar undergoes repeated degradation and resynthesis. If collagen synthesis and lysis aren't in balance, scar tissue will either overgrow or weaken and rupture easily. Differentiation is the longest phase of wound healing. It usually begins at about day 21.

In primary healing, collagen formation is complete by day 42, when equilibrium is established between collagen synthesis and collagen lysis. Next, the collagen fibers and fibrils become dehydrated and reweave into a tight pattern. The scar becomes less and less bulky and continues to gain tensile strength for 2 years. Granulation tissue retracts, and the scar fades from a deep red to a silvery white as the granulation buds retract.

The tensile strength of the scar increases during the differentiation phase. Between the 1st and the 14th day of this phase, the tissues regain approximately 30% to 50% of their original strength. Tensile strength continues to increase, eventually reaching approximately 80% of normal tissue strength. Wounds never completely regain the tensile strength of unwounded tissue.

The differentiation phase includes growth and development of new tissue and strengthening of the scar. Maximum possible healing during the differentiation phase requires adequate nutrition — vitamins to support cellular activity and amino acids for tissue regeneration.

Intrinsic factors affecting healing

Many conditions — and their effects — can compromise wound healing. (See *Factors that compromise wound healing*.) Healing is influenced by systemic conditions or by local conditions in the wound, such as tissue oxygenation, stress, nutrition, and infection. Specific interventions can modify or correct a number of these conditions.

Factors that compromise wound healing

The conditions listed below produce effects that hamper tissue healing.

Condition	Effects
Advanced age	Hypoxia, anemia
Arteriosclerosis	Hypoxia
Cardiac insufficiency	Hypoxia
Collagen vascular disease	Chronic vasculitis
Diabetes mellitus	Thickened capillary membrane
Immunocompromise	Impaired immune response
Malnutrition	Anemia, edema, impaired protein stores
Medications	Steroids (alter inflammatory response)
Smoking	Vasoconstriction, hypoxia

Tissue oxygenation

Oxygen is essential for wound healing, and oxygen tension at the wound site correlates directly with the rate of healing. Neutrophils and macrophages use it to destroy bacteria; amino acids use it to form new protein during regeneration. Collagen synthesis and fibroblast differentiation cannot occur without it. Healing slows or stops when blood oxygen levels or flow causes hypoxia. Unobstructed blood flow not only supplies the wound with oxygen and nutrients, it removes carbon dioxide and metabolic by-products. Any condition that reduces blood flow to a wound, such as arterial occlusion, vasoconstriction, or external pressure, can impede healing.

Any of four major factors can contribute to wound hypoxia: vessel occlusion, hypotension, edema, or anemia. Atherosclerosis is the most common cause of arterial vessel occlusion. Atherosclerosis and hypotension prevent adequate blood from reaching the peripheral tissues. Edema increases the diffusion distance from the capillary to the cell and decreases the pO_2 by as much as 50%. In anemia, decreased blood volume limits the availability of hemoglobin-carrying red blood cells. Even temporary anoxia may impair the production of stable collagen fibers.

Wound healing requires tissue-fluid oxygen tensions of 30 to 40 mm Hg. As long as oxygen tension remains in this critical range, the relative hypoxia of ischemic wounds stimulates macrophages to produce angiogenesis and growth factors, and the angiogenesis factor initiates formation of the new blood vessels of granulation tissue. Below 30 mm Hg, metabolic functions associated with the healing process can't take place.

It appears that lactate mediates both neovascularization and collagen synthesis. The anaerobic process of increased glucose consumption and lactate production is the major source of energy for metabolism in granulation tissue. Lactate stimulates production of angiogenesis factor whether oxygen is present or not. Fibroblasts grow best at low partial pressure of oxygen, and hypoxia also causes fibroblasts to activate the enzymes for collagen synthesis. Chronic tissue hypoxia also stimulates capillary growth from the wound edge to the more hypoxic center. The process stops when oxygen levels rise. Local hypoxia also stimulates macrophages to release growth factors. Poor wound healing is most likely in patients who are hypoxic, are hypotensive, have certain medical conditions (such as diabetes or atherosclerosis), or are critically ill with anemia or edema. Topical application of oxygen, even under pressure, does not improve wound healing.

Stress

Sympathetic nervous system and adrenal responses to stress include neural, hormonal, and metabolic changes that impair wound healing. The exact mechanism isn't clearly understood. During stress, the adrenal glands produce norepinephrine and epinephrine. Norepinephrine causes peripheral vasoconstriction, thereby decreasing oxygen delivery. One of epinephrine's many actions is to enhance epidermal production of the protein chalone, which depresses the regeneration of epidermal tissue. During sleep or relaxation, epinephrine and chalone production fall, the rate of epidermal cell division and maturation increases, and wounds heal more rapidly. Therefore, a plan that provides sleep and rest for the patient with a pressure ulcer will promote wound healing.

Advanced age

Aging affects almost all aspects of the healing response. Slowing epidermal turnover and increasing skin fragility together reduce wound healing by a factor of four. The repair rate declines with falling rates of cell proliferation, lack of development of wound tensile strength, impaired collagen deposition and wound contraction, and reduced healing of experimentally induced blisters. The combination of medical conditions that occur in many elderly persons adversely affects healing. Also, older people tend to be malnourished and poorly hydrated and to have compromised respiratory and immune functions. An age-related decrease in the number of dermal blood vessels dramatically increases the risk of ischemic injury. Loss of dermal and subcutaneous mass further increases the risk for pressure-induced tissue injury.

Malnutrition

Wound healing and the immune response both require an adequate supply of various nutrients, including protein, vitamins, and minerals. A deficiency of dietary protein interferes with neovascularization, lymph formation, fibroblastic proliferation, collagen synthesis, and wound remodeling. Loss of more than 15% of lean body mass interferes with wound healing. The edema that results from hypoalbuminemia further impairs fibroplasia. In addition, the loss of immune function doesn't only slow or prevent the inflammatory phase of healing, it also increases the risk of wound infection.

Patients with chronic wounds may need more protein and calories than the recommended daily allowances and dietary supplements to build body mass and improve healing. Emaciated patients with chronic nonhealing wounds may respond to anabolic steroids to increase weight gain, but the adverse effects are significant.

Protein
A diagnosis of clinically significant malnutrition requires at least one of the following:
■ serum albumin <3.5 g/dl
■ total lymphocyte count <1,500/mm^3
■ recent weight loss >15%.

Low serum albumin levels are a late manifestation of protein deficiency. Serum concentrations below 3.0 g/dl are a recognized screening indicator of poor nutritional status, and those below 2.5 g/dl reflect severe protein depletion.

Persons with extensive pressure ulcers are often protein deficient. Patients with wounds require additional calories and protein (30 to 35 calories per kilogram of body weight per day and 1.25 to 1.50 grams of protein per kilogram of body weight per day) to build new tissue for wound healing. Curiously, despite the established correlation between hypoproteinemia and development of pressure ulcers, no randomized clinical trials have shown that hypoproteinemia predicts the prognosis for healing.

Severe trauma and systemic infection enhance protein metabolism, which is clinically reflected by increased urinary excretion of nitrogen. In addition, protein intake is commonly insufficient in the hospitalized elderly, immobile, or critically ill person. Protein malnutrition plays a greater role in development of pressure ulcers in the elderly than among the neurologically impaired, where pressure is more significant.

Vitamins
Vitamins, particularly vitamin C and vitamin A, appear to be necessary for wound healing. Vitamin C (ascorbic acid) deficiency is associated with impaired fibroblastic function and decreased collagen synthesis, which combine to delay healing and contribute to breakdown of old wounds. An age-associated decrease in ascorbic acid levels may increase the fragility of vessels and connective tissue and lower the threshold for pressure-induced injury. Vitamin C deficiency also causes loss of resistance to infection associated with impaired immune function. Because vitamin C is water-soluble and can't be stored in the body, inadequate intake can quickly produce vitamin deficiency.

Deficiency of vitamin A (retinol) has been associated with retarded epithelialization and decreased collagen synthesis. Deficiency is uncommon because this fat-soluble vitamin is stored in the liver. Chronic dietary deficiency and prolonged severe stress are the major risk factors for vitamin A deficiency.

Other vitamins, such as thiamine and riboflavin, are also necessary for collagen organization and the resultant tensile strength of the wound.

Minerals

Various minerals — such as iron, copper, manganese, and magnesium — play a role in wound healing, but the nature of their influence is unclear. Zinc deficiency appears to delay healing by reducing the rate of epithelialization and fibroblast proliferation. Deficiencies require replacement, but there is no indication that supplemental zinc is useful if a deficiency doesn't exist. Indeed, excess zinc may interfere with wound healing by inhibiting both copper absorption and the action of an enzyme that catalyzes collagen cross-linking.

Corticosteroids

Corticosteroids suppress the inflammatory response in a wound. Inflammation is necessary to trigger the wound-healing cascade, and healing is slow in many patients taking steroids. Use of steroids also does the following:
■ increases the risk of wound complications, including infection, delayed healing, and wound dehiscence
■ inhibits capillary budding, fibroblast proliferation, protein synthesis, and epithelial growth
■ causes depletion of vitamin A from the liver, plasma, adrenals, and thymus and thereby interferes with collagen synthesis and resistance to infection.

Steroid therapy begun after the inflammatory phase of healing (usually 4 to 5 days after wounding) has a minimal effect on wound healing. Clinicians planning steroid or chemotherapy treatment schedules must consider the effect of timing on wound healing. Vitamin A may counteract the anti-inflammatory effect of steroids by its effect on lysosomes in inflammatory cells. Although the optimal dosage has not been determined, it may support early wound healing in patients who require steroid therapy.

Smoking

Nicotine interferes with blood flow in two ways: it is a vasoconstrictor, and it increases platelet adhesiveness, thereby causing clot formation. Cigarette smoke also exerts effects that are independent of its nicotine content:
■ It's a potent vasoconstrictor.
■ The carbon monoxide it contains prevents oxygen from binding to the hemoglobin molecule.

■ By unknown mechanisms, cigarette smoke may cause changes in the vessel endothelium and increase platelet adhesiveness, which may further limit blood flow.

■ Hydrogen cyanide in the smoke inhibits enzymes needed for oxygen transport and oxidative metabolism.

Patients who smoke cigarettes and are preparing for surgical repair of pressure ulcers or other chronic wounds should be told of their higher risk for skin or muscle graft failure and should be supported in their attempts to stop smoking.

Diabetes

Diabetes influences wound healing through mechanical and metabolic effects. Studies in animals suggest that chronic hyperglycemia may be both the cause and the effect of poor wound healing for the following reasons:

■ High levels of glucose compete with transport of ascorbic acid into cells; as mentioned, vitamin C is necessary for the deposition of collagen.

■ Tensile strength and connective tissue production are significantly lower in diabetic than nondiabetic rats.

■ Treatment with insulin reverses the effects of diabetes on wound healing.

Arterial occlusive disease — a common condition in diabetic patients — can impair healing. The reduced sensation of diabetic neuropathy frequently leaves traumatic wounds undetected.

Diabetes impairs the function of leukocytes in a way that decreases their effect on bacteria. The results include impairment of the inflammatory response and the healing cascade, as well as diminished resistance to infection. Infection is a common complication of both diabetes and pressure ulceration. Patients with diabetes have more difficulty resisting infection and their wounds heal more slowly than those of patients without diabetes.

Infection

Infectious complications of pressure ulcers include sepsis and osteomyelitis. Debridement, drainage, and removal of the necrotic tissue alone controls most infections. Many organisms inhabit the surface of a chronic open wound, and topical antibiotic treatments are widely used without a scientifically solid reason. Open wounds do not have to be sterile to heal. Identified infections should be treated with antibiotics, but the mere presence of organisms in the wound may represent colonization, not infection.

The combination of local tissue response to infection and the accumulation of bacterial metabolic end products prolongs the inflammatory phase of healing and interferes with neovascularization and collagen synthesis. Devitalized tissue and extravasated blood provide a source of nutrients for bacteria and increase the risk of infection.

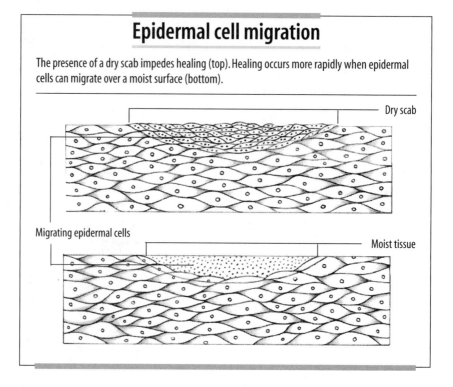

Epidermal cell migration

The presence of a dry scab impedes healing (top). Healing occurs more rapidly when epidermal cells can migrate over a moist surface (bottom).

Dry scab

Migrating epidermal cells

Moist tissue

Neutrophils and monocytes destroy invading bacteria, but they consume oxygen as they control the organisms. Hypoxia inhibits the defensive action of the leukocytes and supports bacterial growth. Thus, sufficient oxygenation is necessary to support the defense against wound infection.

The presence of necrotic tissue prevents the wound from granulating and forming epithelial tissue, and moist necrotic tissue is a medium for bacterial growth. Healing cannot proceed until all necrotic tissue has been removed from the wound.

Wounds with tissue loss, such as pressure ulcers, rapidly become contaminated with bacteria. This contamination becomes significant and interferes with wound healing — that is, it's considered to be infection — when the colony count exceeds 105 organisms per gram of tissue. When local defense mechanisms no longer contain the infection, cellulitis, purulence, and fever ensue.

Systemic antibiotics cannot reduce the bacterial load of the pressure ulcer wound bed because blood flow to the local tissues is poor. Use of parenteral antibiotics is indicated only when signs and symptoms suggest cellulitis, sepsis, or osteomyelitis. Topical antibiotics may kill all but resistant strains of organisms and thereby render the individual insensitive to the antibiotic. A way to determine the presence of true wound infection and guide the treatment decision remains to be determined.

Wound dehydration

Wound healing occurs more rapidly when dehydration is prevented. Epidermal cells migrate faster and cover the wound surface sooner in a moist environment than under a scab. (See *Epidermal cell migration.*) Under experimental conditions, wound fluid promotes fibroblast proliferation. Dressings designed to retain moisture at the wound surface support the healing process.

Evaluation of healing

Restoration of tissue integrity and function are clinical markers of a healed wound. Evaluation of healing requires the analysis of wound assessments. The simplest and most obvious method is to examine the wound and compare the observation with previous observations or reports of the wound. The method should be systematic and consistent. Examination should include:

■ measurement of the wound's length, width, and depth
■ observation of inflammation, wound contraction, granulation, and epithelialization.

Wound-healing times are variable. Etiology, patient characteristics, and wound management all affect the healing rate. See Chapter 5 for measurements of wound healing.

Summary

The wound-healing sequence follows an expected course if intrinsic and extrinsic conditions are optimal. Wounds go through inflammatory, proliferative, and differentiation phases. Whenever possible, the body should be allowed to heal itself. The factors that can interfere with wound healing include malnutrition, infection, stress, and concomitant illness. Dressings can either enhance or impede wound healing. All products that go on or into a wound should be nontraumatic.

Careful monitoring of the wound-healing process without too much interference seems to serve the wound best. The best treatment is to support conditions that promote optimum healing — such as protection from trauma and provision of a moist environment. New techniques for wound care must stand up to scientific scrutiny that confirms their impact on wound management.

Selected references

Ayello, E.A., et al. "Educational assessment and teaching of older clients with pressure ulcers," *Clinics in Geriatric Medicine* 13:483-496, 1997.
Bolton, L.L., et al. "Quality wound care equals cost-effective wound care – A clinical model," *Nursing Management* 27(7);30,32,33-37, 1996.

Eager, C.A. "Monitoring wound healing in the home health arena," *Advances in Wound Care* 10(5):54-57, 1997.

Eaglstein, W.H., and Falanga, V. "Chronic wounds," *Surgical Clinics of North Amercia* 77:689-700, 1997.

Hansson, C. "Interactive wound dressings: A practical guide to their use in older patients," *Drugs Aging* 11:271-284, 1997.

Hess, C.T. "Fundamental strategies for skin care," *Ostomy/Wound Management* 43:32-34,36,38,40-1, 1997.

James, H. "Preventing pressure sores in patient's homes," *Professional Nurse Supplement 1997* 12:12-14, 1997.

Kerstein, M.D. "The scientific basis of healing," *Advances in Wound Care* 10(3):30-36, 1997.

Pieper, B., et al. "Developing collaborative multi-site research in home care," *Home Healthcare Nurse* 16:311-318, 1998.

Wise, L.C., et al. "Nursing wound care survey: Sterile and nonsterile glove choice," *Journal of Wound Ostomy Continence Nursing* 24:144-150, 1997.

Chapter 5

Assessment

Nursing assessment of pressure ulcers is not restricted to the bedfast patient who already has a pressure ulcer; every patient is at some degree of risk. A good assessment considers the entire patient. Data to be gathered include a complete history and physical examination, including psychosocial assessment, evaluation of risk factors, a thorough examination of the skin, and a precise description of any existing pressure ulcer.

Assessing the patient

Assessing the individual with a pressure ulcer includes evaluating the patient's physical and psychosocial health, mental status, learning ability, stress level, depression, social support, medication use, smoking habit, alcohol or drug use, goals, values, lifestyle, sexuality, culture and ethnicity, pressure ulcer risk factors, nutritional status, and any pressure ulcer—related pain or complications. After a complete health history and physical examination, the ulcer itself must be thoroughly assessed. Any pain associated with either the pressure ulcer or the pressure ulcer treatment regimen also should be assessed, using a visual analogue scale. If necessary, topical, oral, or parenteral pain medication should be administered before pressure ulcer examination or treatment is begun.

Assessing risk

Patients who are at risk for developing pressure ulcers can be identified by assessing the following variables:
- number and type of medical diagnoses
- presence of chronic health problems
- chronologic age
- immobility/ability to move independently

- mental status/level of consciousness
- malnutrition/nutritional status
- incontinence/bladder and bowel control
- presence of infection and/or fever
- adequacy of circulation.

Risk increases as the number of problems in each category increases. Approximately two-thirds of elderly patients admitted to hospitals for fractured femur and one-third of patients in intensive care units develop pressure ulcers. Patients with chronic underlying pathology — such as diabetes mellitus, Alzheimer's disease, arteriosclerosis, and spinal cord injury — commonly have more than one risk factor. All health care professionals should be aware of the risk factors for pressure ulcerations, so that the clinician directly responsible for the patient's care can take appropriate prophylactic measures. (See Chapter 6.)

Mobility

Immobility probably is the greatest threat of all for patients with pressure ulceration. Taken together, the patient's reflexive body adjustment in bed and wheelchair, his active bed mobility, active wheelchair repositioning, level of activity, frequency of transfers, ambulation ability, and tolerance of distance/endurance provide a good assessment of mobility.

Mental status

Mental status impairment may limit the patient's ability for self-care. Such a patient may not:
- be able to feel discomfort from pressure
- be alert enough to move spontaneously
- be motivated to move
- remember to move
- respond to commands to move
- be physically capable of changing position.

Patients with impaired mental status may be restrained for their own safety or given sedatives to "calm them down." Clearly, a restrained or sedated patient has fewer spontaneous movements and is less likely to change position. The result: unrelieved pressure over bony prominences and high risk for pressure ulceration of soft tissue.

Nutritional status

Malnutrition is a widespread problem in America and is becoming even more of a problem as our society ages. At the opposite end of the spectrum are the overly fed. Many ill patients who enter the hospital are already malnourished, and well-nourished patients may become malnourished while hospitalized. (See *Physical signs of malnutrition*.)

Physical signs of malnutrition

Signs	Possible causes
Hair	
Dull, dry, lack of natural shine	Protein-energy deficiency
Thin, sparse, loss of curl	Zinc deficiency
Color changes, depigmentation, easily plucked	Other nutrient deficiencies: manganese, copper
Eyes	
Small, yellowish lumps around eyes, white rings around both eyes	Hyperlipidemia
Pale eye membranes	Vitamin B_{12}, folacin, or iron deficiency
Night blindness, dry membranes, dull or soft cornea	Vitamin A or zinc deficiency
Redness and fissures of eyelid corners	Niacin deficiency
Angular inflammation of eyelids	Riboflavin deficiency
Ring of fine blood vessels around cornea	Generally poor nutrition
Lips	
Redness and swelling	Niacin, riboflavin, iron, or pyridoxine deficiency
Gums	
Spongy, swollen, red, bleed easily	Vitamin C deficiency
Gingivitis	Vitamin A, niacin, or riboflavin deficiency
Mouth	
Cheilosis, angular scars	Riboflavin or folic acid deficiency
Tongue	
Swollen, scarlet, raw; sores	Folacin or niacin deficiency
Smooth with papillae (small projections)	Riboflavin, vitamin B_{12}, or pyridoxine deficiency
Glossitis	Iron or zinc deficiency
Purplish	Riboflavin deficiency
Taste	
Diminished	Zinc deficiency
Teeth	
Gray-brown spots	Increased fluoride intake
Missing or erupting abnormally	Generally poor nutrition
Face	
Skin color loss, dark cheeks and eyes, enlarged parotid glands, scaling of skin around nostrils	Protein-energy deficiency, specifically niacin, riboflavin, or pyridoxine deficiency
Pallor	Iron, folacin, vitamin B_{12}, or vitamin C deficiency
Hyperpigmentation	Niacin deficiency
Neck	
Thyroid enlargement	Iodine deficiency
Symptoms of hypothyroidism	

Adapted with permission from Niebert, K.C., ed. *Nutrition Care of the Older Adult.* Chicago, Ill.: American Dietetic Association, 1998.

Oral and cutaneous signs of vitamin or mineral deficiencies

The oral and cutaneous signs listed here may appear in a variety of diseases. However, if they're caused by a vitamin or mineral deficiency, they should begin to improve 4 weeks after supplementation begins.

Clinical signs by site	Deficiency
Oral cavity	
Cheilosis and angular stomatitis	Vitamin B_2
Glossitis (pink or magenta discoloration with loss of villi)	Multiple B vitamins
Eyes	
Scleral changes	Vitamin A
Bilot's spots	Vitamin A
Face	
Seborrhea-like dryness and redness of nasolabial fold, and eyebrows	Zinc
Upper extremities	
Purplish blotches on lightly traumatized areas (due to capillary fragility and subepithelial hemorrhage)	Vitamin C
Extreme transparency of skin on hands ("cellophane skin")	Vitamin C
Abdomen and buttocks	
Waxy, perifollicular hyperkeratosis	Vitamin A
Lower extremities	
Superficial flaking of epidermis, large flakes of dandruff	Essential fatty acids
Cracks in skin between islands of hyperkeratosis:	Nicotinamide (niacinamide)
• Pigmented	Vitamin A
• Nonpigmented	

Source: Bergstrom, N., et al. "Treatment of Pressure Ulcers," Clinical Practice Guideline, No. 15. AHCPR Publication No. 95-0652. Rockville, Md.: U.S. Department of Health and Human Services, Public Health Service, Agency for Health Care Policy and Research, December 1994.

The Nutrition Screening Initiative is a broad multidisciplinary effort led by the American Academy of Family Physicians, the American Diatetic Association, the National Council on the Aging, Inc., and a diverse coalition of over 25 national health, aging, and medical organizations. It recommends use of nutrition screening tools to provide an important frame of reference for individuals and health care providers. Nutritional assessment should include documentation of dental health, oral and gastrointestinal history, chewing and swallowing ability, quality and frequency of foods eaten, his-

Serum albumin deficit levels

Deficit levels of serum albumin can be classified as mild, moderate, or severe.

Mild	3.0 to 3.5 g/dl
Moderate	2.5 to 3.0 g/dl
Severe	<2.5 g/dl

tory of involuntary weight loss or gain, serum albumin levels, nutritionally pertinent medications, and any psychosocial factors affecting nutritional intake. (See *Oral and cutaneous signs of vitamin or mineral deficiencies*.)

Other important factors include a person's ability to acquire and pay for food, food preferences, cultural and lifestyle influences on food selection, ability to cook, facilities for cooking, and environment for eating. Nutritional screening assessments should be repeated at least every 3 months if initial assessment reveals a high risk for malnutrition.

Laboratory tests

No single biochemical or physical measure indicates a person's nutritional health. Depressed serum protein, serum albumin, and transferrin levels together indicate poor nutritional status. In general, the longer the starvation period, the greater the drop in standard plasma levels of these substances. Significant hypoproteinemia causes interstitial edema, which interposes fluid between the cells and consequently reduces tissue oxygenation. This edema may play a role in the genesis of pressure ulceration in elderly, malnourished patients.

Serum albumin concentration in the serum is a gross indicator of nutritional status. Serum albumin has a relatively long half-life of about 20 days, and so concentrations fall slowly during malnutrition. (See *Serum albumin deficit levels*.) A subnormal serum albumin level represents late manifestation of protein deficiency, an established risk factor for pressure ulceration. A low serum transferrin level or low lymphocyte count represent current poor nutritional status.

Body weight

At-risk patients should be weighed weekly. The combination of weight loss and onset of illness is a valuable indicator of nutritional status. A history of unintentional weight loss or weight-height ratio of less than 85% of standard has been related to functional consequences of malnutrition. (See *Assessment recommendations for determining proper weight, caloric levels, and degree of nutritional depletion,* page 46.)

Assessment recommendations for determining proper weight, caloric levels, and degree of nutritional depletion

Wayne State University
DMC Harper Hospital

Food and Nutrition Services
Nutritional Assessment

Recommended weight for height:
  Female: 100 lbs. per 5 ft. + 5 lbs. per inch > 5 ft.
  Males: 106 lbs. per 5 ft. + 6 lbs. per inch > 5 ft.

*Basal energy expenditure
  Female: 655 + (9.6 X wt. in kg) + (1.8 X ht. in cm) - (4.7 X age in years)
  Male: 66 + (13.7 X wt. in kg) + (5.0 X ht. in cm) - (6.8 X age in years)

> Estimated daily calorie levels are determined by multiplying the BEE* and the appropriate stress** and/or activity*** factor.

**Stress factor:

	Stress factor	g protein per kg ideal body weight (IBW)
Surgery:	1.1 to 1.3	1.5 to 2.0
Infection:	1.3 to 1.5	1.5 to 2.5
Maintenance:	1.3	0.8 to 1.2
Repletion:	1.5	1.2 to 2.0
Pulmonary:	1.0 to 1.6	1.0 to 2.0
Cancer:	1.3 to 1.5	0.8 to 2.0
AIDS:	1.3 to 1.5	1.0 to 2.0
Liver failure:	1.5 to 1.75	0.5 to 1.5
Cardiac failure:	1.0 to 1.2	1.2 to 1.5
Renal failure:	1.3 to 1.8	0.5 to 1.0
Hemodialysis:		1.0 to 1.2
Peritoneal dialysis:		1.2 to 1.5
Cystic fibrosis:	1.5 to 2.0	1.5 to 2.0

Activity factor:

Bed rest:	1.0
Active without stress:	1.3
Cardiac failure:	1.2 to 1.3

Fluid requirements:
  <50 years old: 1,500 ml for first 20 kg
  20 ml per kg for remaining kg ABW
  >50 years old: 1,500 ml for first 20 kg
  15 ml per kg for remaining kg ABW

Degree of nutritional depletion/risk/needs:

	Mild	Moderate	Severe
Age:	18 yrs to 64 yrs	<18 yrs or >64 yrs	<18 yrs or >64 yrs
Weight:	<5% loss/6 mos.	5% to 10% loss in 1 to 6 mos.	>5% loss in 1 mo. >10% loss in 6 mos.
	<5% to 10% of IBW with no hx. of unplanned wt. loss in past yr 85% to 90% usual body weight	10% to 20% above or 20% to 30% below IBW 75% to 84% UBW	>20% IBW <70% IBW <74% UBW
Feeding regimen:	Decreased oral intake	Poor intake or NPO for 5 days Parenteral/enteral	Poor intake or NPO for 5 days Parenteral/enteral
Albumin:	2.8 to 3.5	2.1 to 2.7	<2.1
Total lymphocyte count:	1,500 to 1,800	900 to 1,500	<900
Transferrin:	150 to 200	100 to 150	<100
Diagnosis:	Minor surgery/Minor infection	High-risk diagnosis/Problems*****	High-risk diagnosis/Problems*****

*****High-risk diagnosis/Problems may include:

Major surgery	Cancer	Decubitus ulcer	Persistent nausea,
Major trauma	AIDS	Inflammatory bowel	vomiting, diarrhea
GI fistula	Respiratory failure	Renal failure/dialysis	
Abdominal surgery or resection	Malabsorption	Substance abuse	

Key: BEE = basal energy expenditure; ABW = actual body weight; IBW = ideal body weight; UBW = under body weight

Guidelines per ASPEN Certified Nutrition Support Review Manual, 1989, 1993; ADA Manual of Clinical Dietetics, 1988; ADA Dietitians in Nutrition Support Conference, 1990.

A physician, nurse, or dietitian should be notified if a patient has an unintended loss of 10 pounds or more during any 6-month period. In patients at risk for malnutrition, an involuntary change of 5% of body weight is predictive of a drop in serum albumin.

Incontinence

Incontinence increases the risk for pressure ulceration because it causes excessively moist skin and chemical irritation. Fecal or urinary incontinence keeps the skin so soft that even ordinary skin care or movement across bed linen will rub the outer layer away. Of the two types of incontinence, fecal incontinence makes the greater contribution to pressure ulceration, perhaps because the stool contains bacteria and toxins, and urine, which normally is sterile, contains only chemical irritants. However, in patients with both fecal and urinary incontinence, a chemical reaction between the urine and the stool produces substances that further compromise the skin. Vigorous mechanical skin cleansing and use of multiple products for incontinence may contribute to further skin breakdown.

Never accept incontinence as a normal part of aging. It always has a cause. Assessment includes evaluation of reversible causes, including urinary tract infection, medications, confusion, fecal impaction, polyuria related to glycosuria or hypercalcemia, and restricted mobility. The incontinent patient may be confused about the location of an unfamiliar bathroom, too embarrassed to ask for a bedpan, or lacking in the functional skills to perform self-toileting. (See *Assessing urinary incontinence,* page 48.) Tracking the amount and frequency of urination and defecation is important for determining an appropriate incontinence management plan.

Psychological factors

A paraplegic or quadriplegic patient's self-concept may determine whether he develops pressure ulcers. Health care professionals must be vigilant with regard to the emotional status of patients who are at risk for pressure ulceration. If depression is a factor, the patient should be referred for psychological counseling.

Young patients with spinal cord injuries commonly become angry at their situation. If they become depressed and disinterested in self-care, apathy and neglect may lead to repeated episodes of tissue breakdown. Depression is also commonly associated with alcoholism and chemical abuse among spinal cord—injured individuals. Occasionally, the patient sees pressure sores as a means to obtain additional attention from family and health professionals.

Chronic emotional stress also contributes to pressure sore susceptibility. During periods of stress, the adrenal glands increase production of glucocorticoids, which inhibit collagen production, and thereby increase the risk of pressure ulceration (see Chapter 1.) While performing the assessment, encourage the patient to discuss stressful situations. Eliciting this extra infor-

Assessing urinary incontinence

Name _____ Room number _____
Age _____ Sex _____ Race _____ Date of admission _____

History of the incontinence
- Approximate date of onset of incontinence _____
- How frequent are the incontinent episodes over 24 hours? _____
- How often does the patient urinate (continent and incontinent) over 24 hours? _____
- Does the patient urinate regularly? ❑ Yes ❑ No
- Does the patient urinate at night? ❑ Yes ❑ No
- Is the patient incontinent at night? ❑ Yes ❑ No
- Is the patient incontinent during the day? ❑ Yes ❑ No
- What is the usual amount of urine passed?
  ❑ Small ❑ Moderate ❑ Large ❑ Varies
- Is the patient's fluid intake regular? _____
- What is the patient's fluid intake in 24 hours? ❑ Yes ❑ No
  ❑ Small ❑ Moderate ❑ Large ❑ Varies

Cognitive abilities
- Does the patient ask to go to the toilet? ❑ Yes ❑ No
- oes the patient ever go to the toilet for himself? ❑ Yes ❑ No
- Does the patient know where the bathroom is? ❑ Yes ❑ No
- If placed on a toilet, does the patient urinate? ❑ Yes ❑ No
- Does the patient seem aware of being wet? ❑ Yes ❑ No
- Is the patient restless before an incontinent episode? ❑ Yes ❑ No
- Is the patient more confused before an incontinent episode? ❑ Yes ❑ No
- Is the patient concerned after an incontinent episode? ❑ Yes ❑ No

Mobility
- Can the patient get into and out of a chair alone? ❑ Yes ❑ No
- Can the patient walk to the bathroom alone? ❑ Yes ❑ No
- Can the patient walk with the assistance of one person? ❑ Yes ❑ No
- Must the patient be lifted onto the toilet? ❑ Yes ❑ No
- Can the patient maintain balance without holding on? ❑ Yes ❑ No
- Is the patient free to move about at will? ❑ Yes ❑ No
- Does the patient walk very slowly? ❑ Yes ❑ No

Activities of daily living
- Is the patient able to manipulate clothing? ❑ Yes ❑ No
- Is the patient able to button and zipper clothing? ❑ Yes ❑ No
- Does the patient perform hygiene activities for himself? ❑ Yes ❑ No
- Does the patient use a diaper that can be removed?
  ❑ None used ❑ Easily removed ❑ Difficult to remove

Used with permission from Jirovec, M., et al. "Functional assessment of a patient with urinary incontinence," *Nursing Clinics of North America* 23(1):224-225, 1988.

mation may require careful questioning from a health care professional who specializes in psychological assessments.

Risk assessment scales

An experienced clinician may be able to readily identify patients who are at risk for pressure ulcers. It may be more difficult for her to explain exactly *why* a particular patient is at risk. Nurse researchers have created risk assessment tools to objectively rate contributing factors. Most pressure ulcer risk assessment scales are based on the original work of Doreen Norton in Great Britain. Gosnell and Braden based their risk assessment scales on the findings and limitations of existing tools. Most pressure ulcer risk assessment scales identify immobility, inactivity, incontinence, malnutrition, and decreased mental status or decreased sensation as major factors that predispose patients to pressure ulceration. Scoring and summing the variables provides a numeric indicator of a patient's risk, which in turn determines the specificity and intensity of nursing interventions.

The Agency for Healthcare Research and Quality (AHRQ), Guideline for Pressure Ulcer Prediction and Prevention, recommends use of either the Norton or Braden Pressure Sore Risk Assessment Scale. Many health care agencies mandate pressure ulcer risk assessment for every patient. The absolute frequency requirement of reassessment for pressure ulcer risk has not been established scientifically. However, common sense indicates that patients should be reassessed whenever conditions change or when they become chairbound or bedridden. It is important to use a reliable tool because data from assessments of risk are used in the selection of preventive interventions. These interventions are not without cost, and the magnitude of cost is directly related to the number of people defined as "at risk."

Norton Scale

The Norton Scale rates physical condition, mental state, activity level, patient mobility, and incontinence on a scale of 1 to 4. Total scores range from 5 to 20; the lower the score the higher the risk of ulceration. Doreen Norton now places the onset of risk at a score of 16 or below. This scale is simple and easy to use. It has been criticized for not including nutrition, but in fact, nutrition is included as part of the assessment of physical condition in the tool's original form. (For a more detailed look at the Norton Scale, see the Appendices.)

Gosnell Scale

The Gosnell Scale is a refinement of the Norton Scale. The general condition category is called *nutrition*, and the incontinence category is now called *continence*. Gosnell reversed the scoring, so that a score of 5 reflects the lowest risk, and 20 is the highest possible score. The critical cutoff score appears to be 11. (For a more detailed look at the Gosnell Scale, see the Appendices.)

General skin appearance, detailed medication regimen, diet and fluid balance, and intervention categories are included but not rated numerically. Instead, the rater's guide provides descriptors for each numbered risk factor.

Braden Scale

The Braden Scale has six subscales divided into two categories as follows:
■ Intensity and duration of pressure: mobility, activity, and sensory perception
■ Tissue tolerance: moisture, nutrition, and friction/shear.

Each subscale is rated numerically and summed. The risk score can range from 6 to 23, and lower scores signify greater risk.

Previous research on the Braden Scale demonstrated a cutoff score of 16 for classifying pressure ulcer risk. However, a large multisite study evaluated predictive validity and was designed to determine the critical cutoff score and the optimal time for assessing risk in different health care settings. Bergstrom and colleagues found that
■ the critical cutoff score for predicting pressure ulcer risk was 18.
■ risk assessment on admission was highly predictive in all settings but not as predictive as a risk assessment completed within 48 to 72 hours after admission.

They suggested that nurses complete a pressure ulcer risk assessment on admission and develop an initial pressure ulcer prevention plan of care for those at risk. A repeat risk assessment done 48 to 72 hours after admission further defines pressure ulcer risk. At that time, the nurse should revise the plan to address predominant risk factors.

A pilot study by Lyder and colleagues validated the Braden Scale in African-American and Latino/Hispanic elderly patients. They found that a cutoff score of 16 was too conservative for predicting risk in these patients; most of their subjects who developed pressure ulcers scored 17 or 18.

In 1996, Quigley and Curley published a modification of the Braden scale, called the Braden Q, which is used for pediatric pressure ulcer risk assessment.

Inspecting the skin

The skin provides one of the first clues that a patient is at risk for pressure ulceration. One indication of skin condition is response to pressure. Pressure against the soft tissue interrupts blood flow to a localized area and causes pallor to the overlying skin. The pallor reflects tissue ischemia that, when prolonged, can result in extensive tissue damage. When the pressure stops, the skin should quickly return to its normal color as blood flow returns.

Stage I pressure ulcer

Observable pressure-related alteration of intact skin with one or more of the following local changes, compared to the adjacent or opposite area of the body: skin warmth or coolness, firm or boggy feel, or pain or itching. The ulcer presents clinically as a defined area, persistently red in light skin or red, blue, or purple in darker skin.

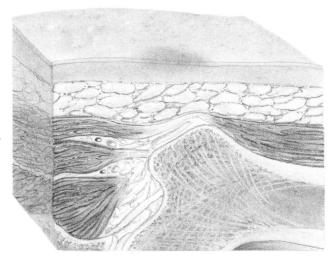

Stage II pressure ulcer

Partial-thickness skin loss involving the epidermis, dermis, or both. The ulcer is superficial and presents clinically as an abrasion, blister, or shallow crater.

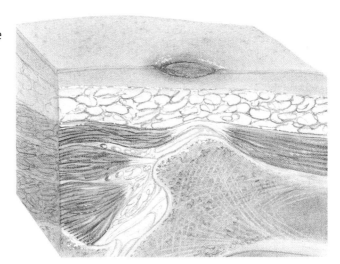

Stage III pressure ulcer

Full-thickness skin loss involving damage or necrosis of subcutaneous tissue, which may extend down to but not through underlying fascia. The ulcer presents clinically as a deep crater with or without undermining of adjacent tissue.

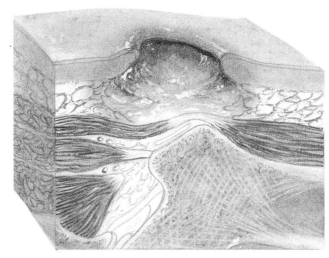

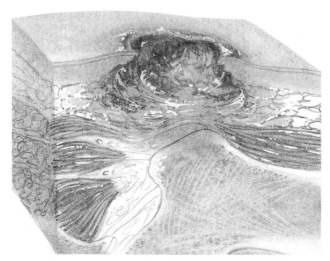

Stage IV pressure ulcer

Full-thickness skin loss with extensive destruction, tissue necrosis, or damage to muscle, bone, or supporting structures (such as tendon or joint capsule). The ulcer may also involve undermining and sinus tracts.

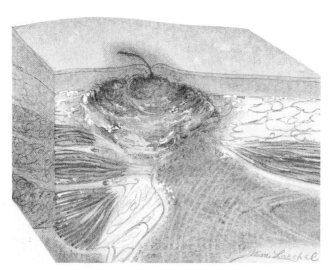

Closed pressure ulcer

Large, walled-off cavity filled with necrotic debris and extending to deep fascia or bone. If intense internal pressure ruptures the skin, the resulting ulcer may present clinically as small and benign, but it drains a large, contaminated base.

Reactive hyperemia

The first external sign of ischemia due to pressure is reactive hyperemia. When skin becomes ischemic under pressure, it becomes reddened, or hyperemic, after the pressure is removed. The bright flush generally lasts from half to three-fourths the duration of ischemia. This protective mechanism dilates the vessels and increases the amount of blood available to nourish and oxygenate the tissue. Increased blood flow to the tissue carries away accumulated waste products. If pressure exceeds tissue tolerance, the mechanism of reactive hyperemia becomes insufficient to meet the demands of the compromised circulation.

Blanchable erythema

Blanchable erythema, the earliest sign of ischemia, appears as a pink to red area of skin. In light-skinned individuals, compressing the reddened area causes the color to blanch or turn pale, and the redness returns immediately after compression is relieved; this is immediate capillary refill. Blanchable erythema causes no long-term effects on the tissue. When the pressure that caused blanchable erythema is totally removed, the tissue should resume its normal color within 24 hours. Blood flow recovery time after relief from pressure reflects risk of ulceration. In the dark-skinned patient, comparing the susceptible area to skin on the contralateral side can help in assessment of subtle color changes.

Nonblanchable erythema

In patients who are debilitated or at extremely high risk for pressure ulcers, skin may become dark red, bluish, or purple and incapable of blanching in response to compression. Nonblanchable erythema may be the first outward sign of tissue destruction. As the tissues are deprived of oxygen beyond the critical period, cells die. Nonblanchable erythema is reversible if it is recognized early and treated.

Shiny erythema

As destruction of the epidermal tissue continues, vesicles appear. A shiny, erythematous base with indistinct borders may be noted. The skin surrounding the shiny base exhibits nonblanchable erythema. Intervention is required to prevent progression of this lesion to a chronic pressure ulcer.

Assessing the ulcer

Pressure ulcers range from nonblanchable erythema of intact skin to deep destruction and loss of tissue. A chronic pressure ulcer has a well-defined border with surrounding nonblanchable erythema. Induration may extend far beyond the open wound. Inspection alone may not reveal the extent of the ulcer, which may have spread extensively beneath the skin, undermin-

Remembering what to assess

The word *assessment* is a useful mnemonic for remembering the parameters for pressure ulcer assessment and documentation. The letters in the word serve as the first letters of data elements included in comprehensive pressure ulcer evaluation.

A = Anatomic location, age of ulcer
S = Size, stage
S = Sepsis
E = Exudate type and amount, erythema
S = Surrounding skin color, swelling, saturation of dressing
S = Sinus tracts (undermining)
M = Maceration
E = Edges, epithelialization
N = Nose (odor), necrotic tissue type and amount, neovascularization
T = Tenderness to touch, tension (induration), tautness, tissue bed (granulation tissue)

ing along fascial planes. Tunnels may connect sacral ulcers to ulcers over the trochanter of the femur or the ischial tuberosities.

Assessment of the pressure ulcer should include:
■ history: etiology, duration, prior treatment
■ anatomic location
■ stage
■ size: length, width, and depth measured in centimeters
■ extent: edges, sinus tracts, undermining, tunneling
■ exudate or drainage
■ necrotic tissue: slough and eschar
■ granulation tissue
■ epithelialization or new skin growth.

The borders of the ulcer can provide clues to healing potential. Intact skin surrounding the ulcer should be assessed for redness, warmth, induration or hardness, swelling, and any obvious signs of clinical infection. Wound edges should be attached or even with the ulcer base. If the skin edges are rolled under, this will inhibit wound closure. (See *Remembering what to assess*.)

Measuring

Pressure ulcers can be measured with simple or sophisticated methods. The simplest way to determine wound size in the clinical setting is to take linear measurements of length and width in centimeters or millimeters. Some clinicians prefer to trace the wound perimeter and then transfer a copy to the medical record.

To determine gross wound depth, insert a gloved finger into the ulcer at the deepest part and then measure how far the finger reaches. Placing cotton-

Closed pressure ulcers

The closed pressure ulcer presents a special challenge. It's not included in any of the four-stage classification systems. Its appearance differs from that of an open lesion but is caused by the same pathophysiologic process. Innocent-appearing and easily overlooked, it conceals a deep and potentially fatal lesion.

A closed pressure ulcer may develop when shear forces cause ischemic necrosis in subcutaneous fat but the skin does not ulcerate (see Chapter 2). The result is a large, walled-off cavity filled with necrotic debris. Normal defense mechanisms, including inflammation, continue to operate, creating intense internal pressure until the skin ruptures. But even then, the deception continues: The resulting small wound appears benign, but it drains a large, contaminated base.

Closed pressure ulcers are most common in the pelvic areas of otherwise healthy people who are chairbound by spinal cord injury. Recognition of chronic closed pressure ulcers is essential.

- Small benign-appearing wounds with drainage or seepage from a deep cavity.
- Small surface area of eschar or open lesion.
- Drainage in small amounts over time or continuous large amount.
- Indurated surrounding tissue possible.

Systemic manifestations of infection are uncommon, and staging is impossible because the extent of tissue destruction isn't apparent until the ulcer is surgically opened.

The only effective treatment for a closed pressure ulcer is wide surgical excision of the ulcer and closure with a muscle rotation flap.

---

tipped applicators and tongue blades into deep wounds or blind tunnels can cause iatrogenic injury.

Clinically, wound volume can be measured by placing an adherent film dressing over the wound cavity and instilling saline through the film via syringe until fluid reaches the film level. The volume of fluid measured in cubic centimeters is the volume of the wound.

Serial color photographs are also useful. Some commercially available film has metric squares superimposed on it, to help determine wound size. The photographer must hold the camera the same distance from the wound bed each time a picture is taken.

Staging

Initial inspection reveals the pressure ulcer's stage, determined by the deepest layer of exposed tissue. Almost universally accepted are the Pressure Ulcer Staging guidelines developed by the National Pressure Ulcer Advisory Panel (NPUAP) and the AHRQ. Although not included in any of the four-stage classification systems, the closed pressure is an extremely serious problem and may contain a deadly lesion. (See *Closed pressure ulcers*.)

■ **Stage I**: An observable pressure-related alteration of intact skin whose indicators, compared to the adjacent or opposite area of the body, may include changes in one or more of the following: skin temperature (warmth or coolness), tissue consistency (firm or boggy feel), or sensation (pain, itching). The ulcer presents as a defined area of persistent redness in lightly pigment skin, whereas, in darker skin tones, it may appear as persistent red, blue, or purplish hues.

■ **Stage II:** Partial-thickness skin loss involving epidermis or dermis, or both. The ulcer is superficial and presents clinically as an abrasion, blister, or shallow crater.

■ **Stage III:** Full-thickness skin loss involving damage or necrosis of subcutaneous tissue, which may extend down to but not through underlying fascia. The ulcer presents clinically as a deep crater with or without undermining of adjacent tissue.

■ **Stage IV:** Full-thickness skin loss with extensive destruction, tissue necrosis, or damage to muscle, bone, or supporting structures (such as tendon or joint capsule). Undermining and sinus tracts also may be associated with stage IV pressure ulcers.

Staging is only a small part of assessing a patient with a pressure ulcer. When assessing pressure ulcers, it is equally important to examine other characteristics, including intact skin surrounding the ulcer. The presence of inflammation, induration, or ischemia may give clues to the prognosis of the ulcer. However, without consideration of the entire person, staging has little value in predicting healing.

Pressure ulcers aren't restaged at each assessment. They're staged only once unless a deeper layer of tissue becomes exposed. Pressure ulcers don't necessarily progress steadily from one stage to the next, and each step may have a different etiology. Likewise, ulcers don't heal by reverse staging. An ulcer grows shallower as it heals, but it doesn't develop new layers of muscle, subcutaneous tissue, and dermis. It heals by growing granulation tissue.

Assessing complications

Complications of pressure ulcers can delay healing and may become life-threatening. Two major medical complications are sepsis and osteomyelitis. Clinically, the difference between colonization and infection may not be readily apparent. Appropriate methods of diagnosing infectious processes are the subject of controversy.

Colonization and infection

All pressure ulcers are colonized with bacteria, and a moderately healthy patient can tolerate some colonization. In most cases, debridement and adequate cleansing prevent the ulcer from becoming infected. In an otherwise healthy individual, bacterial loads of 100,000 (10^5) organisms per gram of tissue are considered to be infection and may delay healing.

Ulcer infection is recognized by the classic signs of rubor, calor, dolor, and tumor. (See *Assessing for infection*.) The cardinal sign of an infected ulcer

Assessing for infection

Certain signs and symptoms may indicate infection in a pressure wound, requiring further assessment.

Erythema (redness, rubor)

A well-defined border of erythema around a wound results from the body's normal response to trauma, but a poorly defined erythemic border may signal infection. Very intense erythema with well-defined borders can also indicate infection, as can red streaking up and down the skin.

Fever (heat, calor)

Systemic fever (along with complaints of malaise) may indicate infection; a local temperature increase may simply result from inflammation, not infection.

Odor

A sweet smell may indicate a *Pseudomonas* infection, and the smell of ammonia may result from a *Proteus* infection. A very foul smell may not signal infection but may instead result from autolytic or enzymatic debridement of necrotic, nonviable tissue.

Edema (swelling, tumor)

Localized edema around the wound that feels warm may signal infection. More generalized edema in an extremity that doesn't feel warm may instead result from another cause, such as chronic heart failure or, in the lower extremities, venous insufficiency.

Drainage

Drainage that accumulates quickly or persists after the wound and surrounding area are cleansed; moderate or copious drainage that persists longer than 5 days after the ulcer initially appears; or drainage that becomes yellow, yellow-green, or green-blue and viscous may signal infection. Red to brown drainage (from blood and fibrin) is normal, as is clear, watery drainage in a healing wound. Make sure you don't confuse drainage with necrotic tissue sloughing off after debridement.

Pain (dolor)

Although subjective, reports of pain may indicate infection. For example, pain in the leg of a patient with arterial insufficiency may simply result from the insufficiency, but severe, persistent wound pain in an otherwise healthy young patient may result from infection.

Confusion

The elderly person with a pressure ulcer may not manifest the expected signs of infection because the immune system has undergone changes associated with normal aging. If an elderly person with a pressure ulcer becomes acutley confused without another obvious reason, the clinician should suspect and assess for infection.

Used with permission. *Topics in Geriatric Rehabilitation* 9(4):37, June 1994.

is advancing cellulitis, which indicates the offending organism has invaded the surrounding tissue.

Sepsis

Sepsis or bacteremia may originate from infected pressure ulcers of any stage. Sepsis often is caused by anaerobes and gram-negative bacteria, such as *Staphylococcus aureus,* gram-negative rods, or *Bacteroides fragilis*. Blood culture is the only way to identify the pathogen.

Osteomyelitis

Osteomyelitis (infection involving the bone) is likely in stage IV pressure ulcers. About 25% of nonhealing ulcers may have underlying osteomyelitis. Osteomyelitis delays healing, causes extensive tissue damage, and is associated with a high mortality rate. A bone biopsy and culture are necessary for diagnosis, although investigators have reported many attempts at noninvasive diagnosis. Bone scans have a high false-positive rate and may lead to inappropriate treatment. If the patient's white blood cell count, erythrocyte sedimentation rate, and plain X-ray are all positive, osteomyelitis is likely. Treatment is provided with long-term systemic antibiotics.

Culturing

Cultures of the pressure ulcer are necessary to identify infecting organisms. Among the commonly used ways of obtaining samples for culture are (see Chapter 9 for a detailed description of obtaining wound swab cultures):

■ wound swab cultures, which merely detect the presence of colonizing bacteria

■ needle aspiration after injection of normal saline, which underestimates the number of organisms isolated from the deep tissue

■ curettage of the ulcer base, which shows good correlation with deep tissue culture

■ deep tissue biopsy and culture, which is the gold standard

■ quantitative cultures of soft tissue and bone when an ulcer does not respond to a course of topical antibiotic therapy.

Healing or deterioration

Assessment of wound status and improvement or deterioration includes description and quantification of many variables. (See Chapter 4 for a detailed discussion of how wounds heal and a description of the stages of wound healing.)

Inferring the rate of healing from successive measurements can be problematic. If the area and perimeter of large and small wounds are measured at intervals,

■ an attempt to calculate absolute reduction in area would erroneously show that large wounds heal faster than small wounds.
■ an attempt to calculate the percentage of reduction in area would erroneously show that small wounds heal faster than large wounds.

The Pressure Sore Status Tool (PSST) identifies location, shape, necrotic tissue amount, exudate type, exudate amount, surrounding skin color, peripheral tissue edema, peripheral tissue induration, granulation tissue, and epithelialization. All items except location and shape are scored on a 5-point scale. The total score — which ranges from 13 to 16 — reflects overall wound status. The tool permits temporal tracking of individual characteristics as well as the total wound. Repeated scoring reveals healing or degeneration of the ulcer. The PSST has been automated and now incorporates graphic capabilities and computerized tracking. (For greater detail, see the Appendices.)

The Sessing Scale is a simple, easy-to-use observational instrument that measures granulation tissue, infection, drainage, necrosis, and eschar on a 7-point scale. The scale is scored by calculating positive or negative changes in numerical values over successive wound assessments. The Sessing Scale is a reliable tool for assessing pressure ulcers in clinical and research settings.

The Pressure Ulcer Scale for Healing (PUSH tool) was developed by NPUAP. The PUSH tool is a research-validated tool that quickly and reliably captures the key assessments necessary to monitor whether a pressure ulcer is getting worse or better over time. The NPUAP advises that assessments be performed at least weekly. (For a more detailed look at the PUSH tool, see the Appendices.)

A qualified health care professional should reassess every patient at least weekly and teach other caregivers to monitor the ulcer for signs of improvement or deterioration each time the dressing is changed.

Summary

Because assessment determines the types of care given to patients with pressure ulcers, it must be comprehensive and orderly. The importance of risk assessment should not be underestimated. Patients must be assessed for pressure ulcer risk on admission to any health care facility and reassessed continually. Pressure ulcer treatment may terminate, but risk assessment and prevention never do.

Staging systems are communication tools that provide information about the type of exposed tissue in the pressure ulcer. Staging only describes tissue involvement. It is not a method for prescribing treatment or measuring pressure ulcer healing. A four-stage pressure ulcer classification system does not address the problem of a closed pressure ulcer. Swab cultures of the wound surface should not be used to identify infecting organisms. Researchers are continually developing tools to describe pressure ulcers and to measure healing or deterioration. The results of this work will improve communication among health care clinicians, educators, researchers, policymakers, regulating bodies, and third-party payers.

Selected references

Bates-Jensen, B. "The pressure sore status tool a few thousand assessments later," *Advances in Wound Care* 109(5):65-73, 1997.

Bergstrom, N., et al. "Treatment of pressure ulcers," Clinical Practice Guideline, no. 15. AHCPR publication No. 95-0652. Rockville, Md.: U.S. Department of Health and Human Services, Public Health Service, Agency for Health Care Policy and Research, December 1994.

Berlowitz, D.R., et al. "Predictors of pressure ulcer healing among long-term care residents," *Journal of the American Geriatric Society* 45:30-34, 1997.

Ferrell, B.A., et al. "The Sessing Scale for assessment of pressure ulcer healing," *Journal of the American Geriatric Society* 43(1):37-40, 1995.

Gosnell, D.J. "An assessment tool to identify pressure sores," *Nursing Research* 22:55, 1973.

Maklebust, J. "Pressure ulcer staging systems: Intent, limitations, expectations," *Advances in Wound Care* 8(4):1995.

Maklebust, J.A., and Margolis, D.J. "Pressure ulcers: Definition and assessment parameters," *Advances in Wound Care* 8(4):6S-7S, 1995.

Norton, D., et al. *An Investigation of Geriatric Nursing Problems in Hospitals.* London: Churchill Livingstone, 1975 (original work published in 1962).

Quigley, S.M., and Curley, M.A.Q. "Skin integrity in the pediatric population: Preventing and managing pressure ulcers," *JSPN* 1(1):April-June 1996.

Stotts, N.A., et al. "Testing the pressure ulcer scale for healing (PUSH) and variations of PUSH." Paper presented at: 11th Annual Symposium on Advanced Wound Care; April 18-22, 1998, Miami Beach, Fla.

Xakellis, G. C., and Frantz, R.A. "Pressure ulcer healing: What is it? What influences it? How is it measured?" *Advances in Wound Care* 10(5):20-26, 1997.

Chapter 6

Prevention

Despite the best hopes of the 1980s, pressure ulcers continue to be a major cause of morbidity and mortality. Health care providers have both an opportunity and a responsibility to help reduce their incidence. Preventing pressure ulcers is not easy, but many interventions are available to help preserve patients' skin and underlying tissue. (See *Preventing pressure ulcers*, pages 60 and 61.) The first step is identifying which patients are at risk for skin breakdown. Only when the clinician knows each patient's internal risk factors can she create a care plan to prevent pressure ulcers. Risk factors are the basis for selecting specific prophylactic interventions. Any change in a patient's condition mandates reevaluation and care-plan revision. Research has confirmed what experienced clinicians know: The amount of care devoted to the prevention of pressure ulcers is significantly reflected in good outcomes.

Goals of care

Any effective plan to prevent pressure ulcers must include both the patient and the family. Teaching may be the most important intervention. Before selecting prevention strategies, the clinician-patient-family team must make decisions about:
- goals of care
- educational needs
- nutritional management
- correct body positions
- turning and repositioning schedules
- support surfaces
- skin care
- monitoring changes in risk status.

Preventing pressure ulcers

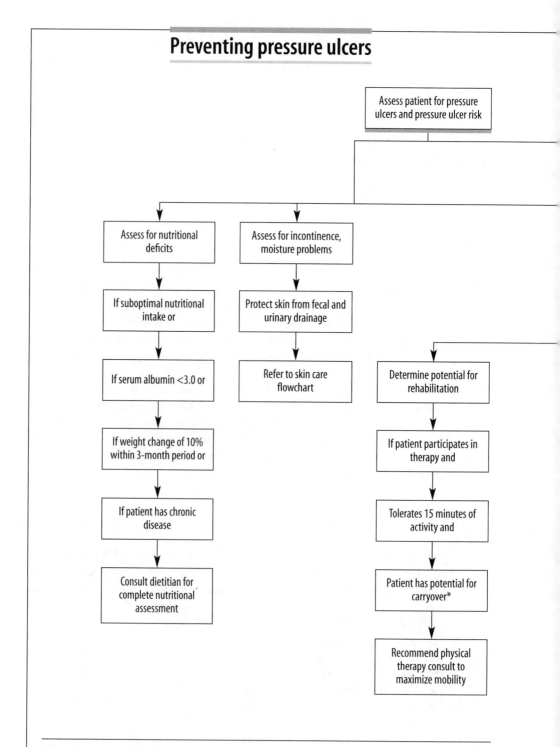

*Observed capacity to learn and follow through with motor skills necessary for increased functional independence.

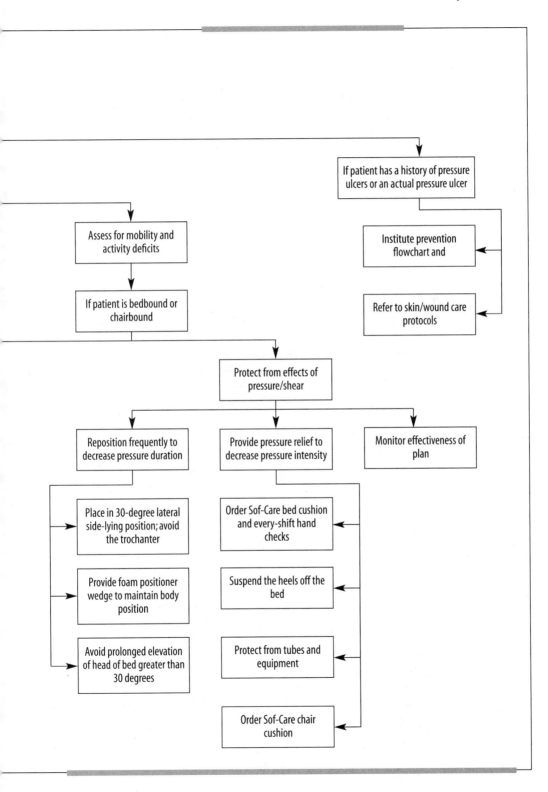

Goals of care, above all, must take into account the patient's desires as well as needs. For example, if a terminally ill patient wants only to be as comfortable as possible and pressure ulcer prevention procedures are painful and burdensome, document the patient's wishes and support them. Some hospice organizations have established standards of care that include both prevention and treatment of pressure ulcers. One of these standards prescribes actions to achieve the goals mutually derived by the patient and the clinician.

Educational needs

Learning needs should be established with the individual or the caregiver. For information on adult learning principles and patient and family education, see Chapter 11.

Nutritional management

The relationship between nutritional status and pressure ulceration is well established, and yet clinicians all too often overlook the patient's nutritional status. Chapter 5 addresses nutritional assessment in detail. Patients and caregivers need to know how important good nutrition is in preventing pressure ulcers. Overall goals of care as well as patient and family preferences should guide decisions for nutritional management.

Dietary intake

Whenever possible, individuals should have a well-balanced diet that includes foods from all four basic food groups. Studies suggest that healthy adults need 0.8 gram of protein per kilogram of body weight, or one to two 3-ounce servings of meat, meal, milk, cheese, or eggs each day.

One of the guiding principles of good nutritional support is maintenance of positive nitrogen balance. An adequate diet provides enough calories for energy needs and additional protein for restoring muscle mass and wound healing. This is anabolic metabolism and positive nitrogen balance. A patient who is not receiving adequate calories will break down glycogen and fat reserves and also will start metabolizing the body's proteins for energy. This is catabolic metabolism and negative nitrogen balance. It is lethal.

Clinicians must monitor both the quantity and quality of food eaten. If intake is questionable, request a dietary consult for complete nutritional evaluation. Cater to patients' food likes and dislikes and any special dietary needs. Involve both bedside caregivers and dietary staff in providing ongoing assistance with meals, monitoring the patients' swallowing ability, and assessing dietary tolerance.

Nutritional goals

The nutritional goal is a diet containing adequate nutrients to maintain tissue integrity. The following actions help achieve that goal:

■ Monitor oral and cutaneous signs of vitamin and mineral deficiencies.

■ Supplement or support the intake of protein, calories, vitamin C, and zinc.

■ Provide a daily high-potency vitamin and mineral supplement if you suspect a vitamin deficiency.

A dietary consult is essential if the patient's intake becomes inadequate, if he has an involuntary weight loss of 5% of body weight, or if the serum albumin level is lower than 3.5 g/dl. If thorough nutritional assessment confirms malnutrition, assisted oral feedings, dietary supplements, or tube feedings may be necessary to achieve positive nitrogen balance. A malnourished patient may require as much as 2 grams of protein per kilogram of body weight per day to reach positive nitrogen balance. (See *Caloric content of various nutritional supplements,* pages 64 and 65.)

Persons at risk for malnutrition need a nutritional screening assessment at least every 3 months. Repeat measurements of protein markers, such as serum albumin, reflect the success or failure of nutritional support.

Managing pressure

Pressure management begins with an understanding of proper body positioning, the importance of turning and repositioning, and the advantages of suitable support surfaces for sleeping (overlays, mattresses, specialty beds) and sitting.

Pressure and body position

A wealth of controlled experiments have confirmed the commonplace observation that lying in one position on a hospital mattress increases the risk of pressure ulceration. Even the usual 2-hour interval is long enough to raise skin temperature significantly. The temperature of a pressure-traumatized area of skin may not return to baseline until long after skin color returns to normal, and visual assessment of erythema does not detect the full extent of damage. It seems that each person's vascular response to normal mechanical forces experienced in the side-lying position is a sensitive measure of susceptibility to pressure ulceration.

A patient who is at risk because of immobility must be repositioned frequently enough to prevent persistent reddening or hyperemia of skin. The temperature response of previously hyperemic areas may provide additional cues to skin recovery from pressure. Repetitive pressure against the skin and underlying tissue, without adequate recovery time, contributes greatly

Caloric content of various nutritional supplements

HARPER HOSPITAL ENTERAL FORMULARY

PRODUCT	ENSURE® Liquid Nutrition	PROMOTE™ High-Protein Liquid Nutrition	OSMOLITE® Isotonic Liquid Nutrition
Calories Liter/Can/Pkg	1,060/254	1,000/237	1,060/254
Protein Liter/Can/Pkg	37.2/8.8	62.4/14.8	37.2/8.8
Fat (g) Liter/Can/Pkg	37.2/8.8	26/6.2	38.5/9.1
CHO (g) Liter/Can/Pkg	145/34.3	130/30.8	145/34.3
Protein source	Sodium and calcium caseinates. Soy protein isolate	Sodium and calcium caseinates. Soy protein isolate	Sodium and calcium caseinates. Soy protein isolate
Fat source	Corn oil	High-oleic safflower oil (50%) *Canola oil (30%) MCT oil (20%)	MCT oil (50%) Corn oil (40%) Soy oil (10%)
Carbohydrate source	Corn syrup, sucrose	Hydrolyzed cornstarch, sucrose	Hydrolyzed cornstarch
Na (mEq/L)	36.8	40.4	27.6
K (mEq/L)	40	50.6	25.9
Osmolality	470	350	300
NP Cal Liter	911	751	911
Amt to meet RDA (ml)	1887	1,250	1887
Cost per 8 oz. serving	.55	.99	.90
Comments	Lactose free. All purpose. Low residue. Can be used on clear liquid diets. Good taste.	High protein. Lactose free. Low residue. *Source of omega 6 F.A.	Isotonic. Low residue. Bland taste. Lactose free.
Tube/oral	Tube/oral	Tube/oral	Tube/oral

to pressure-induced ischemia and necrosis. Both duration and intensity of pressure need to be decreased to reduce risk.

ENSURE PLUS® High-Calorie Liquid Nutrition	PULMOCARE® Specialized Nutrition for Pulmonary Patients	VITAL®HN Nutritionally Complete Partially Hydrolyzed Diet	CARNATION INSTANT BREAKFAST®
1,500/355	1,500/355	1,000/300	1,120/280
55/13	62.6/14.8	41.7/12.5	58/15
53.3/12.6	92.1/21.8	10.8/3.2	35/8
200/47.3	106/25	185/55.4	136/35
Sodium and calcium caseinates. Soy protein isolate	Sodium and calcium caseinates	Partially hydrolyzed whey, meat, and soy. Free amino acids	Nonfat dry milk, calcium caseinate, sweet dairy whey
Corn oil	Corn oil	Safflower oil (55%) MCT oil (45%)	Milk fat
Corn syrup, sucrose	Hydrolyzed cornstarch, sucrose	Hydrolyzed cornstarch, sucrose	Lactose, sucrose corn syrup solids
49.6	57	20.3	11.3/8 oz.
54	48.6	34.1	18.7/8 oz.
690	490	500	720
1,280	1,250	833	888
1,420	947	1,500	1,060
.95	1.22	4.03	.48
Lactose free. High calorie. Low residue. Normal pro. good taste.	55% Fat 28% CHO Good for pulmonary patients Reduce CO_2	Chemically defined. Peptides and free amino acids. Use for malabsorption.	Contains lactose oral. Above analysis when mixed with whole milk.
Tube/oral	Tube/oral	Tube/oral	Oral

Body positioning

Body positioning techniques can be important tools to help minimize pressure on vulnerable soft tissue over bony prominences.

Proper positioning in bed

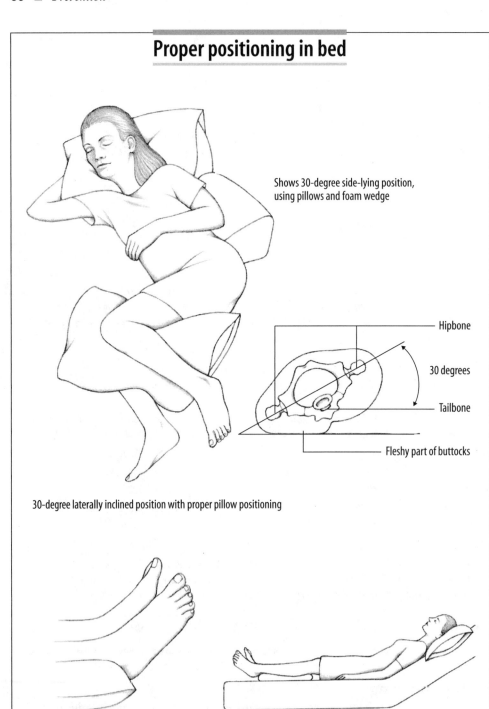

Shows 30-degree side-lying position, using pillows and foam wedge

Hipbone

30 degrees

Tailbone

Fleshy part of buttocks

30-degree laterally inclined position with proper pillow positioning

Proper heel placement

Head of bed elevation limited to 30 degrees or less

In bed

No patient should ever lie on skin that is already reddened by pressure. Donut-shaped products or ring cushions that totally surround an ischemic area tend to reduce the blood flow to an even wider area of tissue. If the reddened area is on an extremity, lifting the extremity onto a pillow reduces pressure to the area. Pillows placed between the legs prevent opposing knees and ankles from exerting pressure on one another. (See *Proper positioning in bed.*) When a patient is resting in the side-lying position, weight should never be placed directly on the greater trochanter of the femur. A 30-degree laterally inclined position simultaneously diverts pressure from the sacrum and trochanter. Pillows or foam positioning wedges can be used to maintain this position. Flexing the legs further reduces pressure over the trochanter. Eliminating the 90-degree side-lying position is the responsibility of every person caring for a patient who is at risk for pressure ulcers.

It is almost impossible to reduce pressure over heels to a level below the capillary closing pressure, even on specialty support surfaces. Consequently, heels should be suspended to avoid pressure on the small surface area of the rounded bony prominence; many commercial products that achieve this are available.

The angle of the supporting bed surface affects the patient's risk for mechanical damage to the skin. As was discussed in detail in Chapter 1, the head of the bed should be raised as little as possible (no more than 30 degrees) so that the patient does not slide down in bed. If the patient must have the head of the bed elevated during meals or tube feedings, lower the head about 1 hour after the meal. If the head must be elevated for other medical reasons, carefully monitor the skin of the sacral region. A physical therapist can offer valuable suggestions when keeping the patient in a safe position becomes a challenge.

Turning and repositioning

The sensory nerves normally detect persistent local pressure before ischemia occurs. A person with an intact nervous system compensates for local pressure by shifting weight frequently while sitting or standing or even during sleep. Healthy people change position as frequently as every 15 minutes. Patients who have mental status changes or spinal cord injuries may not feel pressure and, consequently, do not move to avoid discomfort. Clinicians need to reposition these patients or remind them to turn at least every 2 hours. How often a patient needs to be repositioned depends on how well soft tissue can tolerate the effects of pressure. Patients should move or be repositioned frequently enough to allow any reddened areas of skin to recover from the effects of pressure. A turn clock may be a helpful reminder of correct body positions and appropriate turning times. (See *Using a turn*

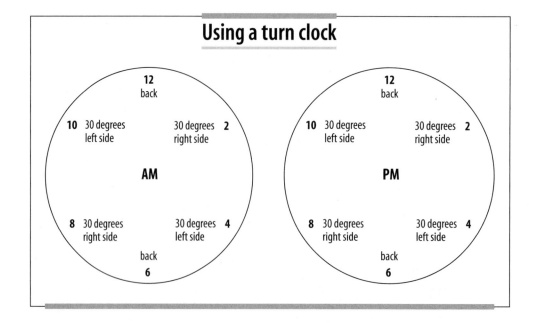

Using a turn clock

clock.) Both patients and caregivers should supplement full body turning schedules with smaller shifts in body weight.

To avoid effects of friction and shear forces,

■ lift patients rather than drag them across the bed surface
■ place film or hydrocolloid dressings on the skin over pressure points
■ have the patient wear socks and long sleeves to protect heels and elbows.

To help avoid the hazards of immobility, patients should be rehabilitated to their maximum level of functioning. Physical therapists should be consulted to teach bed mobility to bedridden patients. Many bedridden patients find side rails helpful in increasing bed mobility. They either turn independently while holding on to side rails or hold them to assist caregivers with turning. An overbed frame with attached trapeze helps some patients who can use upper body strength to lift their buttocks off the bed and avoid abrasive friction burns to the skin.

Sitting

Sitting carries the greatest risk of pressure ulcers. Because of gravitational force, body weight is concentrated over a smaller surface area of the sacral tuberosity. Good body posture and alignment help minimize the pressure on susceptible surfaces. A patient should never sit directly on a reddened area. The thighs should be horizontal so the weight is evenly distributed along the backs of the thighs. If the knees are higher than the hips, body weight concentrates on the ischial tuberosities, placing them at risk for pressure ulceration. Adequate support of the ankles, elbows, forearms, and wrists

Measurements influencing posture and propulsion

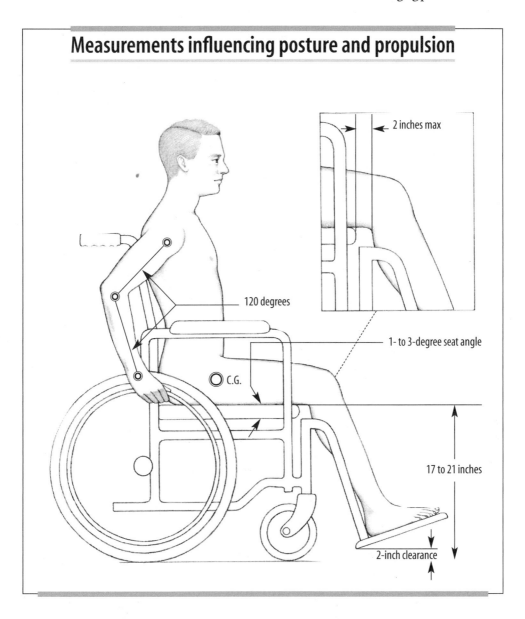

2 inches max

120 degrees

1- to 3-degree seat angle

C.G.

17 to 21 inches

2-inch clearance

in a neutral position reduces the risk, as does separating the knees so they do not rub together.

A wheelchair must match the patient's needs. (See *Measurements influencing posture and propulsion*.) Again the leg must be positioned so that the patient's weight is equally distributed over the length of the thigh. Too great a seat angle, with knees higher than buttocks, increases pressure on the ischial tuberosities and sacrum, causing tissue damage.

Pillow bridging

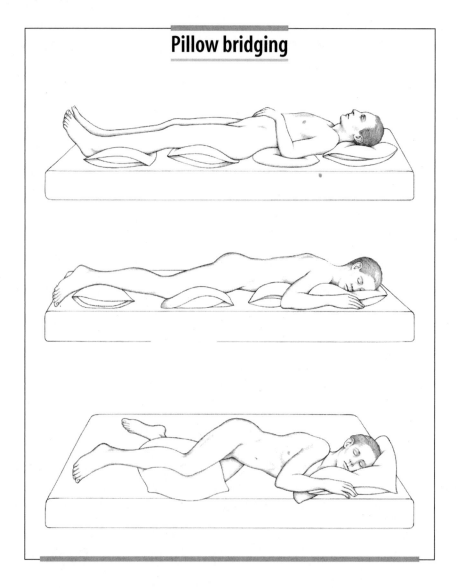

Body posture and orientation can dramatically affect the pressure or shear forces generated between the patient's seat and the chair's seat. If possible, patients need to reposition themselves every 15 minutes. Paraplegic patients can relieve pressure by doing wheelchair push-ups if they have enough upper body strength. If the patient cannot do push-ups to relieve pressure, simply leaning the body forward toward the thighs reduces the pressure over the ischial tuberosities. Clinicians need to evaluate whether an individual patient can safely lean forward. A patient who is unable to lift or shift his weight should be assisted in moving back to bed.

Assistance from bed to chair and then from chair to assisted ambulation gradually reduces the risk created by inactivity. To give the inactive patient incentive, provide such devices as overhead frames, trapezes, walkers, and canes as well as assistance in maneuvering I.V. poles and other equipment.

Support surfaces

Whether at-risk patients are in a bed or on a chair, pressure points require protection. Using pillows to bridge vulnerable areas is an effective way to eliminate pressure. (See *Pillow bridging*.) A growing array of beds, mattresses, and cushions is available to help reduce the intensity of pressure. Pressure-reducing surfaces include:

■ foam, gel, water, and air mattresses
■ alternating pressure pads
■ low-air-loss, high-air-loss, and oscillating beds
■ turning frames

Horizontal support

Horizontal support surfaces include mattress overlays, mattresses, and specialty beds.

Mattress overlays

Foam, air, and gel products are the most commonly used tools to prevent pressure ulcers. Good foam overlay products for a person of average weight are at least 3 to 4 inches thick, have a density of 1.3 pounds per cubic foot, and have 25% indentation load deformation (ILD) of 30 pounds. Density and ILD describe softness and stiffness of foam and determine efficacy and durability. Two-inch foam mattress overlays only increase comfort; they do not reduce risk for pressure ulceration. Solid foam mattress overlays are superior to convoluted foam mattress overlays. Good quality foam

■ allows adequate deformation.
■ provides good support.
■ does not fatigue or wear out as readily as inexpensive foam.

Controlled studies have revealed no evidence that either a foam overlay or an alternating pressure pad is superior in preventing skin breakdown. In a comparison of alternating pressure pad, air mattress overlay, and water mattress overlay in the intensive care unit (ICU), only patients on the alternating pressure pad had unacceptably high sacral and heel pressures.

In another study, an air mattress overlay and an air-fluidized bed had almost the same interface pressures, and both provided better pressure reduction over the sacrum and trochanter than the standard hospital mattress. None of the surfaces reduced heel pressures to below capillary closing pressure. In another study, we found that a three-layered air cushion produced the lowest pressure over the trochanters of healthy subjects. Clinical specialists at a university hospital found that high-risk patients using the same cushion developed far fewer pressure ulcers than patients with the same risk factors reported in the literature.

Some clinicians advocate the use of dynamic rather than static pressure relief mattresses. However, a study comparing the skin microvascular response of healthy persons on a dynamic mattress overlay with those on a static pressure-reducing mattress found no significant differences in trochanteric skin blood perfusion. Both surfaces increased skin temperature and blood flow.

Any pressure-reducing overlay is useless if the weight of the body fully compresses it and rests on the standard mattress, or "bottoms out." A "hand check" will reveal when pressure reduction is adequate and the patient has not bottomed out. In a correctly done hand check, one slides the hand — flat, fingers outstretched, and palm up — between the mattress overlay and the underlying mattress. (See *Hand check to assess pressure relief.*) If the person's body can be felt through the mattress overlay, pressure reduction is inadequate, and the patient needs a support surface with more depth.

Mattresses

Pressure-reducing foam-core mattresses can help reduce the incidence of pressure ulcer and save health care dollars by eliminating costly overlays and specialty beds. Significantly fewer patients develop pressure ulcers when using the foam mattress. However, these mattresses lose both comfort and support over time, and they require close monitoring for signs of deterioration.

If incontinence, wound drainage, or perspiration is increasing the risk for pressure ulceration, a support surface that flows air across the skin helps keep the skin dryer. Many portable low-air-loss mattresses are available.

Specialty beds

A study comparing an air suspension bed with a standard ICU bed and mattress found that patients on the air bed had significantly fewer pressure ulcers than patients who were on a regular mattress. Few well-designed, randomized, controlled studies have compared types of support surfaces. Clinicians need comparative data on the effects of low-air-loss versus air-fluidized surfaces and on low-air-loss overlays versus low-air-loss beds.

Seating support surfaces

Chair cushions designed to reduce pressure on the ischial tuberosities are available. All seem to comparably reduce reactive hyperemia over the ischium.

Hand check to assess pressure relief

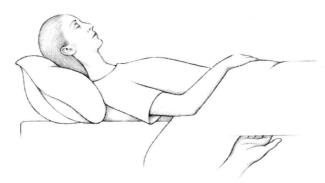

With your palm facing up and your fingers flat, slide your hand under the support surface, directly under the pressure point, as shown above. Don't flex your fingers.

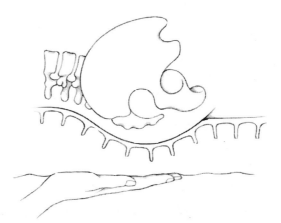

With good support under the patient, you won't feel the bony prominence with a flat hand, even when the patient is lying in a "worst-case" position (that is, with the head of the bed elevated 30 degrees and the patient side-lying on the greater trochanter).

Adapted with permission from Gaymar Industries, Inc.

People who are wheelchair dependent need durable cushions that can withstand everyday use. For patients who weigh between 50 and 300 pounds, the recommended specifications for foam wheelchair cushions are:

- thickness — 3 to 4 inches
- ILD — 25% at 40 to 70 pounds
- density — 1.8 to 2.8 pounds per cubic foot.

Some wheelchair-seating clinics specialize in making custom-fitted chair cushions. They may have computerized mechanisms for assessing patient characteristics as well as for designing seating surfaces. These costly cushions are a justifiable expense, given the alternative of pressure ulceration or enforced bed rest.

For spinal cord–injured patients, wheelchair cushion selection is based on pressure evaluation, lifestyle, postural stability, continence of bladder and bowel, and cost. Patients must be aware that older cushions fatigue and lose the capacity to adequately reduce pressure. A hand check helps determine the pressure-reducing adequacy of a chair cushion. Not replacing a worn-out cushion is false economy.

Choosing support surfaces

There is no scientific evidence that one support surface consistently works better than all others. The best way to match a support surface to a patient's needs is to learn the special characteristics of each type of surface. (See *Selected characteristics for special support surfaces*.) Learn the generic categories of beds, mattresses, and cushions and which commercial products fall into each category. (See *Pressure reduction devices: Advantages and disadvantages,* pages 76 and 77.) The choice of pressure-reducing equipment can be based on the following criteria:

- clinical effectiveness
- financial cost
- ease of use by caregivers
- comfort
- services offered by the supplier
- patient and staff educational materials supplied by the manufacturer.

The VA Healthcare System investigated the use of expensive support surfaces at their facilities nationwide. They then developed an algorithm for selection based on need for pressure ulcer prevention, pressure ulcer treatment, or patient comfort. (See *Specialty support surfaces,* pages 78 and 79.) The Guideline for the Prediction and Prevention of Pressure Ulcers from the Agency for Healthcare Research and Quality (AHRQ) provides the basis for decision nodes in the algorithm. The VA Health Care System emphasizes first-line or low-technology devices to contain expenditures.

Tissue interface pressure measurements reflect the relative effectiveness of pressure-reducing support surfaces, and the suitability of a support sur-

Selected characteristics for special support surfaces

Performance characteristics	Support devices					
	Air-fluidized	Low-air-loss	Alternating air	Static flotation (air or water)	Foam	Standard mattress
Support area	Yes	Yes	Yes	Yes	Yes	No
Low moisture retention	Yes	Yes	No	No	No	No
Reduced heat accumulation	Yes	Yes	No	No	No	No
Shear reduction	Yes	?	Yes	Yes	No	No
Pressure reduction	Yes	Yes	Yes	Yes	Yes	No
Dynamic	Yes	Yes	Yes	No	No	No
Cost per day	High	High	Moderate	Low	Low	Low

Source: "Treatment of Pressure Ulcers," Clinical Practice Guideline, No. 15. AHCPR Publication No. 95-0652. Rockville, Md.: U.S. Dept. of Health and Human Services, Public Health Service, Agency for Health Care Policy and Research, December 1994.

face can vary with the patient environment. Examples, in descending order of tolerable pressure, include:
■ intensive care units — foam overlay used for less than 7 days; the patient lies on a side for <10 minutes and is repositioned hourly
■ acute care settings — foam overlay for <21 days; patient is repositioned every 2 hours
■ long-term care settings, such as homes or nursing homes — turning can be expected only every 6 to 8 hours.

The costs of mattresses, beds, and chair cushions vary considerably, and the most expensive ones are not always the most effective. Some support surfaces are made for single-patient use, and others are rental items used by many people. Charges can range from $24.00 to purchase a foam overlay to a daily rental fee of $125.00 for a highly technical therapy bed. Often, emphasis on decreased resource consumption may give cost an inappropriately greater weight than clinical effectiveness. Caregivers must be vigilant and adamant about the effectiveness of items used for patients.

Institutions rightly require that requests for special support surfaces be justified. (See *Patient criteria for high- and low-air-loss therapies,* page 80, and *Com-*

Pressure reduction devices: Advantages and disadvantages

Description	Advantages	Disadvantages
Overlays *Indications:* Critically ill patient with a Braden score of 18 or less, or who will be on bed rest for longer than 24 hours		
Foam Varying density, convoluted foam	Varying densities provide pressure reduction in high-pressure areas; most patients find foam mattresses comfortable	May be flammable; patients are difficult to reposition due to envelopment; foam may cause increased perspiration; adds height to the bed, which may make it more difficult to get the patient out of bed
Static air mattress Vinyl air mattress that is inflated with a blower	May be more effective than foam with heavier patients	Inflation level must be checked regularly; may cause increased perspiration due to plastic surface; adds height to the bed, which may make it more difficult to get the patient out of bed
Alternating pressure air mattress A pump inflates mattress cells in an alternating fashion	Usually there is no charge for the motor if the mattress is purchased	Alternating air pressure requires a motor and an electrical source; plastic surface may increase perspiration
Low-air-loss beds *Indications:* Immobile patients who are difficult to turn and who exhibit one of the following: decreased serum albumin, anasarca, paralysis and/or sedation, expected prolonged ICU stay, existing skin breakdown, or pain associated with the bed surface, such as patients with cancer or Guillain-Barré		
Bed surface consists of inflated air cushions, each section is adjusted for optimal pressure relief for patient's body size	Provides pressure relief in any position; most models have built-in scales; surface fabrics are made of low-friction material	Must use incontinence pads recommended by manufacturer; air cushions may make it difficult to transfer patients into and out of bed; patients still must be turned frequently for pulmonary toilet
Air-fluidized beds *Indications:* Immobility associated with posterior surgical grafts, flaps, or burns		
Air is blown through glass beads to "float" the patient	Relieves pressure and reduces shear, friction, and moisture	Extremely heavy and difficult to move; foam wedge is required to elevate the head of the bed, which negates the relief of pressure, shear, friction, and moisture on the upper back and head; difficult to transfer patient; increased airflow may increase evaporative fluid loss, leading to dehydration

Pressure reduction devices: Advantages and disadvantages *(continued)*

Description	Advantages	Disadvantages
Pulsating beds Air cushions that alternately inflate and deflate, providing continuous pulsating action	Pulsation may improve peripheral venous return	Not yet well defined
Oscillating, low-air-loss beds *Indications:* Severe immobility, such as hemodynamically unstable patients who do not tolerate turning and/or with documented pulmonary pathophysiology requiring frequent position changes for secretion mobilization		
Bed surface consists of air cushions that are programmed to alternately inflate and deflate sections so the patient is rotated from side to side; in some models, the bed frame rotates	Pressure relief and low-friction surface are provided with gentle repositioning; most models have built-in scales	Patients must be positioned correctly for effective turning; conscious patients may not tolerate the movement of the bed; patients must have stable spines
Oscillating support surfaces Entire bed frame and surface rotate in an arc	Pressure reduction may be provided; frequent turning of patients with unstable spines is possible	Conscious patients may not tolerate the bed movement; bed rotation increases the risk of shearing forces on the tissue; contact with support surfaces during rotation may lead to pressure ulcer development; may be difficult to maintain lines and other invasive devices with bed frame rotation

Note: Due to the cost of specialty beds, the need for the bed should be evaluated daily; when mobility is improved and other indications for the specialty bed no longer exist, the patient should be moved to a regular bed, with an overlay device if needed.

Adapted with permission from AACN Clinical Issues in Critical Care Nursing, Vol 1, No 3, 1990.

paring high- and low-air-loss therapies, page 81.) In some settings, a particular product may not be available because of reimbursement restrictions, or a health care agency may carry only certain products. Even if a preferred type of support surface is unavailable, document the patient's needs.

A pressure-reducing surface on the bed or chair may give caregivers a false sense of security. Special equipment is certainly helpful as part of the overall management plan, but it is never a substitute for attentive care. Every patient requires an individual turning schedule, which must be based on assessment of the patient's tissue tolerance to pressure.

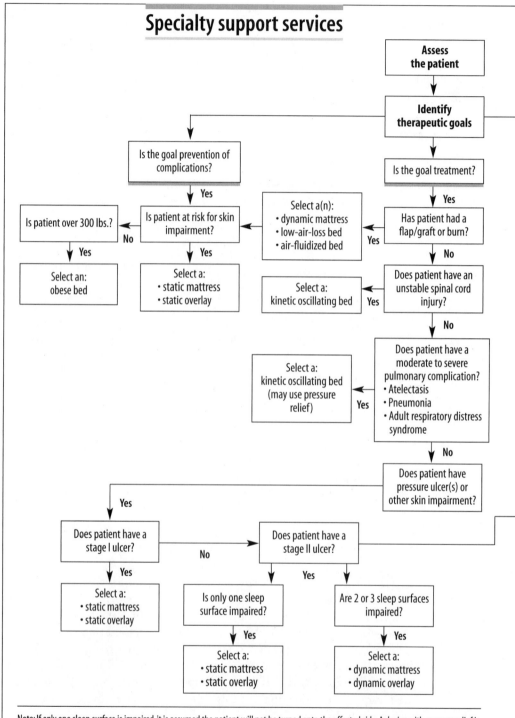

Specialty support services

Assess the patient

↓

Identify therapeutic goals

↓

Is the goal treatment?

↓ Yes

Has patient had a flap/graft or burn? → Yes → Select a(n):
• dynamic mattress
• low-air-loss bed
• air-fluidized bed

↓ No

Does patient have an unstable spinal cord injury? → Yes → Select a: kinetic oscillating bed

↓ No

Does patient have a moderate to severe pulmonary complication?
• Atelectasis
• Pneumonia
• Adult respiratory distress syndrome
→ Yes → Select a: kinetic oscillating bed (may use pressure relief)

↓ No

Does patient have pressure ulcer(s) or other skin impairment?

Is the goal prevention of complications?

↓ Yes

Is patient at risk for skin impairment? → No → Is patient over 300 lbs.?
↓ Yes → Select an: obese bed

↓ Yes

Select a:
• static mattress
• static overlay

Does patient have a stage I ulcer?

↓ Yes

Select a:
• static mattress
• static overlay

No →

Does patient have a stage II ulcer?

↓ Yes

Is only one sleep surface impaired?

↓ Yes

Select a:
• static mattress
• static overlay

Yes →

Are 2 or 3 sleep surfaces impaired?

↓ Yes

Select a:
• dynamic mattress
• dynamic overlay

Note: If only one sleep surface is impaired, it is assumed the patient will not be turned onto the affected side. A device with pressure relief is indicated if two or three sleep surfaces are impaired.

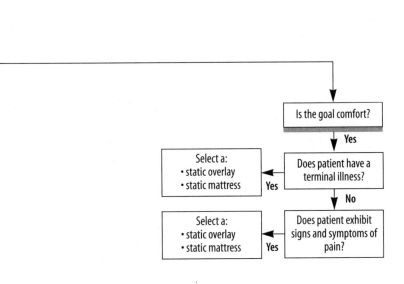

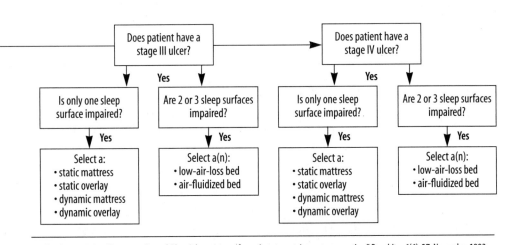

Used with permission. Thomason, S., et al. "Special support surfaces: A cost-containment perspective," *Decubitus* 6(6): 37, November 1993.

Patient criteria for high- and low-air-loss therapies

1. For patients who have plastic surgery operations:
   a. Air-loss therapy is necessary for 2 to 3 weeks for patients who have whole buttock/gluteal rotation flaps to the sacrum; wean to air mattress overlay before discharge.
   b. Air-loss therapy is unnecessary for patients who have local/Limberg rotation flaps to the sacrum.
2. Patients with severe or multiple pressure ulcers may be eligible for air-loss therapy after the following criteria have been met:
   a. Other less costly pressure relief devices have been tried first (for example, air mattress overlay) unless patient has had recent plastic surgery and requires air-loss therapy.
   b. The patient was on an air mattress overlay during a previous admission and developed a pressure ulcer, or an existing ulcer deteriorated.
   c. The following plans are in place
      - nutrition
      - incontinence management
      - debridement
      - topical wound management plan
3. Patients with bone metastasis/pathologic fractures are eligible for air-loss therapy when severe pain is unrelieved by pain medication and prohibits position changes.
4. Patients who have radical vulvectomy operations with imposed immobility require high-air-loss therapy for approximately 10 days postoperatively because of the necessity to do wound irrigations without repositioning the person.
5. Patients who have massive edema leading to generalized weeping and/or sloughing skin may require high-air-loss therapy because of its drying effect.

Harper Hospital–Detroit Medical Center
Detroit, Michigan

Skin care

No patient is exempt from regular examination for pressure areas, the timing based on the clinician's assessment of risk for pressure ulceration and of the patient's ability to tolerate pressure. Many clinicians were taught to massage reddened areas of skin over bony prominences. To the contrary, recent studies show that massage may reduce blood flow and cause tissue damage.

Older adults have special needs for skin care. As their skin loses elasticity and epidermal proliferation slows, its functional effectiveness as a barrier diminishes. Also, as the epidermal-dermal junction flattens, the epidermis loses its anchor points to the dermis. Gentle handling can reduce the likelihood of skin tears caused by epidermis sliding across dermis.

Comparing high- and low-air-loss therapies

High-air-loss therapy (air-fluidized bed) may be more efficacious than low-air-loss therapy in the following circumstances:
1. *Uncontrolled incontinence* because the increased drying effect of air-fluidized beds reduces maceration of tissue.
2. *Repeated extensive dressing changes* because air-fluidized beds increase the ease of positioning.
3. *Positioning restrictions* — Patients who have severe trochanteric ulcers and hip contractures are more easily positioned on air-fluidized beds.

Low-air-loss therapy may be more efficacious than high-air-loss therapy in the following circumstances:
1. *Flotation disorientation* — With low-air-loss therapy, elderly patients may have less disorientation than with high-air-loss therapy.
2. *Continuous moist dressings* — If saline soaks are ordered, low-air-loss therapy may be preferred because high air loss can dry the dressings too rapidly.
3. *Risk of aspiration* — Patients who require tube feedings are at less risk for aspiration with low-air-loss therapy because the head of the bed can be elevated without decreasing pressure relief capability. Air-fluidized beds require the use of foam back wedges to elevate the head — this may decrease the pressure-relieving capability of the air-fluidized bed.
4. *Out-of-bed activity* — Patients who need to be out of bed are more easily moved/ambulated from low-air-loss surfaces. The low-air-loss surfaces deflate in the seat area. The air-fluidized bed has a permanent railing over which patients must be lifted.

Note: If all other factors are equal, be aware that the Harper Hospital Department of Epidemiology requires that patients on air-fluidized beds be in private rooms. Patients on low-air-loss surfaces may be placed in semiprivate rooms.

Harper Hospital–Detroit Medical Center
Detroit, Michigan

Advancing age is closely associated with progressive skin dryness, which can reduce pliability and initiate cracking of the epidermis. Investigators have found an association between dry, flaking skin and risk for pressure ulcers. Lack of moisture in the air is a major environmental contribution to dry skin. Relatively low humidity is common in overheated hospitals, long-term care facilities, and the homes of many elderly people. Central or room humidifiers can significantly reduce the detrimental effect of low humidity.

Cleansing the skin

The skin needs to be cleansed only when soiled. This is especially important for people with dry, aged, or at-risk skin, in whom frequent bathing may remove the natural barrier and increase skin dryness. There are many ways to maintain adequate hygiene without a daily shower or tub bath. When possible, the patient should make his own choice of frequency and type of bathing. Most patients at risk for pressure ulcers require only occasional full-body bathing. Often this means routine "face and fanny care" with cleansing of the axilla and perineal area when soiling from perspiration, urine, feces, or wound drainage makes it necessary.

The skin's protective acid mantle should be maintained with nonalkaline cleansing agents, such as a mild, synthetic detergent bar. The temperature of bath water should be slightly warm. When skin is very dry, the most prudent choice may be warm water without any cleansing agents. Minimal force always should be used during skin cleansing; this means gentle washing with a soft cloth and patting the skin dry with a soft towel. Vigorous rubbing is contraindicated.

Moisturizing the skin

It is important to keep the skin well lubricated without saturating the epidermis. Loss of moisture from the stratum corneum causes dryness, which, in turn, decreases pliability. Topical agents relieve the signs and symptoms of dry skin. These come in a variety of preparations, such as lotions, creams, and ointments. A pharmacy consult can provide information about products that are commercially available.

The Pressure Ulcer Committee at Harper Hospital developed a skin care flowchart that lists the products carried by the hospital and indicates the decisions that lead to an appropriate choice. The flowchart is now automated so that clinicians can independently order products from the pharmacy or central supply via computer. (See *Skin care flowchart,* pages 84 and 85.)

Lotions

Of all the moisturizers, lotions have the highest water content, evaporate the most quickly and, therefore, need to be reapplied the most frequently. Lotions are composed of powder crystals dissolved in water and held in suspension by surfactants. They may be more aesthetically pleasing than creams or ointments because they are easy to apply, have a cooling effect, are nonocclusive, and do not leave a greasy film on the skin. Some dermatologists recommend using lotions in a low-humidity environment, believing that the high water content adds more moisture to the skin.

Creams

Creams are preparations of oil in water, so they are more occlusive than lotions. They need to be applied about four times daily for maximum effectiveness.

Ointments

Ointments are mixtures of water in oil and, hence, are the most occlusive. The oil component of ointments can be lanolin or petrolatum. Petrolatum is more effective on dry skin than lanolin. Ointments provide a longer lasting effect on skin moisture than either lotions or creams.

Protecting the skin

Skin that is waterlogged from constant wetness is more easily eroded by friction, more permeable to irritants, and more readily colonized by microorganisms than normal skin. Urinary and fecal incontinence create problems from excessive moisture and chemical irritation. Fecal incontinence may be more damaging to the skin than urinary incontinence because the feces contain bacteria. When both types of incontinence coexist, the urea in urine interacts with chemical enzymes in the stool to cause diaper dermatitis.

Incontinence is not a normal part of aging. Patients may be incontinent for any number of reasons. Fecal impaction or tube feedings may precipitate diarrhea. In urinary incontinence, medication may be the culprit, or the patient may have a urinary tract infection, may be unable to reach the bathroom in time, or may be confused or too embarrassed to ask for the bedpan.

Once the cause of incontinence is determined, a care plan must be developed to manage the problem. Incontinence alone is not an indication for an indwelling urinary catheter. If the cause of incontinence is reversible, patients should be given frequent voiding opportunities with positive reinforcement for requesting toileting assistance or staying dry. A prompted timed voiding regimen can decrease the frequency of incontinence episodes in elderly patients.

Incontinence collectors

For continuing incontinence, several external urinary and fecal collection devices are available. Many incontinent men use condom catheters connected to dependent drainage. External urinary collection devices for women are less successful. Fecal incontinence collectors are made of pectin skin barriers with attached drainable pouches, much like colostomy pouching systems. A regular schedule for changing these collectors is useful. It is much easier to change an intact fecal collector than a leaking appliance on a patient with diarrhea. A caregiver who is unfamiliar with these incontinence collectors should ask an enterostomal therapy or wound care specialist to demonstrate their application. Rectal tubes are a poor choice for managing fecal incontinence because they may cause such complications as vasovagal responses and anal-tissue ischemia.

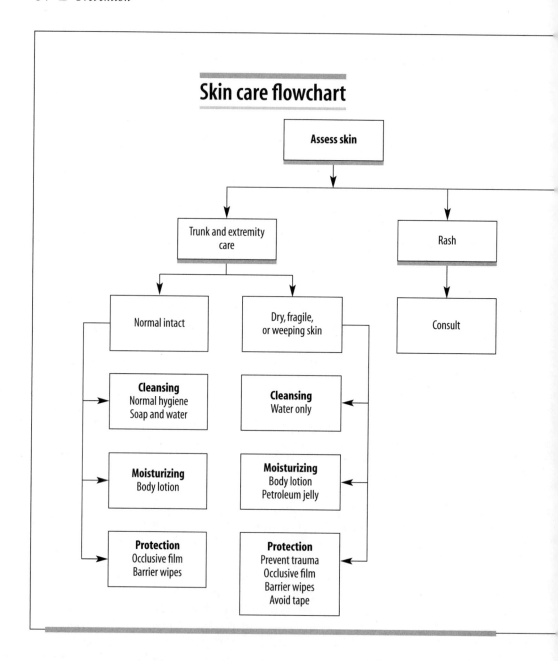

Skin care flowchart

Assess skin

Trunk and extremity care

Rash

Normal intact

Dry, fragile, or weeping skin

Consult

Cleansing
Normal hygiene
Soap and water

Cleansing
Water only

Moisturizing
Body lotion

Moisturizing
Body lotion
Petroleum jelly

Protection
Occlusive film
Barrier wipes

Protection
Prevent trauma
Occlusive film
Barrier wipes
Avoid tape

Underpads

If a patient is not a candidate for an external collection device, hygiene must be provided immediately after soiling. Absorptive underpads wick moisture away and provide a quick-drying surface for the skin. Infants wearing disposable absorbent gel diapers have significantly less skin wetness, closer to

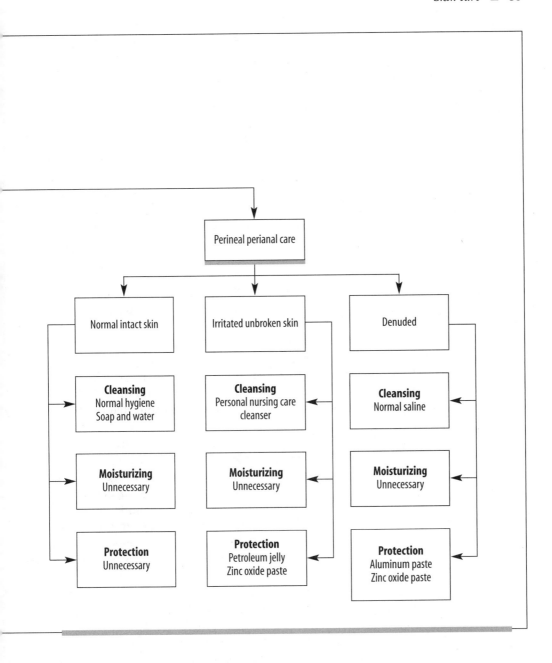

normal skin pH, and less contact dermatitis than those wearing disposable cellulose core diapers or laundered cloth diapers. Nevertheless, many health care facilities will not stock disposable underpads if their cost outweighs that of washable, reusable underpads. Clinicians must remain vigilant about the effectiveness of various types of underpads used by health care facilities.

Plastic and paper linen savers should never be placed next to the patient because they hold moisture, which irritates the skin surface. Support staff sometimes place linen on top of incontinence underpads to avoid completely changing the bed when a patient voids. This practice nullifies the purpose of the underpad, which is to protect the skin, not the bed. Likewise, securing an incontinence underpad around the patient like a diaper defeats the purpose of the underpad. The patient is served by lying on top of the pad and letting the uncovered areas of skin air-dry. When the patient is repositioned, another skin surface can be air-drying.

Diapers and incontinence underpads do not eliminate the need for vigilance on the part of caregivers. An established schedule should determine the time for automatically checking patients who are likely to be incontinent.

Topical barriers

Liquid copolymer film barriers can offer protection for unbroken at-risk skin. These liquid barriers come in multiuse spray canisters or foil packets of single copolymer-saturated wipes. The alcohol content of some liquid barriers may sting irritated or denuded skin. The purpose of the liquid barrier is to create a plastic-like film that protects the skin from moisture, so it is important to use a barrier that is not water soluble. After applying the liquid barrier, fan the area and separate opposing parts until the skin is completely dry and nontacky. Cleansing does not have to completely remove the barrier before the next application.

Areas of intact skin around open wounds need to be protected from drainage and maceration. Petroleum jelly is effective if the moisture is from water or saline. If the moisture or drainage contains irritants, a paste may be necessary to protect the skin. A paste is composed of ointment with powder added for thickness and durability. Zinc oxide is a common ingredient of commercially available protective barrier pastes. Paste is an excellent skin barrier that is purposely difficult to remove so that it will remain effective. Its tenacity makes it more impermeable to irritants. Paste is best removed with mineral oil.

Avoid using a topical barrier that leaves oil on the skin if an adhesive product, such as a hydrocolloid, will be used. Hydrocolloid wafers are useful physical barriers to protect skin from moisture or drainage. Moist dressings can be placed directly on top of hydrocolloid wafers. The skin under the wafer will remain dry as long as the wafer remains intact.

Monitoring changes in risk status

Risk factors determine which interventions the clinician includes in each patient's care plan. (See *Preventing pressure ulcers: Risk factors and interventions*.)

Preventing pressure ulcers: Risk factors and interventions

The table below summarizes the risk factors and illustrates prophylactic interventions to reduce pressure ulcer risk.

Risk factors	Interventions
Immobility	Provide pressure-relief surface Establish turning schedule Reduce shear and friction Consult physical therapist
Inactivity	Provide assistive devices to increase activity
Incontinence	Cleanse and dry skin after elimination Assess etiology of incontinence Apply protective skin barriers
Decreased mental status	Assess patient/family ability to provide care Educate caregiver regarding pressure ulcer prevention
Malnutrition	Provide adequate nutritional and fluid intake Consult dietitian for nutritional evaluation
Impaired skin integrity	Avoid pressure, friction, shear, excessive wetness Moisturize skin Don't massage red areas Don't use donuts Don't use heat lamps

The interventions can be used as a basis for a generic standard protocol for pressure ulcer prevention. Changes in patient risk status require a revision of the plan of care.

Once you have developed the pressure ulcer prevention plan, consider all the factors that may influence patient outcomes, write realistic and measurable goals, and then solicit support from other health care professionals. Try to communicate the importance of consistent care to peers, for if a plan is to be fairly evaluated, all caregivers must implement care in the same manner.

If, despite everyone's best efforts, the patient develops a pressure ulcer, the prevention plan must be intensified. The pressure area cannot heal while the area remains ischemic. Prevention efforts will fail unless pressure relief is adequate and the patient's risk factors, such as malnutrition, are corrected.

Summary

To prevent pressure ulcers in their patients, clinicians must develop comprehensive plans of care. Crafting one where prevention measures figure heavily increases the chances of a successful outcome. Collaboration with the patient and the patient's family to establish a preventive care plan is essential. This plan of care must include discussions and decisions on educational needs, nutritional management, correct body positions, turning and repositioning schedules, appropriate support surfaces and skin care, and monitoring changes in risk status. By implementing an intensive pressure ulcer prevention care plan, clinicians can alleviate the pain and discomfort that accompany pressure ulcers, thus improving the patient's outlook and quality of life.

Selected references

Macklebust, J. "Preventing pressure ulcers in home care patients," *Home Health Care Nurse* 17(4):229-238, 1999.

Macklebust, J. "An update on horizontal patient support surfaces," *Ostomy/Wound Management* 45(1A Suppl):70S-77S, January 1999.

Stotts, N. "Risk of pressure ulcer development in surgical patients: A review of the literature," *Advances in Wound Care* 12(3):127-136, 1999.

Chapter 7

Treatment

The extracellular environment of the wound greatly influences the healing process. Clinicians often have the opportunity to manipulate environmental factors that support healing. Significant interventions include protecting the wound and providing a physiologic environment by

■ relieving pressure (body positioning, repositioning, and use of support surfaces)
■ providing adequate nutrients
■ providing local wound care (including wound debridement, adequate cleansing, and selection of appropriate wound dressing materials)
■ minimizing pressure ulcer risk factors.

See also Chapters 5 and 6 for detailed discussions of assessing risk factors and preventing ulceration by providing good body positions, repositioning, support surfaces, and nutrition. In general, the same conditions that put the patient at risk for pressure ulceration also impede healing.

Support surfaces

If pressure is not removed or reduced, all other efforts toward healing the pressure ulcer will be futile. Pressure-reducing devices work by redistributing pressure at bony prominences over the larger surface area of the entire body. An effective support surface must mold to the body to maximize contact, redistribute the patient's weight as evenly as possible, and consequently raise the pressure over less prominent areas of the body. The amount of pressure directed to the new area is usually trivial in comparison with the original pressure on bony prominences and is clinically inconsequential as long as it remains below capillary closing pressure.

The number of patient support or sleep surfaces marketed as pressure-reducing devices has escalated during recent years. There are specialized mattresses and beds to support the entire body in order to more evenly distribute the pressure. Slabs of polyurethane, foam pads, and mattresses are made in numerous densities, thicknesses, and convolution patterns. Mattress over-lays are made of gel, sheepskin, and water- or air-filled vinyl cushions. So-phisticated electronic buoyant support systems have been designed to float, turn, and independently move the patient into and out of bed.

Many studies report intermediate outcomes, such as interface pressure measurements or changes in ulcer surface area, rather than patient outcomes, such as healing. Intermediate outcomes are useful for decision making when randomized controlled studies on patient outcomes are not available. How-ever, effective care in today's health care marketplace requires a shift of fo-cus to clinical measurement, such as treatment outcomes. Manufacturers must collaborate on this research effort to make a difference for patients. Clinicians who are called on to be more cost-effective will select support sur-faces according to cost in the absence of compelling evidence of compara-tive clinical effectiveness.

The practical considerations for selecting support surfaces are unchanged from those published in the *Clinical Practice Guidelines: Treatment of Pressure Ulcers* from the Agency for Healthcare Research and Quality (AHRQ). The algorithm on management of tissue loads published there remains useful for providing clinical guidance. When a clinician matches the condition of the patient to the therapeutic benefits of support surfaces, a variety of sur-faces will likely meet the patient's needs.

Nutrition

Elderly, hospitalized patients frequently become extremely malnourished. This greatly increases their chances of complications and death. Because the consequences can be so serious, health care providers must take active steps to make sure older patients receive adequate nutrition; those with pressure ulcers should receive aggressive nutritional support. Tissue repair requires both energy (calories) and adequate amounts of vitamins, minerals, and oth-er nutrients. The role of nutrition in healing pressure ulcers and preventing their recurrence is well accepted clinically, but the research data are incom-plete and contradictory. Studies are in progress to determine if weight gain induced by anabolic androgenic steroid use enhances wound healing.

A sound principle of nutrition in wound care is to provide the substrates essential for healing. (See *Role of selected nutrients in wound healing.*) Proteins are needed for repair and regeneration, angiogenesis, fibroblast activity, col-lagen synthesis, and scar formation. Adequate carbohydrate and fat intake is needed to prevent amino acids from being used for energy expenditure. It seems that patients with pressure ulcers preferentially use their energy in-take for wound healing. One study found that, in malnourished patients with stage IV pressure ulcers who consumed 40 kcal/kg body weight (2,800 calories for an approximately 150-pound person), the ulcers healed and the patients did not gain a significant amount of weight. Vitamins and miner-

Role of selected nutrients in wound healing

Nutrient	Role	Recommendation
Calories	• Fuel for cell energy • "Protein protection"	• 30 to 35 kcal/kg/day or enough to maintain positive nitrogen balance
Protein	• Building block for cells and tissues	• 1.25 to 1.50 g/kg/day or enough to maintain positive nitrogen balance
Vitamin C (Ascorbic acid)	• Hydroxylation of proline and lysine in collagen synthesis	• RDA = 60 mg supplement • If deficient, 500 mg b.i.d. • Need long time to develop clinical scurvy from vitamin C deficiency • Low toxicity
Vitamin A	• Enhances epithelialization, collagen synthesis, and cross-linking • Can reverse steroid effects on skin and delayed healing	• RDA = 4,000 IU supplement • If deficient, 20,000 U x 10 days
Vitamin E	• No known role in wound healing	• None
Zinc	• Cell mitosis & cell proliferation	• RDA 12 to 15 mg • Correct deficiencies • No improvement in wound healing with supplementation unless zinc deficient • Use with caution! Large doses can be toxic and may inhibit copper metabolism and impair immune function
Fluid	• Essential fluid environment for all cell function	• 30 to 35 ml/kg/day • Increase by another 10 to 15 ml/kg if patient is on an air-fluidized bed • Use noncaffeine, nonalcoholic fluids without sugar • Water is best (6 to 8 glasses/day)

Adapted with permission from "Nutritional aspects of wound healing," *Home Healthcare Nurse* 17(11):719–730, 1999.

als should be increased, but specific requirements for wound healing are not known. (See Chapter 6 for more information about nutrition and supplements.)

Staging nutritional intervention

Level I

1. Estimate nutritional needs.
2. Monitor ability to self-feed; consider use of finger foods, adaptive utensils, refeeding programs, increased time, or feeding assistance.
3. Pay attention to food preferences and tolerances; optimize the eating environment by individualizing meal times and patterns as much as possible; ensure good food quality and variety.
4. Monitor food and fluid intake.
5. Consider an interdisciplinary assessment of chewing and swallowing ability.
6. Add medical nutritional products to supplement intake.
7. Limit use of unsupplemented liquid diets or other restrictive diets.
8. Routinely reassess nutritional status and response to nutrition intervention.
9. Document and reevaluate the plan of care.

Level II

1. Institute tube feedings to meet nutritional needs if this is compatible with overall goals of care.
2. Take precautions to prevent pulmonary aspiration and other complications.
3. Monitor nutritional intake through counting calories.
4. Routinely reassess nutritional status and response to nutrition intervention.
5. Document and reevaluate the plan of care.

Adapted with permission from Ross Products Division, Abbott Laboratories, Columbus, Ohio, from Campbell, S.M. *Pressure Ulcer Prevention and Intervention: A Role for Nutrition,* May 1994, pp. 14-15.

Early identification of malnutrition and subsequent intervention can alter the healing trajectory in patients with wounds. (See *Staging nutritional intervention.*) A nutritional plan should be comprehensive and individualized. Because there is no such thing as a standard patient, there can be no such thing as a standard formula. Nutritional support of patients with wounds includes participation of the dietitian, physician, clinician, pharmacist, patient, and family. Principles of nutritional therapy include:

■ a multidisciplinary approach
■ early and regular assessment of nutritional status
■ goal setting
■ meeting the patient's metabolic needs.

Nutrition intervention begins with a nutritional assessment, which serves as a basis for planning. Chapter 5 discusses nutritional assessment in detail. Treatment, including feeding, must incorporate overall patient goals. More research is needed to identify markers that predict healing and to establish the precise relationship between various elements of nutrition and pressure ulcer healing.

Local care

Local pressure ulcer care involves wound debridement, wound cleansing, appropriate dressing materials, and selected adjuvant therapy.

Debridement

Although debridement is the cornerstone of wound management, no randomized controlled studies have been conducted to determine its effectiveness. However, clinical experience shows that removing all necrotic tissue, exudate, and metabolic wastes from the wound increases the chances for healing and diminishes the risk of infection. Wound healing cannot occur in the presence of necrotic tissue. Necrotic tissue may present as moist yellow or gray tissue that is in the process of separating from viable tissue. If the necrotic tissue becomes dry, it presents as thick, hard, leathery black eschar. Areas of necrotic or devitalized tissue may mask underlying fluid collections or abscesses.

Debridement of nonviable tissue is considered the most important factor in the management of contaminated wounds. Methods of debridement are classified as sharp, mechanical, chemical, and autolytic. The clinician's choice depends on the type of wound, the amount of necrotic tissue, the condition of the patient, the setting, and the caregiver's clinical experience. Combining debridement methods may increase effectiveness.

Sharp debridement

The most rapid and efficient method of debridement is sharp surgical debridement. The clinician uses a cutting tool, such as a scalpel, scissors, or laser, to remove macroscopically identified necrotic tissue from the wound bed. In randomized, controlled studies, sharp debridement of diabetic foot ulcers correlated with improved wound healing. Similar studies need to be conducted on patients with pressure ulcers.

A scalpel can be used to separate the edges of eschar from the necrotic wound bed. Scissors can be used to snip black, brown, gray, or yellow necrotic tissue from the pressure ulcer. If the patient has advancing cellulitis, sharp debridement of devitalized tissue is urgent. The main benefit of sharp debridement is the rapidity with which dead tissue can be removed. Sharp debridement is imprecise and may remove some viable tissue. It requires particular caution when used on patients who have low platelet counts or who are taking anticoagulants.

A physician, physician's assistant, physical therapist, or advanced practice clinician determines the need for this type of debridement. State laws and community standards provide the requirements for performing this procedure.

Mechanical debridement

Mechanical debridement removes dead tissue by applying a mechanical scrubbing force or use of wet-to-dry dressings (see "Gauze dressings" later in this chapter). Mechanical debridement is nonselective, can harm healthy granulation tissue or epithelial cells, and may be painful. If a wound contains granulation tissue, the caregiver should moisten the gauze with enough normal saline to avoid tearing away new tissue as the dressing is removed. Superficial wounds or wounds with small amounts of necrotic tissue can be more effectively treated with other debridement techniques.

Chemical debridement

Chemical debridement with enzymatic agents is a selective method of debridement. The various types of enzymes target specific necrotic tissues, such as protein, fibrin, and collagen. The type of enzyme chosen depends on the type of necrotic tissue in the wound. Enzymes are generally categorized as proteolytic, fibrinolytic, and collagenase. Necrotic fibrins and proteins are located in the wound bed more superficially than is devitalized collagen.

During the inflammatory process of wound healing, one of the more important enzymes released is endogenous collagenase. Because collagen makes up at least 75% of the dry weight of skin, the action of endogenous collagenase is one of the rate-limiting steps in tissue remodeling. The collagenase used to debride wounds is derived from *Clostridium histolyticum*. At physiologic pH (range of 6 to 8), collagenase dissolves and liquefies necrotic wound debris.

In a recent randomized controlled trial of 21 patients, Alvarez and colleagues compared collagenase and papain/urea formulations for chemical debridement. Papain/urea was more effective than collagenase in reducing the amount of nonviable tissue and in raising 50% granulation tissue. However, time to healing or bacterial burden did not differ between the pressure ulcers treated with either ointment.

Enzymes can be inactivated with either topical anti-infective agents containing heavy metals or acidic solutions that alter the pH. Debilitated patients who undergo enzymatic debridement should be closely monitored for systemic bacterial infections.

Autolytic debridement

Autolytic debridement makes use of the body's own enzymes to digest devitalized tissue. Moisture-retentive dressings allow endogenous enzymes in the wound fluid to liquefy necrotic tissue. The wound fluid contains macrophages and neutrophils that digest and solubilize necrotic tissue. Autolytic debridement is the most selective form of debridement but requires additional time to remove devitalized tissue. Autolytic debridement is generally not painful. During autolytic debridement, frequent cleansing is essential to wash out the partially degraded tissue fragments.

Cleansing

Optimal wound healing cannot proceed until all foreign material is removed from the wound. Removal of inflammatory material from the wound surface is best done using pressure irrigation. Wound irrigation has two components: a cleansing solution and a mechanical means of delivering the solution to the wound bed.

Cleansing agents

The most common and cost-effective wound-cleansing solution is isotonic saline (0.9% sodium chloride). Skin cleansers never should be used on open wounds; they are much more toxic than wound cleansers. Tests that directly compare the toxicity of cleansing solutions can provide useful information on their relative safety. (See *Relative toxicity indexes of nonantimicrobial and antimicrobial wound cleansers,* page 96.) This toxicity index does not mean to imply that the toxic solutions can be diluted and then used for wound cleansing. The cleansing efficacy of any cleansing solution should be balanced against its potential to damage macrophages and fibroblasts within the wound tissue.

Irrigation techniques

Wounds need to be irrigated with enough force to enhance cleansing without traumatizing the wound bed. To be effective, the irrigation force must be greater than the adhesion forces holding the debris to the wound bed. An ideal pressure for flushing necrotic tissue from a wound is 8 psi. Cleansing the wound with a steady stream from a piston syringe is more beneficial than using a bulb syringe or gravity drip.

Several studies have demonstrated that increasing the pressure of the irrigating stream enhances removal of bacteria and soil from wounds. Wound inflammation and wound infection occur significantly less often in wounds cleansed with the syringe and needle irrigation system than in those cleansed with the bulb syringe.

Increasing the pressure of an irrigation stream can increase the cleansing efficiency of the irrigation process to a point. Too high an irrigation pressure can cause trauma to the soft tissue. Commercial dental cleansing devices deliver too much pressure, are needlessly traumatizing, and should be avoided.

Clinical practicalities

Use of a 35-ml syringe and a 19-gauge needle delivers a stream of irrigant to the wound surface at an effective irrigation pressure. However, needles used for wound lavage can become contaminated with blood, exudate, and other body fluids. A major concern is transmission of hepatitis B, hepatitis C, hepatitis E, and human immunodeficiency virus. Alternative delivery systems can reduce danger from needle sticks to care providers. For example, a

Relative toxicity indexes of nonantimicrobial and antimicrobial wound cleansers

Product	Manufacturer	Toxicity Index
Dermagran®	Derma Sciences, Inc.	10
Shur-Clens® Wound Cleanser	ConvaTec®	10
Biolex™ Wound Cleanser	Bard Medical Division, C.R. Bard, Inc.	100
Carra-Klenz™	Carrington Laboratories, Inc.	100
Saf-Clens® Chronic Wound Cleanser	ConvaTec®	100
Clinswound™	Sage Laboratories, Inc.	1,000
Constant-Clens Dermal Wound Cleanser		
Curaklense™ Wound Cleanser	Kendall Healthcare Products Company	1,000
Ultra-Klenz™	Carrington Laboratories, Inc.	1,000
Clinical Care® Dermal Wound Cleanser	Care-Tech® Laboratories, Inc.	1,000
MicroKlenz™ Antimicrobial Wound Cleanser	Smith & Nephew United, Inc.	10,000
SeptiCare™ Antimicrobial Wound Cleanser	Sage Laboratories, Inc.	10,000

Adapted with permission from *Wounds* 9(1):15-20, 1997. © 1997. Health Management Publications, Inc.

19-gauge angiocatheter attached to a 35-ml syringe delivers the right amount of pressure and eliminates unnecessary use of a needle. This is an expensive but effective clinical method of irrigating wounds.

As part of a quality improvement initiative, Harper Hospital adopted an alternative cost-effective wound irrigation system: a 250-ml soft plastic bottle of sterile normal saline attached to a Baxter screw cap with irrigating tip. When squeezed with full force, this irrigation system delivers an irrigating stream with impact pressures of approximately 4.5 to 5 psi. This system has become part of the Harper Skin/Wound Care Protocol. Compliance with wound cleansing and infection control policies has improved, and clinicians appreciate the user-friendly approach. One bottle provides adequate cleansing solution for irrigating a large wound, or enough solution for three dressing changes per 24 hours on a smaller wound. The bottle and cap are discarded 24 hours after being opened. As with any pressurized irrigation method, clinicians should be aware of splashback and use appropriate precautions. (See *AHRQ guidelines on pressure ulcer treatment: Irrigation pressures.*)

AHRQ guidelines on pressure ulcer treatment: Irrigation pressures

Device	Irrigation Impact Pressure (psi)
Spray Bottle — Ultra Klenz™a (Carrington Laboratories, Inc., Dallas, TX)	1.2
Bulb Syringea (Davol Inc., Cranston, RI)	2.0
Piston Irrigation Syringe (60-ml) with catheter tip (Premium Plastics, Inc., Chicago, IL)	4.2
Saline Squeeze Bottle (250-ml) with irrigation cap (Baxter Healthcare Corp., Deerfield, IL)	6.0
Water Pik® at lowest setting (#1) (Teledyne Water Pik, Fort Collins, CO)	7.6
Irrijet® DS Syringe with tip (Ackrad Laboratories, Inc., Cranford, NJ)	8.0
35-ml syringe with 19-gauge needle or angiocatheter	42.0
Water-Pik® at middle setting (#3)b (Teledyne Water Pik, Fort Collins, CO)	>50.0
Water-Pik® at highest setting (#5)b (Teledyne Water Pik, Fort Collins, CO)	>50.0
Pressurized Cannister-Dey-Wash™b (Dey Laboratories, Inc., Napa, CA)	

aThese devices may not deliver enough pressure to adequately cleanse wounds.

bThese devices may cause trauma and drive bacteria into wounds. They are not recommended for cleansing of soft-tissue wounds.

Source: Beltran, Thacker, and Rodeheaver, 1994.

Whirlpool cleansing

Whirlpool baths have been used for wound cleansing since their development by French surgeons during World War I. The vigorous whirling and agitation of the water contributes to its cleansing action. The turbulence of the water is thought to assist in removing surface debris. Investigators caution that the use of whirlpool with even moderate water agitation can damage granulation tissue and migrating epidermal cells. Once a wound has been cleansed of foreign debris, the potential for harm to regenerating tissues outweighs the whirlpool's benefits. Therefore, the use of a whirlpool bath to cleanse granulating wounds is not recommended.

Dressings

Humidity is of prime importance, affecting both the rate of epithelialization and the amount of scar formation (see Chapter 4 for a discussion of moisture and wound healing). A wound bed is kept hydrated with the use of appropriate dressings. Moisture-retentive dressings prevent desiccation and promote formation of granulation tissue. If the wound bed is exposed to the air, it dehydrates and cells die.

Open wounds, such as pressure ulcers, require dressings that protect and maintain their physiologic integrity. The ideal dressing keeps the wound surface moist without allowing excessive fluid accumulation, macerated skin, and bacterial proliferation. Some of the occlusive dressings designed to keep wounds moist have caused concern about the possibility of promoting bacterial growth under the dressing. However, these dressings may protect wounds from pathogenic bacteria. (See *Wound dressing guidelines,* pages 100 to 103.)

Selection

Many materials have been used through the ages to cover wounds — from hot oils and waxes to animal membranes and feces. Many useful dressing materials are now available for care of chronic wounds, such as pressure ulcers. The basic purpose of the dressing must be considered before one is selected. Functions of a dressing are:
- to protect the wound from contamination
- to protect the wound from trauma
- to provide compression if bleeding or swelling is anticipated
- to apply medications
- to absorb drainage or debride necrotic tissue.

The condition of the wound and the desired function determine the type of dressing that is used. The pressure ulcer must be evaluated and a treatment plan determined before the most suitable dressing can be selected. Clinicians should choose dressing techniques that keep the wound bed moist and the surrounding intact skin dry.

Types of dressings

No single type of dressing can provide an optimum environment for all wounds. Each product has its advantages and disadvantages.

Gauze dressings

Gauze dressings are made of cotton or synthetic fabric that is absorptive and permeable to water, water vapor, and oxygen. Gauze may be used dry, moist, or impregnated with petrolatum, antiseptics, or other agents. It is made in varying weaves and with different size interstices. It may be used in special dressing techniques.

Dry. A dry dressing protects the wound from trauma and infection. On a primarily closed wound, the dressing is placed on the wound dry and is removed dry. On an open wound, dry dressings should be used only to wick the exudate from the ulcer. The dressing is changed as needed to control the exudate.

Wet-to-dry. Wet-to-dry saline gauze dressings are used to debride necrotic tissue. Saline-moistened gauze is wrung until it is just damp, opened, placed on the wound surface, and allowed to dry until it adheres to the necrotic tissue. It is then pulled away from the wound, removing debris that adheres to the interstices of the dressing. This method of debridement is nonselective and may damage new tissue.

Continuously moist. Continuously moist saline gauze dressings keep the wound moist and promote healing when frequent inspection is necessary. It is used for wounds that do not contain large amounts of necrotic tissue. This dressing should be placed in the wound moist and be remoistened or changed frequently enough to keep the wound tissue continuously moist. Care must be taken that the moist gauze dressing is not placed on the surrounding intact skin, where it causes maceration. A thin layer of petrolatum or hydrocolloid on the surrounding intact skin protects it from the moist dressing.

Polyurethane film

Polyurethane film dressings are synthetic, semipermeable, transparent, and adhesive. They allow free flow of oxygen from the air to the wound, and of water vapor from the wound to the air, but they are impermeable to bacteria and to particles in the environment. These dressings enhance epithelial migration by preventing a scab from forming. Polyurethane dressings have adhesive backings that allow them to adhere to dry skin, but some film dressings adhere to the base of the ulcer and, when removed, strip away new epidermis. On skin surface areas at risk for abrasion, polyurethane film can be used prophylactically to decrease the amount of friction between the patient's skin and the sheets. It also may be used to protect the skin from fecal and urinary incontinence.

Film dressings seem to carry relatively little risk of wound infection and to provide faster healing and lower cost than wet-to-dry techniques for stage II ulcers. They should not be used for stage III ulcers because the ulcer depth usually requires packing. They are as effective as other moist wound-heal-

Wound dressing guidelines

Dressing Generic Category	Description/Composition	Trade Name
Transparent Film	Polyurethane or copolymer with porous adhesive layer that allows oxygen to pass through the membrane and moisture vapor to escape	Bioclusive; Flexifilm; Opsite; Tegaderm; Polyskin
Hydrocolloid	Hydrophilic colloid particles bound to polyurethane foam, impermeable to bacteria and other contaminants; minimal to moderate absorptive properties	Comfeel; Cutinova; Hydro; Curaderm; Duoderm; Intrasite; Restore; RepliCare; Tegasorb; Hydrocol; Ultec
Hydrogen	Water-or glycerin-based, nonadherent, cross-linked polymer; variable absorptive properties; contains 80%–99% water	Biolex; Curafil; Curasol; Carrsyn Gel; Hypergel; lamin; IntraSite; Flexaderm; MPM Hydrogel; Nu-gel; SoloSite; Restore; Hydrogel; Tegagel; Vigalon
Foams	Hydrophilic polyurethane or gel film—coated foam, nonocclusive, nonadherent, absorptive wound dressing	Alleyvn; CarraSmart; Curafoam; Cutinova Foam; Flexzan; Hydrosorb; Lyofoam; Polyderm; Border; Teille
Calcium Alginate	Nonwoven composite of fibers from calcium alginate, a cellulose-like polysaccharide, highly absorptive dressing manufactured from brown seaweed. Forms a soft gel when mixed with wound fluid	Algiderm; AlgiSite; CarraSorb; Curasorb; Dermacea Alginate; Kaltostat; PolyMem Alginate; Restore CalciCare; Sorbsan; Tegagen HI; HG Alginate

Adapted with permission from Baranoski, S. "Wound dressings: Challenging decisions," *Home Healthcare Nurse* 17(1):22-23, January 1999.

Indications For Use	Advantages and Benefits	Disadvantages
Donor sites; partial-thickness wounds; stage I–II pressure ulcers; superficial burns; secondary dressing	Wound inspection; impermeable to external fluids & bacteria; conformable; promote autolytic debridement; prevention/reduces friction; change daily or p.r.n. if leakage noted; numerous sizes available	Nonabsorptive; may adhere to some wounds; not for draining wounds; fluid retention may lead to maceration of periwound area
Stage I–IV pressure ulcers; partial- and full-thickness wounds; dermal ulcers; under compression wraps/stockings; necrotic wounds; can be used as a preventive dressing for high-risk friction areas; use as a secondary dressing or under taping procedures; numerous sizes, shapes, forms, and thicknesses	Facilitates autolytic debridement; self-adherent/some may adhere to wound bed; impermeable to fluids/bacteria; conformable; reduction of pain; thermal insulation; absorptive — minimal to moderate; long wear time — 3 to 5 days, decreases frequency of dressing changes	Opaque; not recommended for heavily draining wounds, sinus tracts, or fragile skin; some contraindicated for full-thickness wounds and/or with infections (check package inserts); some may be difficult to remove; leakage can be a problem/edges roll up; foul odor noted with removal can be confused with infection; some may leave a residue in wound bed
Stage II–IV pressure ulcers; partial- and full-thickness wounds; dermabrasion; painful wounds; dermal ulcers; radiation burns; donor sites; necrotic wounds	Nonadherent; trauma-free removal/soothing to patient; rehydrates the wound bed; reduces wound pain; can be used with topical medications; can be used in infected wounds; softens and loosens necrosis, slough to aid debridement; daily dressing change; available in sheets and gels	Some require secondary dressing to secure; may macerate periwound skin; not recommended for heavily draining wounds
Partial- and full-thickness wounds with minimal to heavy amount of drainage; stage II–IV pressure ulcers; surgical wounds; dermal ulcers; under compression wraps/stockings; infected and noninfected wounds (varies, check package insert); tunneling and cavity wounds (varies, check package insert)	Nonadherent; trauma-free removal; conformable; many sizes, shapes, and forms available; absorptive, minimal to heavy drainage; easy to apply and remove; frequency of dressing change depends on the amount of drainage	Not recommended for nondraining wounds; not recommended for dry eschar; not all foams recommended for infected wounds and for use in tunnels and tracts (check package insert); may require secondary dressing or tape to secure; may macerate periwound area if not changed appropriately
Partial- and full-thickness wounds; moderate to heavy draining wounds; stage III–IV pressure ulcers; dermal wounds; surgical incision/dehisced wounds; post-op wounds for hemostasis; sinus tracts, tunnels, or cavities; infected wounds; donor sites	Highly absorbent and nonocclusive; trauma-free removal; can be used on infected wounds; hemostatic properties for minor bleeding; reduced frequency of dressing changes; available in sheets, ropes, and within other composite-type dressings	Contraindicated for dry eschar, third-degree burns, surgical implantation, and heavy bleeding; may require secondary dressing to secure; gel may have foul odor during dressing change

(continued)

Wound dressing guidelines *(continued)*

Dressing Generic Category	Description/Composition	Trade Name
Composites	Combination of two or more physically distinct products manufactured as a single dressing that provides multiple functions. Features may include a bacterial barrier, absorptive layer, foam, hydrocolloid, or hydrogel; semiadherent or nonadherent	Alldress; Covaderm Plus; Epigard; MPM Multi-layered; Telfa Island; Telfa Plus; Tegaderm Absorbent Pad
Collagens	Collagen is a major protein of the body. Dressing stimulates cellular migration and contributes to new tissue development and wound debridement	Fibracol; Medifil Particles/Gel/Pads; Skin Temp Sheets
Enzymatic Debriders	Proteolytic, chemical agent that breaks down devitalized tissue	Accuzyme; Collagenase/Santyl; Elase
Gauze Dressings	Manufactured in many forms: woven and non-woven, impregnated, and nonadherent	Manufacturers and distributors of gauze products: Kendall Healthcare Products; Johnson & Johnson Medical; DeRoyal Industries; Sherwood, Davis & Geck; SOA Molnfycke; Derma Sciences; MPM Medical

ing techniques. Additionally, film dressings result in a significant savings in time compared with techniques employing saline gauze.

Hydrocolloids

Hydrocolloid dressings are adhesive, moldable wafers made of carbohydrate-based materials, usually with a waterproof backing. Most are impermeable to oxygen, water, and water vapor. These dressings contain hydroactive particles that interact with moisture to form a gel. They adhere to the dry, surrounding, undamaged skin to contain the wound exudate and prevent wound contamination. Keeping the wound bathed in serous exudate enhances healing and permits removal of the dressing without damaging the newly formed epithelium. Some researchers believe that interactive dressings need to have a porous backing to allow for a more controlled evaporation of wound exudate. Those with an occlusive backing should not be used on clinically infected wounds.

Indications For Use	Advantages and Benefits	Disadvantages
Primary and secondary dressings for partial- and full-thickness wounds; stage I–IV pressure ulcers, varies with each product; minimal to heavy draining wounds; dermal ulcers; surgical incisions	Facilitate autolytic debridement; conformable; multiple sizes and shapes available; easy to apply and remove; most include adhesive border; frequency of dressing change dependent on wound type (check package insert)	Adhesive borders may limit use on fragile skin; some contraindicated for stage IV ulcers (check package insert)
Partial- and full-thickness wounds; stage III and some stage IV pressure ulcers (check package insert); dermal ulcers; donor sites; surgical wounds	Absorbent, nonadherent; conforms well; may be used in combination with topical agents	Contraindicated for third-degree burns and sensitivities to bovine products; not recommended for necrotic wounds; requires secondary dressing to secure; may require rehydration
To debride full-thickness necrotic wounds, pressure ulcers, dermal ulcers, post-op wounds, infected wounds	Nonsurgical method of debridement; requires daily and/or twice-daily dressing changes (check package insert)	Inactivated by soaps, detergents, acidic solutions, and metallic ions; must be covered by secondary dressing; some enzymatics can damage healthy tissue
Indications vary with individual gauze product; draining wounds; necrotic wounds; wounds requiring debridement, packing, or management of tunnels, tracts, dead space; surgical incisions; post-op wounds, burns; dermal ulcers; pressure ulcers	Readily available in many sizes and forms; can be used on infected wounds, in combination with other topical products; effective as a packing agent in tracts, tunnels, undermining areas	May disrupt wound healing if allowed to dry out or changed inappropriately; fibers may shed and/or adhere to wound bed; requires secondary dressing often; not recommended for effective moist wound therapy treatment; frequent dressing changes

Hydrocolloids are effective for stage II, III, and IV pressure ulcers. The rate of ulcer healing varies with initial ulcer depth. Patients with debilitating cancer or diabetes and those with deeper ulcers seem to have poor results with hydrocolloid dressings.

Controlled trials have not supported the claim that hydrocolloid dressings are likely to cause wound infection. However, it should be noted that most of the controlled trials *excluded* subjects whose ulcers, at initial assessment, were clinically judged to be infected. Patients have reported less pain or discomfort with hydrocolloid dressings compared with previous treatments. Controlled studies have shown that treatment with hydrocolloid dressings saved a significant amount of time when compared with saline gauze treatment.

Gels/hydrogels

Hydrogel dressings are water-based, nonadherent, polymer-based dressings with some absorptive properties. These dressings maintain a moist environment and may be used with a topical medication if indicated. One property of gel dressings is the ability to cool the wound by as much as 5° F. This may increase comfort for patients with painful wounds.

Some hydrogels are fluid-donating agents and others can either donate or absorb liquid, depending on the wound's moisture content. Future gel dressings may be able to "read" the moisture content of a wound and deliver or absorb the necessary amount of fluid to maintain an ideal environment. Also, it is possible that they will be used as carriers for growth factors and biologically active molecules.

Currently, gels/hydrogels appear to be effective for treating pressure ulcers. Their relative benefits over other types of moist wound-healing techniques for pressure ulcer treatment remain to be determined.

Foam dressings

Foam dressings are made from a spongelike polymer that may be adherent. Foam may be impregnated or coated with other materials, such as topical medication. It has some absorptive properties. Foam dressings create a moist environment and provide thermal insulation of the wound. If a foam dressing has hydrophilic properties, this allows for some absorption of wound drainage.

Alginate dressings

Alginate dressings are made from a naturally occurring polysaccharide found in brown seaweed. The principal constituent is alginic acid, converted to mixed calcium and sodium salts. This dressing is a nonwoven twisted fiber rope or fibrous mat. The mat is placed in the wound and held in place with a secondary dressing. As the dressing absorbs wound fluid, it forms a soft hydrogel. The dressing is capable of absorbing up to 20 times its own weight in exudate, and its primary use is with moderately to heavily exudating wounds.

Subjective evaluations have reported that dressings were effective for exudate control, odor control, and pain control. Alginates appeared to be associated with minimal pain on dressing changes and less pain than historical control treatments.

Pastes, powders, and beads

Paste, powder, and bead dressing materials are formulated primarily to fill wound cavities. Most can absorb wound exudate, which then converts the dressing to a gelatinous mass, which can be irrigated from the wound. One gram of hydrophilic beads can absorb up to 4 grams of water. The granules do not digest bacteria or necrotic tissue, but they draw bacteria away from the wound bed.

Composite dressings

Composite dressings are two or more different products combined by the manufacturer. They may be used when the features of each dressing are desired.

Selecting dressings

Some dressings claim to have enhanced capabilities or lower complication rates than other types of dressings. Controlled studies are needed to support such claims. (See also Chapter 12.)

The persistent mistaken belief that dressings heal wounds encourages clinicians to try multiple dressings without considering other, more important factors. Harper Hospital developed skin/wound care decision-making flowcharts to assist clinicians with selection of appropriate dressing materials (see Appendices). These flowcharts have improved and standardized the care of specific types of wounds.

Infection control

Infection is a major concern in the care of a patient with a pressure ulcer. Bacteria normally cover the body surface and the gut; however, when skin is damaged and the immune system is compromised, these same bacteria can become virulent. Acute wounds generally are more susceptible to bacterial invasion than chronic wounds. All chronic wound surfaces are colonized with bacteria. It is only when conditions are favorable that infection occurs.

Number and type of organism, wound type, and general condition of the patient affect the patient's ability to resist infection. The most common sites for infection are the lungs, urinary tract, skin, and abdomen. All sites must be evaluated when the patient presents with a fever and a high white blood cell count. When infection of an ulcer is suspected, a culture should be obtained. The AHRQ Pressure Ulcer Treatment Guideline recommends that quantitative bacterial cultures also be obtained when clean ulcers are not healing.

Open wounds do not have to be sterile to heal. However, healing may be impaired when the bacterial count in an ulcer exceeds 10^5 organisms per gram of tissue. The most accurate method of determining bacterial load is by tissue biopsy or by fluid from needle aspiration. But not all facilities have staff members who can obtain tissue with a scalpel or punch biopsy. Nor do they have the laboratory facilities to process the tissue. Use of a swab technique for obtaining a specimen cannot be relied on to accurately document the bioburden in the tissues because the swabbing is done in a variety of ways. However, if a standardized method is used, a quantitative swab technique can document the bioburden in pressure ulcers. The technique for obtaining the specimen should include bacteria from the tissue rather than from the surface of the wound. The results of the swab culture must reveal more than just presence or absence of bacteria. Reports on the bioburden must be presented in a quantitative or semiquantitative manner for the information to be useful. (See also Chapter 9 for a current Policy and Procedure form.)

If a pressure ulcer is infected, antimicrobial therapy should begin as soon as possible. Antibiotic selection is based on the most likely pathogen, the organism's antimicrobial susceptibility, the efficacy of the drugs, potential adverse effects, and cost.

Antibiotics are biologically derived products that have a specific method of inhibiting microbial function. It appears that silver sulfadiazine exerts its toxic effects on bacteria through heavy metal poisoning, which also accounts for the toxic effects on human fibroblasts. These findings may explain the clinical observation of delayed wound healing with the use of silver sulfadiazine. The effect of various topical agents on bacterial counts and on the viability of healthy tissue is not clear. Also, the emergence of allergy and sensitivity to topical treatments is of concern.

Topical antimicrobials
Topical antimicrobial agents include both antibiotics and antiseptics. The use of antimicrobials on open wounds is highly controversial, and several studies report adverse effects. Patients with chronic wounds may develop allergies to topical agents, such as bacitracin and neomycin, and should be monitored for sensitivity. The AHRQ Pressure Ulcer Treatment Guideline recommends initiating a 2-week trial of topical antibiotics for clean pressure ulcers that are resistant to healing or are continuing to produce exudate after 2 to 4 weeks of optimal care. Prolonged use may create resistant organisms. Research studies show topical antibiotics are effective in reducing the bacterial levels in pressure ulcers to 10^5 organisms per gram of tissue.

Antiseptics
Antiseptics are highly reactive chemicals that indiscriminately destroy cell function. Povidone-iodine, acetic acid, sodium hypochlorite, and hydrogen peroxide are cytotoxic to fibroblasts. Their use to decrease the bacterial count in open wounds is contraindicated. Antiseptics indiscriminately damage tissue, interfere with tissue function, increase injury, and delay wound healing. Pressure ulcers should be managed by aggressive attention with conservative agents.

Adjunctive therapy
Clinicians often seek adjunctive therapies in their effort to support or stimulate healing of a nonhealing pressure ulcer. It is difficult for practitioners

to remain abreast of all the new wound care technology and products being introduced to the marketplace as the science of wound healing evolves.

Emerging adjunctive therapies for the treatment of pressure ulcers include growth factors, electrical stimulation, hyperbaric oxygen, bioengineered skin, and ultrasound therapy as well as warmth therapy and vacuum-assisted devices. Research supporting these therapies is limited. Electrical stimulation was the only adjunctive therapy recommended in the 1994 AHRQ Clinical Practice Guideline.

Growth factors

In the past, the rate of wound healing was set by nature, and there was little one could do except create optimal conditions to assist the body's own healing mechanisms. Advances have been made in the understanding of wound repair as topical growth factor research continues. Growth factors are polypeptide molecules that control the growth, differentiation, and metabolism of cells during wound healing. They are purported to promote new granulation tissue and the growth of new skin to cover the wound. They appear to act within a network of interacting factors to produce the biologic response. Growth factors interact with cells at the local level to stimulate or accelerate the repair of chronic, nonhealing wounds.

One type of platelet-derived growth factor is extracted from the patient's own blood. The laboratory dispenses the growth factor solution to the patient for topical administration by the patient or a caregiver. The growth factor solution is believed to stimulate initial wound healing, but the underlying cause of the ulcer must be treated as well to prevent recurrence. The rate of healing varies with the disease underlying the ulceration.

Chronic wounds treated with growth factors have been reported to improve. Outcome studies documenting the benefits of growth factors on pressure ulcers are lacking. Preliminary research shows encouraging results on pressure ulcer healing. However, a number of unanswered concerns remain, including:

■ too few clinical trials with demonstrated clinical efficacy
■ the lack of FDA standards against which the effects of growth factors can be measured
■ the need to demonstrate lack of adverse effects, such as tissue overgrowth resulting in excessive scarring
■ the need to determine dosages and methods of delivering the growth factors to the wound.

It may be that different growth factors are beneficial at different phases of wound healing. It is anticipated that continued growth factor research will more fully explain the action of growth factors in healing wounds.

Electrical stimulation

Traditionally, electrical stimulation has been used for conditions treated by physical therapists, such as muscle spasms and injuries, but there is an increasing interest in this method of treatment for accelerating closure of chronic wounds. In clinical trials, electrotherapy has enhanced the healing rate of pressure ulcers unresponsive to conventional therapy. Three types of electrical waveforms have been applied to wound healing: low-intensity direct current, high-voltage pulsed current, and pulsed electrical stimulation. Physiologic changes occur at the tissue and cellular levels in a wound exposed to exogenous electrical stimulation.

Pulsed high-frequency high-peak power electromagnetic energy has been studied in wound healing. The treatment is noninvasive and can be applied through clothing and surgical dressings. The biologic effects that enhance wound healing include increased blood flow, stimulation of collagen formation, and phagocytosis. Low-intensity pulsed direct current is thought to enhance the growth of fibroblasts and keratinocytes. The finding that it produced a significant improvement in healing of stage II pressure ulcers in spinal cord—injured men suggests that this may be a cost-effective treatment.

Hyperbaric oxygen

Hyperbaric oxygen (HBO) has been used as adjunctive therapy for conditions in which the underlying pathophysiology is local tissue hypoxia. HBO therapy is the administration of 100% oxygen under pressure greater than 1 atmosphere. HBO is administered in chambers that accommodate a single patient or many. The patient breathes oxygen as gradually rising atmospheric pressure causes oxygen to dissolve in the plasma at a higher concentration than would occur at sea level. The hemoglobin becomes supersaturated and delivers a greater supply of oxygen to the tissues.

HBO therapy was first used in the 1930s to treat the decompression sickness of undersea divers. HBO therapy also has been shown to be effective for carbon monoxide poisoning as it is the most rapid way of displacing carbon monoxide bound to hemoglobin. Research demonstrating the effectiveness of HBO therapy for wound healing has been less well documented.

The immune system, vascular tone, and wound healing all are affected by oxygen. It has been proposed that intermittent HBO treatments stimulate the oxidative functions of wound healing, providing greater availability of oxygen to fibroblasts, leukocytes, and endothelial cells. Conditions that reduce oxygen supply, such as anemia and chronic pulmonary disorders, decrease metabolic functions. Increasing the oxygen level allows restoration of these activities. Wound healing is optimal when periods of oxygenation alternate with relative hypoxia.

Topical HBO is not recommended for treatment of pressure ulcers as it does not increase tissue oxygen tension beyond the superficial dermis. Wounds that are poorly perfused owing to arterial insufficiency require surgical intervention to restore blood flow to the tissue. Oxygen, even under pressure, cannot get to tissues that have insufficient arterial inflow.

HBO treatment requires specialized equipment and highly trained personnel. Most patients with chronic wounds are unlikely to have access to this treatment unless a nearby facility has an HBO chamber already in place for treatment of decompression and carbon monoxide poisoning. More research is needed to find out whether the effects of HBO on chronic wounds are worth the time and expense required.

Bioengineered skin

The use of bioengineered skin in wound management is likely to increase significantly over the next decade. Cell culture techniques now permit the successful cultivation of cells in vitro to produce viable epithelial sheets. Applications include the successful treatment of skin ulcers. Long-term results in burn wounds appear to be comparable to those with split-thickness skin grafting.

Two bioengineered products have been studied in humans. One, composed of an epidermis and a dermis, is made with human keratinocytes and fibroblasts and type 1 bovine collagen. The other is made from human fibroblasts grown in a mesh of absorbable polymer. Both are intended to function as dressings and tissue replacements. It is not clear whether tissue takes permanently, but it does not seem to be rejected. Controlled studies are needed in patients with pressure ulcers.

Ultrasound

Ultrasound therapy is the use of high-frequency sound waves generated by oscillation of a crystal in a transducer. The oscillation can be produced continuously or in pulsed interrupted mode. Ultrasound is available with both thermal and nonthermal effects. The passage of the sound wave across the cell wall is thought to cause a change in diffusion rate and cell membrane permeability and thereby influence wound healing. In one clinical study, the use of ultrasound was associated with an accelerated rate of the inflammatory phase of wound healing. Mixed results of ultrasound studies indicate the need for more research to support the use of ultrasound in treatment of pressure ulcers.

Noncontact radiant heat bandage

A newer wound therapy unit uses a noncontact bandage with a warming unit. The bandage is an adhesive foam collar dressing covered with transparent film. A warming device incorporating infrared heating elements fits into a pocket in the film dressing. The unit warms to 38° C (100.4° F) and maintains 100% relative humidity, raising both periwound and wound temperatures to normal. The idea behind the device is that all cellular physiologic functions proceed best at normal skin temperature and that restoring normal temperature enhances blood flow and oxygenation. The Food and Drug Administration has approved warmth therapy for wound treatment.

Controlled negative pressure

Negative pressure wound therapy, also known as vacuum-assisted closure, may support wound closure when healing is delayed or impeded. If wound fluid is trapped in the area around the wound bed, negative pressure can evacuate the stagnant fluid. This reduction of edema improves blood flow to the wound.

A foam dressing is placed in the wound bed and sealed with an adhesive occlusive dressing. A computerized vacuum pump with a disposable collection chamber transmits subatmospheric pressure through an evacuation tube. The controlled negative pressure is maintained until the wound closes by secondary intention or the wound bed is ready for surgical closure.

Negative pressure creates a vacuum in the wound bed that stretches the cells and pulls them together. The beneficial consequences include:
- release of biochemical mediators of cellular proliferation from the stretched cell membrane
- formation of new blood vessels and granulation tissue
- reduction of bacterial load and cleansing of the wound bed.

Operative repair

Operative repair is an option for clean stage III and stage IV ulcers that do not respond to more conservative care. With surgical intervention, skin closure and tissue coverage are rapid. Criteria need to be standardized to determine patient eligibility. Before operative repair, the clinician needs to consider the patient's medical stability, nutritional status, and ability to tolerate the operative procedure/postoperative recovery as well as the likelihood that an operation will improve functional status. Included in the discussion are patient concerns regarding quality of life, personal preferences, treatment goals, risk of recurrence, and anticipated rehabilitative outcomes.

Operative procedures indicated for pressure ulcer repair include one or more of the following: direct closure, skin grafting, skin flaps, musculocutaneous flaps, and free flaps. Selection of a specific reconstructive technique is individualized for each patient. The location of the ulcer, prior ulceration and/or surgery, and the patient's mobility status, daily habits, and other associated medical problems are factored into the decision.

A good perioperative program includes comprehensive preoperative assessment and planning for postoperative care and follow-up. Because patients often enter the hospital on the operative day, it is helpful if the clinician can meet with the patient beforehand to provide teaching about postoperative care. Patients are informed of factors within their control that may impair wound healing, including smoking, diet, activity, and pressure relief.

Clinicians should help patients develop postoperative plans to reduce risk factors and increase the chance of operative success. The patient's commitment to the success of the program often can be determined at this time.

Surgical repair of the pressure ulcer may include skin grafts or muscle flaps. A muscle rotation flap is created by lifting nearby healthy tissue from the fascia and rotating the tissues to cover the defect caused by the pressure ulcer. Blood vessels that are carried over within the muscle flap nourish the tissues. This type of wound closure is beneficial for ulcers with major tissue loss because the muscle adds padding to dissipate pressure. A skin graft to the donor site may be necessary if the rotation causes a large tissue defect. The surgeon often has to remove an exposed bony prominence to prevent recurrence of the problem.

Postoperative care for patients is crucial to the success of the operation. In any situation in which skin grafts or muscle rotation flaps are used, care focuses on maintaining circulation and preventing infection.

■ At the time of the operation, wound drains are placed to remove air, serum, or fluid that collects beneath the flap. These drains should be checked to ensure that they are functioning properly.

■ Hematoma formation seriously compromises circulation and may result in flap necrosis. Flap circulation must be assessed carefully, and measures must be taken to assist in protecting the healing tissue.

After the operation, patients are kept immobile for about 2 weeks. The use of an air-fluidized or low-air-loss bed allows the patient to lie on the flap without undue pressure. Caution in turning the patient from side to side, even when using a specialty bed, is essential to avoid tension on the suture line and friction and shear on the flap.

■ Use extra personnel to move the patient in order to reduce the risk of tension on the new suture line.

■ Lift the patient's body to change the patient's position.

■ Under no circumstances should the patient be allowed to slide across the bed.

Protection of the grafted blood supply is critical for the first 14 days until the new capillaries are formed within the flap.

■ Inspect the graft area routinely for pallor or cyanosis indicating tissue ischemia. A healthy flap looks like the patient's normal skin.

■ Report color changes to the surgeon immediately.

■ Avoid activity that increases pressure on the flap. This includes the use of a bedpan if it places pressure on the newly grafted area. The patient can defecate onto a plastic pad until the graft is healed enough to tolerate brief periods of pressure. Fecal contamination can be avoided by using constipating medications and a low-fiber diet. Controlled bowel evacuation is accomplished with scheduled suppository insertion.

In addition to maintaining circulation, care focuses on measures to prevent infection. Because the vascular reserve of a flap is never normal, infection must be prevented at all costs. The vasculature may be able to cope with normal metabolic needs; however, the added burden of an inflammatory reaction may predispose the flap to necrosis. Infection at the graft site may result in loss of all or part of the graft.

■ Because infection threatens the viability of the flap, cleanse the incision areas carefully.

■ Remove crusts and dried fluids from the incision lines with sterile cotton-tipped applicators and sterile saline.

■ Cleanse the flap incisions carefully until all sutures are removed.

Steps can be taken throughout all phases of hospitalization to promote healing and prevent infection in skin grafts and flaps used primarily to close pressure ulcers.

Approximately 2 weeks after the operation, the patient begins sitting for progressively longer periods of time. After each sitting period, the caregiver must inspect the flap (unless the patient can do so with a mirror) for redness or pallor. Ongoing management of the repaired wound emphasizes education about pressure reduction and routine skin inspection.

Operative repair is only the beginning of a long-term recovery and maintenance process. Recurrence rates for pressure ulcers after operative repair vary, but the results often are dependent on patient selection. Risk factors for recurrence include noncompliance and carelessness. Pressure ulcers may recur because the patient chooses not to comply or because he has inadequate access to assistance and equipment that would allow continuous prevention of ulcers. Perioperative patient education programs are necessary regardless of the operative method chosen. Long-term follow-up is essential to determine adherence to recommended protocols.

Evaluating outcomes of care

All pressure ulcers should be reevaluated weekly. Plentiful evidence shows that weeks of ineffective treatment can be avoided if appropriate clinical assessments are done at least once a week. Given optimal care, the pressure ulcer should show signs of healing within 2 weeks. If the ulcer does not show progress, the entire plan of care must be revisited.

Exudative ulcers take longer to heal than nonexudative ulcers. One study showed that most full-thickness ulcers can heal in 6 to 7 weeks. None of the baseline characteristics were predictive of healing. However, differences in patient characteristics were substantial. Good prognostic factors include:

■ mental acuity

■ mobility

■ good nutritional status

■ percent reduction in ulcer size after 2 weeks of treatment.

Healing of partial-thickness pressure ulcers can be assessed clinically by observing epithelialization. Epithelial maturation occurs approximately 10 to 14 days after resurfacing. Epithelial migration, cell division, and differentiation constitute epidermal healing. At this time, the visual appearance is that of blending into the surrounding undamaged epidermis.

Tracking variances from expected outcomes

Good practice is supported when the clinician "maps" optimal care and then tracks variances from these expected outcomes. Pressure ulcer reassessment should be done weekly, and progress toward healing should be seen within 2 weeks. A logical course of care emerges (see Chapter 8 for a discussion of care maps). Case management of patients with pressure ulcers involves optimizing care, charting progress toward healing, and controlling variances with aggressive intervention.

Summary

Wound care practitioners must make treatment decisions based on the knowledge and strength of available evidence. Evidence-based practice focuses on using the most recent and valid literature to direct the care provided. Published studies on wound cleansing, debridement, dressings, and support surfaces provide a foundation for treatment decisions based on clear evidence. Before making treatment decisions, practitioners should seek evidence of the treatment's effectiveness. By practicing this way, the clinician will waste less time on ineffective treatments and will generate more evidence for treatments that work.

The wound-healing sequence follows an expected course if intrinsic and extrinsic conditions are optimal. Optimum healing is promoted by allowing the body's own healing mechanisms to occur. Routine wound cleansing should be accomplished with a minimum of chemical and mechanical trauma. The benefits of obtaining a clean wound must be weighed against potential for trauma to the wound bed. Indiscriminate use of antiseptics inhibits healing. Dressings provide an immediate environment that can support or impede wound healing. All dressings that support moist healing have equally good effects. New techniques for wound care must stand up to scientific scrutiny.

Selected references

Alvarez, O. M., et al. "Chemical debridement of pressure ulcers: A prospective randomized comparative trial of collagenase and papain/urea formulations," *Wounds 2000:*12(2):15-25, 2000

Anjello, E. A., et al. "Nutritional aspects of wound healing," *Home Healthcare Nurse* 17(11):719-730, Nov/Dec 1999.

Argenta, L.C., and Morykwa, M.J. "Vacuum-assisted closure: A new method for wound control and treatment; clinical experience," *Annals of Plastic Surgery* 38:563-576, 1997.

Baranoski, S. "Wound dressings: Challenging decisions," *Home Healthcare Nurse* 17(1):19-26, January 1999.

Brown, D.L., and Smith, D.J. "Bacterial colonization/infection and the surgical management of pressure ulcers," *Ostomy/Wound Management* 45(1A suppl):1095-1205, Jan 1999.

Frantz, R.A. "Adjunctive therapy for ulcer care," *Clinics in Geriatric Medicine* 13(3):553-564, August 1997.

Goode, P.S., and Thomas, D.R. "Pressure ulcers: Local care," *Clinics in Geriatric Medicine* 13:543-552, 1997.

Krasner, D., and Sibbald, R.G. "Moving beyond the AHCPR guidelines: Wound care evolution over the last five years," *Ostomy/Wound Management* 45(1A):1S-120S, 1999.

Maklebust, J. "Using wound care products to promote a healing environment," *Critical Care Clinics of North America* 8(2):125-158, 1996.

Maklebust, J. "An update on horizontal patient support surfaces," Ostomy/Wound Management 45(1A):70S-77S, 1999.

McGuckin, M. "The case for evidence based practice standards," *Advances in Wound Care* 11:46, 1998.

Mendez-Eastman, S., and Black, J. "Surgical alternatives for wounds," *Nursing Clinics of North America* 34(4):873-893, Dec 1999.

Niazi, L.P.M., and Salzberg, C.A. "Operative repair of pressure ulcers," *Clinics in Geriatric Medicine* 13(3):587-597, August 1997.

Ovington, L.G. "Dressings and adjunctive therapies: AHCPR guidelines revisited," *Ostomy/Wound Management* 45(1A):94S-106S, 1999.

Ovington, L.G. "The well-dressed wound: An overview of dressing types," *Wounds* 10(suppl A):1A-11A, 1998.

Robson, M.C. "Wound infection: A failure of wound healing caused by an imbalance of bacteria," *Surgical Clinics of North America* 77:637-650, 1997

Rodeheaver, G. "Pressure ulcer debridement and cleansing: A review of current literature," *Ostomy/Wound Management* 45(1A):80S-85S, 1999.

Senecal, S.J. "Pain management of wound care," *Nursing Clinics of North America* 34(4):847-860, Dec 1999.

Sieggreen, M., and Maklebust, J. "Debridement: Choices and challenges," *Advances in Wound Care* 10(2):32-37, March/April 1997.

Steed, D.L. "The role of growth factor in wound healing," *Surgical Clinics of North America* 77(3):575-586, June 1997.

Stotts, N.A., and Cavanaugh, C.E. "Assessing the patient with a wound," *Home Healthcare Nurse* 17(1):27-36, Jan 1999.

Stotts, N.A., and Hunt, T.R. "Pressure ulcers: Managing bacterial colonization and infection," *Clinics in Geriatric Medicine* 13:565-573, 1997.

Stotts, N.A. "Evidence-based practice: What is it and how is it used in wound care," *Nursing Clinics of North America* 34(4):955-963, 1999.

Strauss, S.E. "Evidence based medicine as a tool," *Hospital Medicine* 59:762-765, 1998.

van Rijswijk, L., and Broder, B. "Pressure ulcer patient assessment and wound assessment: An AHCPR clinical practice guideline update," *Ostomy/Wound Management* 45(1A suppl):565-655, Jan 1999.

Chapter 8

Care maps

After a systematic approach is initiated for assessing the degree of pressure ulcer risk, an institutional protocol should be developed to guide the caregiver in planning individual care. Clinicians frequently ask for a "recipe" for pressure ulcer care. If the ideal treatment were known, the pressure ulcer problem could be solved. To date, there is no recipe or ideal treatment.

Most clinicians base their care map on the patient's diagnosis and risk for developing pressure ulcers. Patients at risk for pressure ulcers have a diagnosis of "risk for impaired skin integrity," and those with pressure ulcers have a diagnosis of "impaired skin integrity" or "impaired tissue integrity." Interventions are directed toward resolving these clearly defined problems, and standardized care maps for impaired skin integrity have been published.

Harper Hospital model

The Pharmacy and Therapeutics (P&T) and Pressure Ulcer Committees at Detroit Medical Center's Harper Hospital collaborated to increase the quality and decrease the cost of topical pressure ulcer treatment. Members of the Pressure Ulcer Committee developed a decision-tree and a care map for skin and wound care to guide the staff in caring for patients. (See *Decision tree: Local wound care*, pages 116 and 117, and *Care map for pressure ulcer management*, pages 118 to 141.) Physicians, pharmacists, and nurses on the P&T Committee approved the charts as a standard hospital protocol. Physicians now write an order for "Skin and Wound Care Protocol," and clinicians use the items to independently order products from either the pharmacy or the central supply department.

Before implementation, the collaborators provided hospital-wide education to physicians, physician assistants, nurses, nurse practitioners, physical therapists, dieticians, pharmacists, and others interested in skin or wound care. The charts represent only topical treatment and not total care. (See Ap-

(Text continues on page 142.)

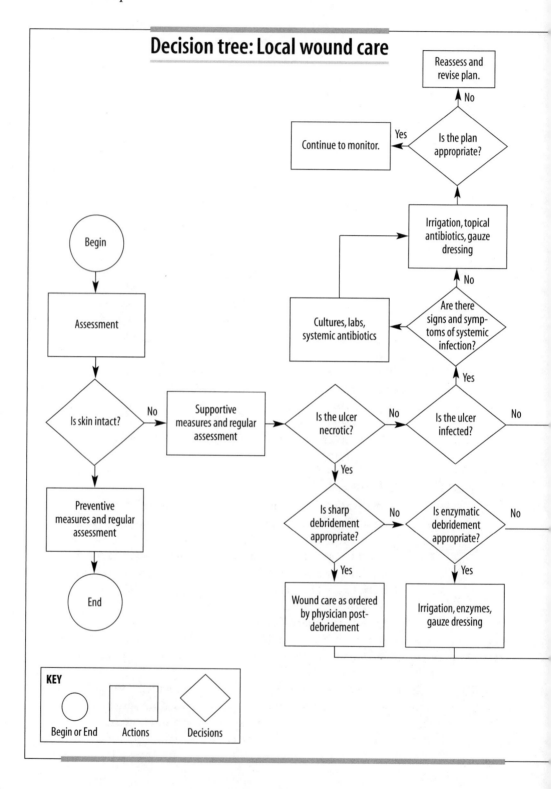

Decision tree: Local wound care

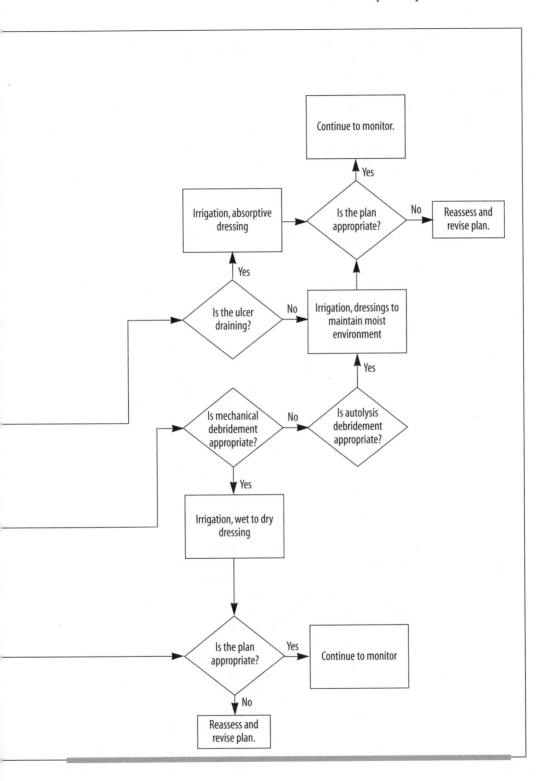

Care map for pressure ulcer management

Assessment	Plan	Rationale	Evaluation
Diagnosis: Risk factors	Care orders	Key rationale for care orders	Expected outcome
Risk for impaired skin integrity related to specific external and/or internal factors	Assess pressure ulcer risk on admission, daily, and when condition changes.	Prevention begins with identifying patients at risk for pressure ulcers.	Intact skin with absence of non-blanchable erythema.
	Assess patient's general health status:		
	• Age	Aging process is associated with arteriosclerotic change in vessels, loss of subcutaneous tissue, and decreased skin elasticity.	
	• Nutrition	Poor nutrition, as evidenced by unintentional weight loss, iron-deficiency anemia, hypoproteinemia, and vitamin deficiency, predisposes patients to tissue breakdown and is detrimental to wound healing.	
	• Mobility	Pressure for prolonged periods of time can lead to tissue destruction from anoxia.	
	• Sensory deficits	Sensory deficits may include absent or decreased awareness of pain and pressure. Sensory deficits may be due to physical impairment or altered mental status.	
	• Presence of excessive moisture	Moist skin at pressure points may lead to maceration. Macerated skin is easily rubbed away by friction.	
	• Diaphoresis or bowel or bladder incontinence	Moisture from perspiration or incontinence of urine/feces also reduces the resistance of skin to bacteria. Bacteria and toxins in the stool increase risk of skin breakdown.	
	• Use of excess lotion	Extra lotion adds excess moisture, which can macerate the skin.	
	• Bed protectors or "blue pads" next to skin	Blue pads hold moisture next to the skin. They are not absorbent and serve only as bed protectors.	

Care map for pressure ulcer management *(continued)*

Assessment	Plan	Rationale	Evaluation
Diagnosis: Risk factors	Care orders	Key rationale for care orders	Expected outcome
	• Diabetes mellitus	Diabetics often have neuropathy, impaired circulation, and poor wound healing.	
	• Infection	Infection increases the metabolic rate.	
	Assess for areas of blanchable and nonblanchable erythema, especially over bony prominences and pressure points.	Blanchable erythema indicates temporary ischemia or temporarily interrupted blood flow. Reactive hyperemia is the first response to temporary ischemia. It is characterized by a bright red flush caused by excessive blood flow to the area following a temporarily arrested blood flow. The flush shouldn't last longer than one-half to three-fourths the ischemic time. Nonblanchable erythema is redness of the skin that doesn't pale when gentle pressure is applied, indicating that tissue damage isn't yet ulcerated; this is classified as a stage I pressure ulcer.	
Diagnosis: Knowledge deficit	Care orders	Key rationale for care orders	Expected outcome
Knowledge deficit: Pressure ulcer prevention techniques as evidenced by inability of patient or significant other to state or demonstrate techniques of prevention	Assess patient or significant other's understanding of factors that contribute to pressure ulcers.	Level of knowledge and motivation of the patient must be assessed in order to develop a teaching plan.	Verbalization or demonstration of pressure ulcer prevention techniques, such as: • Correct positioning • Movement • Skin care • Nutrition • Early recognition of tissue damage

(continued)

Care map for pressure ulcer management *(continued)*

Assessment	Plan	Rationale	Evaluation
Diagnosis: Knowledge deficit	Care orders	Key rationale for care orders	Expected outcome
	Teach patient or significant other appropriate measures to prevent pressure ulcers:		
	• Nutrition	Adequate nutrients maintain positive nitrogen balance, which improves the quality of the soft tissue.	
	• Full-body repositioning	Relieves pressure from major bony prominences.	
	• Small shifts in body weight	Relieve pressure on bony prominences in extremities.	
	• Active and passive range of motion (ROM) exercises	Prevents joint contractures and helps prevent deconditioning.	
	• Skin care	Use of fundamental principles of cleansing, moisturizing, and protecting is essential to healthy skin.	
	• Skin protection from urine and feces	Prevents skin breakdown from maceration or chemical irritation.	
	• Early recognition of tissue damage	Alerts caregiver to avoid turning patient onto areas of nonblanchable erythema.	
Diagnosis: Pressure	Care orders	Key rationale for care orders	Expected outcome
Risk for impaired skin integrity related to pressure from immobility	Encourage highest degree of mobility and activity for patient.	Occlusion of blood vessels due to pressure from lack of normal movement is the basic cause of pressure ulcers. Flow is blocked by pressure on vessel from underlying bony prominences and compressing surfaces.	Intact skin with absence of nonblanchable erythema.
		Severe or prolonged interrupted blood flow will stop nutrients and O_2 from getting to cell and metabolites and CO_2 from leaving cell, thus leading to cell destruction.	Patient repositions self or is repositioned as condition indicates.
	Ambulate as ordered and tolerated.	Increased activity and mobility facilitate circulation and increase the sense of well-being.	

Care map for pressure ulcer management *(continued)*

Assessment	Plan	Rationale	Evaluation
Diagnosis: Pressure	Care orders	Key rationale for care orders	Expected outcome
	Provide assistive devices to increase independent movement.	The greatest risk for the development of pressure ulcers exists when the patient is unable to move.	
	• Bedbound: trapeze, side rails	Assist patient to increase independent mobility.	
	• Impaired ambulatory: canes, walkers, hand rails	Assist patient to increase independent activity.	
	Use active and passive ROM as appropriate.	Physiotherapy relieves pressure, promotes circulation, and decreases risk for joint contracture.	
	Change patient's position when in bed at least every 2 hours around the clock unless there is a medical contraindication as stated in the physician's orders. Shift patient's position every 15 minutes while chair sitting, according to the following guidelines:	The critical time period for tissue change due to pressure is between 1 and 2 hours, after which irreversible changes can occur. Patients having one or more presdisposing factors may need more frequent turning. Low pressure for a long period of time is more detrimental than high pressure for a short period of time. Moderate pressure within normal physiological limits can cause tissue damage if repeated too frequently.	
	• Use the 30-degree, laterally inclined position for bed patients whenever possible.	This position eliminates pressure from the sacrum and trochanter simultaneously.	
	• Position pillows to relieve pressure over bony prominences.	The patient is supported above the surface of the bed with free space between the bony prominence and the bed.	
	• Encourage proper posture in a chair.	Slouching in a chair and improper footstool height can increase pressure on bony prominences.	
	• Limit chair sitting to 1 hour.	Tissue compression is highest in the sitting position.	
	• Supplement full-body repositioning with minor shifts in body weight.	Small shifts in body weight are known to reduce the incidence of pressure ulcers.	

(continued)

Care map for pressure ulcer management *(continued)*

Assessment	Plan	Rationale	Evaluation
Diagnosis: Pressure	Care orders	Key rationale for care orders	Expected outcome
	• Post "turn clock" or repositioning schedule at bedside.	Alerts caregiver to recommended position changes and appropriate time intervals for turning.	
	Increase comfort and reduce mechanical sources of irritation.		
	• Apply 2-inch convoluted foam mattress (for example, "egg crate" foam) for comfort.	Thin foam mattress overlays don't adequately reduce pressure but provide comfort only.	
	• Keep linen smooth.	Wrinkles and foreign objects in the bed or chair may produce pressure or friction.	
	• Remove foreign objects from bed or chair.		
	• Select pressure-reducing devices and measures as appropriate.		
	• Obtain pressure-dispersing mattress or sleep surface.		
	Use air mattress overlay that reduces pressure below capillary closing pressure.	To maintain capillary blood flow	
	Use only one sheet and one lift sheet between patient and mattress:	Excessive linen interferes with pressure dispersion.	
	• Suspend heels to relieve pressure; for example, pillow under calf, egg crate cushion under Achilles tendon, vascular boot.	Vascular boots relieve pressure by suspending the heels. However, vascular boots shouldn't be used in patients who have "foot drop." If there is fixed plantar flexion, the heel won't be in proper position for pressure relief.	
	• Obtain pressure-reducing chair cushion.	To maintain capillary blood flow; tissue compression is highest in sitting position.	
	• Don't use rubber or inflatable rings; that is, "doughnuts."	Doughnuts may impede circulation; they relieve pressure in one area but increase pressure in the surrounding areas.	

Care map for pressure ulcer management *(continued)*

Assessment	Plan	Rationale	Evaluation
Diagnosis: Pressure	Care orders	Key rationale for care orders	Expected outcome
	• Limit time on bedpan.	Bedpans cause pressure and impede circulation.	
	• Avoid massage over bony prominences and hyperemic areas.	Massage over reddened areas may cause breaking of capillaries and traumatize skin. Vigorous massage angulates and tears vessels.	
Diagnosis: Shear	Care orders	Key rationale for care orders	Expected outcome
Risk for impaired skin integrity related to shearing forces	Carefully assist the patient into a sitting position. Avoid sliding patient across bed surface.	Shearing forces damage soft tissue by causing an opposite but parallel sliding motion of the layers of tissue under skin surfaces. This regulates in torn, angulated, or compressed blood vessels.	Intact skin with absence of non-blanchable erythema. Patient is repositioned to minimize shearing forces in reclining and sitting positions.
	Limit Fowler's or high-Fowler's position in high-risk patients. Encourage low semi-Fowler's position when in bed. Position the patient upright while in chair. Limit the use of a geriatric chair. Use pressure-reducing chair cushion while sitting.	When the head of the bed is raised 30 degrees or more, a greater compression force is placed on the posterior sacral tissues. Additional weight from the upper body is transferred to the tissues via the spinal column and sacrum. The body tends to slide downward to the foot of the bed, thereby increasing compression and shearing forces on the posterior sacral tissues, which in turn increases risk for tissue breakdown.	
	Limit sitting time to 1 hour.	Tissue compression is highest in a sitting position.	
	Position hips and knees on an even plane to distribute pressure evenly over back of thighs.	This body alignment will decrease ischial pressure and shear while chair sitting. Elevating knees higher than hips transfers pressure to ischial tuberosities.	

(continued)

Care map for pressure ulcer management *(continued)*

Assessment	Plan	Rationale	Evaluation
Diagnosis: Shear	Care orders	Key rationale for care orders	Expected outcome
	Avoid use of "knee gatch."	Pressure behind the knees may reduce blood flow to the lower extremities, thereby increasing risk for tissue ischemia.	
Risk for impaired skin integrity related to friction	Lift patient carefully when positioning; use lift sheet.	Friction can cause abrasion by rubbing away outer layers of skin. Use of lift or draw sheet will minimize friction on skin.	Intact skin with absence of abrasion.
	Encourage patient to assist as much as possible when moving in bed. Obtain overhead trapeze if indicated.	Use of trapeze facilitates self-care in positioning. Lifting buttocks from bed may reduce friction.	Patient is repositioned or moved to avoid frictional forces.
	Use long sleeves and cotton or wool socks to prevent friction over elbows or heels.	These devices decrease friction but don't relieve pressure.	
	Avoid devices, such as heel and elbow protectors, that require strapping tightly around an extremity.	Any device that is secured with a tight strap impedes blood flow and increases the risk of pressure ulcer formation.	
	May use a sheepskin pad under back/buttocks to decrease friction.	A genuine sheepskin minimizes friction but doesn't relieve pressure. Sheepskin may retain body heat and lead to increased perspiration. Synthetic orlon pile doesn't have properties that reduce pressure or friction.	
Diagnosis: Nutrition-fluid	Care orders	Key rationale for care orders	Expected outcome
Risk for impaired skin integrity related to inadequate nutritional and/or fluid intake	Obtain patient's dietary history.	Provides baseline data.	Intact skin with absence of non-blanchable erythema.
			Patient maintains stable body weight.
			Serum albumin level will be 3.0 or higher.

Care map for pressure ulcer management *(continued)*

Assessment	Plan	Rationale	Evaluation
Diagnosis: Nutrition-fluid	Care orders	Key rationale for care orders	Expected outcome
	Assess patient's nutritional status.	Poor general nutrition is frequently associated with loss of weight and muscle atrophy. The reduction in subcutaneous tissue and muscle reduces the mechanical padding between the skin and underlying bony prominences and increases susceptibility to pressure ulcers. Poor nutrition also leads to decreased resistance to infection and interferes with wound healing.	
	Consult dietician if patient has problems with nutrition.	Nutritional deficit is a known risk factor for the development of pressure ulcers.	
	Weigh patient on admission.	Initial weight provides baseline data.	
	Weigh patient two times per week.	Weight loss or gain serves as a guide for nutritional and fluid status.	
	Dietary intake: • Specify amounts and types of foods.	Adequate calories don't necessarily reflect a healthy diet.	
	• Indicate calorie count if indicated.	Caloric count, when assessed along with the amount and quality of dietary intake, provides objective data.	
	• Supplement meals if indicated. Request vitamin supplement if indicated.	Commercial liquid formula may be easily tolerated by patients and usually is well absorbed by the gut.	
	Factors limiting intake: • Ability to feed self • Physical impairment • Dentition • Nothing-by-mouth status • Nausea/vomiting • Psychosocial factors	Patient may be able to increase oral intake if limiting factors are decreased.	
	Monitor lab values:	Hemoglobin (Hb) and serum albumin may be indicators of general nutritional status.	
	• Hemoglobin	Hb is needed to transport O_2 to cell.	

(continued)

Care map for pressure ulcer management *(continued)*

Assessment	Plan	Rationale	Evaluation
Diagnosis: Nutrition-fluid	Care orders	Key rationale for care orders	Expected outcome
	• Albumin 3.0 to 3.5 indicates mild protein malnutrition 2.5 to 3.0 indicates moderate protein malnutrition <2.5 indicates severe malnutrition.	Protein is necessary for new tissue synthesis. Serum albumin level is a gross indicator of protein available for use in the body. Albumin levels may be decreased due to inadequate protein intake or loss of protein from a draining ulcer.	
	• Serum transferrin	Because it reflects a more specific and current nutritional status, serum transferrin level may be indicated.	
	• Total lymphocyte count <1,800/mm^3	Lymphocyte count reflects the body's ability to mobilize an inflammatory response.	
	• Edema	Decreased colloid osmotic pressure due to low levels of albumin will result in edema, which interferes with the supply of nutrients to the cell and exerts pressure on the vasculature, making edematous tissue fragile and prone to breakdown.	
	Assess patient's fluid history, including oral intake and urine output. Assess patient's current fluid status. Fluid overload:		Urine output approximates fluid intake.
	• Sacral edema • Lower extremity edema	Fluid collects in the most dependent body part.	
	• Pulmonary edema	Fluid overload in a patient with compromised cardiopulmonary status will result in pulmonary edema.	
	Fluid deficit:	Dehydration may lead to hypovolemia, causing decreased oxygenation to the tissue. It may also lead to cracking of the skin and increased susceptibility to breakdown.	

Care map for pressure ulcer management *(continued)*

Assessment	Plan	Rationale	Evaluation
Diagnosis: Nutrition-fluid	Care orders	Key rationale for care orders	Expected outcome
	• Poor skin turgor	Skin turgor may be an inaccurate indicator of dehydration in the elderly due to normal loss of subcutaneous tissue and decrease in skin elasticity with age.	
	• Dry mucous membranes		
	• Dry tongue		
	Consult with physician and dietician for individualized assessment of fluid and nutritional status.	Fluid intake of 2,000 mL in 24 hours will maintain tissue hydration. Fluid intake may, however, be contraindicated in some patients.	
Diagnosis: Risk factors	Care orders	Key rationale for care orders	Expected outcome
Impaired skin integrity related to presence of pressure ulcer	Assess pressure ulcer characteristics.	Use a clockwise orientation to describe location of ulcer characteristics. The patient's head signifies the 12 o'clock position.	
	Assess dimensions of ulcer base in centimeters.	Initial measurements serve as baseline data and provide a basis for comparison of healing or deterioration of tissue.	
	• Length		
	• Width		
	• Depth		
	• Undermining		
	• Sinus tracts or fistulae		
	• Tunneling		
	Color		
	Granulation		
	Epithelialization		
	Drainage	Exudative wounds take longer to heal.	
	Necrosis		
	• Slough		
	• Eschar		
	Odor		

(continued)

Care map for pressure ulcer management *(continued)*

Assessment	Plan	Rationale	Evaluation
Diagnosis: Risk factors	Care orders	Key rationale for care orders	Expected outcome
	Wound margins		
	Assess surrounding intact skin		
	Surrounding erythema		
	Induration		
	Maceration		
	Determine stage of pressure ulcer.		
	Determine presence of individual risk factors that may affect the healing process.	Specific risk factors vary in individuals. The care plan is directed toward compensating for the risk factors.	
	Determine goal of care.	The goal for the patient directs the care plan.	
	Develop an individual care plan based on characteristics of pressure ulcer, presence of related risk factors, and goal of care.		
	Communicate the importance of consistent care throughout the course of treatment.	Consistency is the key to effectiveness. A treatment regimen can't be critically evaluated unless all caregivers implement the plan in the same manner.	

STAGE I PRESSURE ULCERS

Diagnosis: Impaired skin integrity	Care orders	Key rationale for care orders	Expected outcome
Observable pressure-related alteration of intact skin with skin warmth or coolness, firm or boggy feel, or pain or itching. The ulcer presents clinically as a defined area, persistently red in light skin or red, blue, or purple in darker skin.	Reduce individual risk with special emphasis on relief of pressure. Avoid pressure to the affected area.	Risk assessment applies to every individual with a pressure ulcer.	Intact skin with absence of non-blanchable erythema.
	Assess and record skin characteristics. Document changes.	Change in pressure areas can develop rapidly and requires appropriate changes in care plan. Measurements should be taken at least weekly and documented in the progress notes.	
	Keep area clean: • Use plain water. Soap should be avoided.	Commercial soaps contain alkalis, which dry the surface layer of the skin.	

Care map for pressure ulcer management *(continued)*

Assessment	Plan	Rationale	Evaluation
STAGE I PRESSURE ULCERS *(continued)*			
Diagnosis: Impaired skin integrity	Care orders	Key rationale for care orders	Expected outcome
	• Consult with pharmacist for special cleansing agents that don't alter skin pH.	Use cleansing agents only if needed (i.e., if skin can't be cleaned by saline or water)	
	• Use emollients judiciously if skin is dry.	Dry skin can lead to cracking, which alters the body's first line of defense. Excessive use of emollients can lead to maceration.	
	May apply transparent film or hydrocolloid over reddened bony prominence. Frequency of dressing change is determined by clinician's judgment.	Dressing reduces friction by acting as a protective layer over skin.	
	Avoid massaging over bony prominences.	Massage of soft tissue over the area of hyperemia is contraindicated because it may facilitate additional breakdown of tissue.	
STAGE II PRESSURE ULCERS			
Diagnosis: Impaired skin integrity	Care orders	Key rationale for care orders	Expected outcome
Partial-thickness skin loss involving epidermis and/or dermis. The ulcer is superficial and presents clinically as an abrasion, blister, or shallow crater.	Reduce individual risk with special emphasis on relief of pressure. Avoid pressure to affected area.	Risk assessment applies to every individual with a pressure ulcer.	Progressive healing as evidenced by increasing amounts of epithelium.
	Assess and document dimensions of ulcer base in centimeters. • Length • Width • Depth • Undermining • Sinus tracts or fistulae	Change in pressure areas can develop rapidly and requires appropriate changes in care plan. Measurements should be taken at least weekly and documented in the clinician's progress notes.	

(continued)

Care map for pressure ulcer management *(continued)*

Assessment	Plan	Rationale	Evaluation
STAGE II PRESSURE ULCERS *(continued)*			
Diagnosis: Impaired skin integrity	Care orders	Key rationale for care orders	Expected outcome
	• Tunneling		
	Color		
	Granulation		
	Epithelialization		
	Drainage		
	Necrosis		
	• Slough		
	• Eschar		
	Odor		
	Wound margins		
	Assess surrounding intact skin.		
	• Surrounding erythema		
	• Induration		
	• Maceration		
	Cleanse ulcer with normal saline.	Cleansing is necessary because broken skin is an interruption in the body's first line of defense against infection.	
	Cover pressure ulcer with a dressing that maintains a moist environment over the ulcer.	Wound healing occurs best in a moist environment. Maintenance of adequate wound hydration minimizes scab formation so that epithelial migration can proceed unimpeded.	
	• Semipermeable polyurethane dressing	Maintains a moist environment because it is permeable to water vapor and oxygen yet acts as a barrier to fluid and bacteria.	
	• Hydrocolloid dressing	Interacts with wound fluid to form a moist protective gel that allows moist wound healing while remaining adherent to intact skin.	
	• Moist normal saline dressing over ulcer base only	Moisture mechanically softens tissue while it absorbs and reduces drainage. Maceration of intact skin surrounding the ulcer could lead to further breakdown.	

Care map for pressure ulcer management *(continued)*

Assessment	Plan	Rationale	Evaluation
STAGE II PRESSURE ULCERS *(continued)*			
Diagnosis: Impaired skin integrity	Care orders	Key rationale for care orders	Expected outcome
	Avoid drying agents or treatments; for example, heat lamps, Maalox, milk of magnesia.	Wound healing is delayed in a dry environment, which promotes scab formation and impedes epithelial migration. Heat increases demand for oxygen and is injurious to ischemic tissues. Antacids alter the protective acid mantle of the skin.	
STAGE III PRESSURE ULCERS			
Diagnosis: Impaired skin integrity	Care orders	Key rationale for care orders	Expected outcome
Full-thickness skin loss involving damage or necrosis of subcutaneous tissue, which may extend down to, but not through, underlying fascia. The ulcer presents clinically as a deep crater with or without undermining of adjacent tissues.	Reduce individual risk with special emphasis on relief of pressure. Avoid pressure to affected area.	Risk assessment applies to every individual with a pressure ulcer.	Progressive healing as evidenced by decreasing dimensions of ulcer base and presence of granulation tissue.
	Assess and document dimensions of ulcer base in centimeters. • Length • Width • Depth • Undermining • Sinus tracts or fistulae • Tunneling Color	Change in pressure areas can develop rapidly and requires appropriate changes in care plan. Measurements should be taken at least weekly and documented in the clinician's progress notes.	
	Granulation	Indicates new blood vessel growth.	
	Epithelialization	Indicates new skin growth.	
	Drainage		
	Necrosis	Indicates dead tissue in wound.	
	• Slough • Eschar		
	Odor		

(continued)

Care map for pressure ulcer management *(continued)*

Assessment	Plan	Rationale	Evaluation
STAGE III PRESSURE ULCERS *(continued)*			
Diagnosis: Impaired skin integrity	Care orders	Key rationale for care orders	Expected outcome

Wound margins

Assess surrounding intact skin.

- Surrounding erythema — Indicates inflammation.
- Induration — Indicates chronic venous congestion.
- Maceration

Aspirate blister to decrease fluid pressure. — The blister acts as a protective barrier against infection and provides a moist medium for epithelialization.

If blister is broken, gently cleanse with normal saline. — Cleansing is necessary because broken skin is an interruption in the body's first line of defense against infection.

Cover ulcer base with a dressing that maintains a moist environment over the ulcer. — Wound healing occurs best in a moist environment. Maintenance of adequate hydration minimizes scab formation so that epithelial migration can proceed unimpeded.

- Semipermeable polyurethane dressing — Maintains a moist environment because it is permeable to water vapor and oxygen but impermeable to fluids and bacteria.

- Hydrocolloid dressing — Allows moist wound healing while remaining adherent to intact skin. Because of the ability to absorb fluid, these dressings may be effective for draining noninfected wounds. Shouldn't be used for clinically apparent infection.

- Moist normal saline dressing over ulcer base only — Maceration of intact skin surrounding the ulcer could lead to further breakdown.

Don't cover a wound cavity with an occlusive dressing. — Open wounds must be allowed to drain to the surface to avoid abscess formation.

Care map for pressure ulcer management *(continued)*

Assessment	Plan	Rationale	Evaluation
STAGE III PRESSURE ULCERS *(continued)*			
Diagnosis: Impaired skin integrity	Care orders	Key rationale for care orders	Expected outcome
	Avoid drying agents or treatments; for example, heat lamps, Maalox, milk of magnesia.	Wound healing is delayed in a dry environment that promotes scab formation and impedes epithelial migration. Antacids alter the protective acid mantle of the skin.	
STAGE III/IV PRESSURE ULCERS WITHOUT NECROSIS OR INFECTION			
Diagnosis: Impaired skin integrity	Care orders	Key rationale for care orders	Expected outcome
Stage III: Full-thickness skin loss involving damage to subcutaneous tissue, which may extend down to, but not through, underlying fascia. The ulcer presents clinically as a deep crater with or without undermining of adjacent tissues. Stage IV: Full-thickness skin loss with extensive destruction or damage to muscle, bone, or supporting structures (for example, tendon or joint capsule)	Reduce individual risk with special emphasis on relief of pressure. Avoid pressure to affected area. Assess and document dimensions of ulcer base in centimeters. • Length • Width • Depth • Undermining • Sinus tracts or fistulae • Tunneling Color Granulation Epithelialization Drainage Necrosis • Slough • Eschar	Risk assessment applies to every individual with a pressure ulcer. Change in pressure areas can develop rapidly and requires appropriate changes in care plan. Measurements should be taken at least weekly and documented in the clinician's progress notes. Indicates extension of ulcer that can't be seen. Indicates connection of deep ulcer to surface tissue. Indicates new blood vessel growth. Indicates new skin growth. Indicates dead tissue in wound.	Progressive healing as evidenced by presence of granulation tissue and progressive decrease in diameter and depth.

(continued)

Care map for pressure ulcer management *(continued)*

Assessment	Plan	Rationale	Evaluation
STAGE III/IV PRESSURE ULCERS WITHOUT NECROSIS OR INFECTION *(continued)*			
Diagnosis: Impaired skin integrity	Care orders	Key rationale for care orders	Expected outcome

	Odor		
	Wound margins		
	Assess surrounding intact skin.		
	• Surrounding erythema	Indicates inflammation.	
	• Induration	Indicates chronic venous congestion.	
	• Maceration		
	Develop wound management plan:		
	• Irrigate wound with normal saline. Use enough irrigation pressure to cleanse the wound without causing trauma.	Irrigation with normal saline may assist in removing dead cells and reducing bacteria count. Safe, effective irrigation pressures range from 4 to 15 psi. Forceful irrigation greater than 15 psi shouldn't be used.	
	• Examine sinus tracts and undermined areas of wound for retained dressing materials.	Use of a dressing with cotton filler is contraindicated for wound packing because the filling as a foreign substance may retard healing.	
	• Fill wound loosely with dressing materials.		
	For a nondraining ulcer, use dressings such as:		
	• Plain gauze impregnated with saline, gel, Vaseline, or bismuth	Moist dressings provide a physiological environment for formulation of granulation tissue.	
	• Foam	A wound is filled to reduce dead space, decreasing the risk of abscess formation. Packing shouldn't be so tight as to compress tissue and interfere with circulation.	
	For a draining ulcer, use absorptive dressings such as:	Heavily exudative wounds heal more slowly than nonexudative wounds. Absorption of exudate will prevent maceration of intact skin.	
	• Dry gauze		
	• Alginates		
	• Hydrogels		

Care map for pressure ulcer management *(continued)*

Assessment	Plan	Rationale	Evaluation

STAGE III/IV PRESSURE ULCERS WITHOUT NECROSIS OR INFECTION *(continued)*

Assessment	Plan	Rationale	Evaluation
Diagnosis: Impaired skin integrity	Care orders	Key rationale for care orders	Expected outcome
	• Pastes		
	• Powders		
	• Beads		
	Cover wound with secondary dressing.	Dressing helps to protect the wound.	
	Consult wound care resource persons to determine suitability of moisture-retentive dressing.	Provides a moist physiological environment for formulation of granulation tissue but may be contraindicated in certain situations. Consult wound care specialist regarding appropriate use.	
	Evaluate care plan and institute changes as appropriate.	Change in the pressure ulcer may necessitate revision of the care plan.	

STAGE III/IV NECROTIC PRESSURE ULCERS

Assessment	Plan	Rationale	Evaluation
Diagnosis: Impaired skin integrity	Care orders	Key rationale for care orders	Expected outcome
Stage III: Full-thickness skin loss involving damage or necrosis of subcutaneous tissue, which may extend down to, but not through, underlying fascia. The ulcer presents clinically as a deep crater with or without undermining of adjacent tissues.	Reduce individual risk with special emphasis on relief of pressure. Avoid pressure to affected area.	Risk assessment applies to every individual with a pressure ulcer.	Pressure ulcer is clean as evidenced by absence of slough or eschar.
	Assess and document dimensions of ulcer base in centimeters. • Length • Width • Depth	Change in pressure areas can develop rapidly and requires appropriate changes in care plan. Measurements should be taken at least weekly and documented in the clinician's progress notes.	
	• Undermining	Indicates extension of ulcer that can't be seen.	
	• Sinus tracts or fistulae • Tunneling	Indicate connection of deep ulcer to surface tissue.	
	Color		
	Granulation	Indicates new blood vessel growth.	*(continued)*

Care map for pressure ulcer management *(continued)*

Assessment	Plan	Rationale	Evaluation
STAGE III/IV NECROTIC PRESSURE ULCERS *(continued)*			
Diagnosis: Impaired skin integrity	Care orders	Key rationale for care orders	Expected outcome
Stage IV: Full-thickness skin loss with extensive destruction, tissue necrosis, or damage to muscle, bone, or supporting structures (for example, tendon or joint capsule)	Epithelialization	Indicates new skin growth.	
	Drainage		
	Necrosis	Indicates dead tissue in wound.	
	• Slough	Moist dead tissue.	
	• Eschar	Dry dead tissue. Depth can't be determined until eschar is removed.	
	Odor		
	Wound margins		
	Assess surrounding intact skin.		
	• Surrounding erythema	Indicates inflammation.	
	• Induration	Indicates chronic venous congestion.	
	• Maceration		
	Cleanse pressure ulcer		
	Irrigate wound forcefully with normal saline every 8 hours or with each dressing change.	Irrigation under pressure reduces bacteria count and removes debris from the wound.	
	Consult with physician regarding use of whirlpool.	Agitation of the water assists in softening and removing wound debris. Avoid placing wounds near water jets, however, as force may be too great.	
	Consult with physician or wound care specialist prior to surgical debridement if eschar or necrosis is present.	Sharp debridement is the most effective method of removing necrotic tissue.	
	If mechanical debridement is indicated, apply moist-to-dry dressing using normal saline.	As gauze dries, it sticks to the necrotic tissue, thereby causing debridement when the dressing is removed. Pulling the dressing from the wound may be painful.	

Care map for pressure ulcer management *(continued)*

Assessment	Plan	Rationale	Evaluation
STAGE III/IV NECTROTIC PRESSURE ULCERS *(continued)*			
Diagnosis: Impaired skin integrity	Care orders	Key rationale for care orders	Expected outcome
	For chemical debridement using enzymes, consult with physician prior to any preliminary removal of slough or eschar via sharp or chemical debridement and prior to crosshatching of eschar with a scalpel.	Debridement time is decreased if eschar and large amounts of slough are first removed. Enzymatic action occurs only on the surface of the wound. Crosshatching of eschar allows penetration of the enzymatic debriding agent into and through the eschar.	
	• Irrigate wound as appropriate for each enzymatic agent.	Irrigation rinses away debris and should be done at least daily because most enzymatic debriding agents lose their effectiveness within 24 hours. The irrigation solution shouldn't interfere with the action of the enzymatic agent. Whirlpools can also provide effective wound irrigation.	
	• Apply the enzymatic debriding agent only to necrotic tissue.	Some enzymatic debriding agents may irritate healthy tissue.	
	• Apply a dressing as directed for the selected enzymatic debriding agent.	Dressing should be applied so that the enzyme is in contact with necrotic tissue. Some enzymatic agents require a moist dressing, whereas others require a dry dressing.	
	• Collaborate with the physician or wound specialist regarding discontinuation of enzymatic agent when wound is no longer necrotic and healthy granulation base is present.		
	For autolytic debridement with moisture-retentive dressings, first consult with a wound care specialist regarding hydrocolloid, film, moist saline gauze, or gel dressings.	Within a moist environment, the body produces lytic enzymes that selectively separate necrotic tissue from healthy tissue.	

(continued)

Care map for pressure ulcer management *(continued)*

Assessment	Plan	Rationale	Evaluation

Stage III/IV nectrotic pressure ulcers *(continued)*

Assessment	Plan	Rationale	Evaluation
Diagnosis: Impaired skin integrity	Care orders	Key rationale for care orders	Expected outcome
		Acts as a barrier to fluid, stool, environmental contaminants; it is permeable to oxygen and moist vapor, thereby keeping wound base moist.	
	• Cleanse wound as directed. • Dry surrounding tissue. • Apply dressing; change as directed.	The amount of time required for effective debridement varies.	

Stage III/IV infected pressure ulcers

Assessment	Plan	Rationale	Evaluation
Diagnosis: Impaired skin integrity	Care orders	Key rationale for care orders	Expected outcome
Impaired skin integrity related to bacterial invasion of surrounding tissue, as evidenced by cellulitis, systemic signs of infection, and/or purulent drainage	Reduce individual risk with special emphasis on relief of pressure. Avoid pressure to affected area.	Risk assessment applies to every individual with a pressure ulcer.	Absence of signs indicating local or systemic infection; for example, swelling, heat, or tenderness.
	Assess and document dimensions of ulcer base in centimeters. • Length • Width • Depth • Undermining	Change in pressure areas can develop rapidly and requires appropriate changes in care plan. Measurements should be taken at least weekly and documented in the clinician's progress notes. Indicates new extension of ulcer that can't be seen.	
	• Sinus tracts or fistulae • Tunneling Color Granulation Epithelialization Drainage Necrosis	Indicate connection of deep ulcer to surface tissue. Indicates new blood vessel growth. Indicates new skin growth. Indicates dead tissue in wound.	

Care map for pressure ulcer management *(continued)*

Assessment	Plan	Rationale	Evaluation
STAGE III/IV INFECTED PRESSURE ULCERS *(continued)*			
Diagnosis: Impaired skin integrity	Care orders	Key rationale for care orders	Expected outcome

	• Slough		
	• Eschar		
	Odor		
	Wound margins		
	Assess surrounding intact skin.		
	• Surrounding erythema	Indicates inflammation.	
	• Induration	Indicates chronic venous congestion.	
	• Maceration		
	Assess for signs of local infection in surrounding tissue:	Erythema, heat, induration, and pain may be evidence of tissue response to bacterial invasion.	
	• Redness		
	• Heat		
	• Induration		
	• Edema		
	• Pain		
	• Purulent drainage		
	Assess for signs of systemic infection:		
	• Elevated temperature	Elevation in body temperature and abnormal rise in WBC count may be signs of systemic infection. Body temperature should be monitored closely after surgical wound debridement because bacteria may enter the bloodstream at this time.	
	• Changes in WBC count		
	• Confusion	Acute confusion may be an indication of sepsis.	
	Notify the physician if there are signs of local or systemic infection.	A deep wound culture or tissue biopsy may be indicated.	
	Implement a wound management plan in collaboration with physician or wound care specialist.		

(continued)

Care map for pressure ulcer management *(continued)*

Assessment	Plan	Rationale	Evaluation
STAGE III/IV INFECTED PRESSURE ULCERS *(continued)*			
Diagnosis: Impaired skin integrity	Care orders	Key rationale for care orders	Expected outcome
	Irrigate wound with normal saline at each dressing change.	Irrigation dilutes the bacteria count and removes debris. Saline is the irrigating solution of choice.	
	Apply topical antibiotics; for example, silvadene, if ordered.	The use of antiseptics is controversial. Iodophors may be toxic to fibroblasts and interfere with wound healing; allergic reactions have occurred in instances of iodophor use. The use of topical antibiotics is also controversial; there is no scientific evidence that they decrease the bacteria count in tissue surrounding a wound. Topical antibiotics may be used to decrease the bacteria count in the wound itself prior to surgical repair of the ulcer.	
	Absorb purulent wound drainage using:		
	• Coarse mesh gauze dressing	Dressings absorb drainage and prevent crust formation, which could interfere with healing.	
	• Moisture-retentive dressings with absorptive properties: dry gauze, alginates, pastes, powders, beads	Dry gauze absorbs drainage.	
		Absorptive. For use in highly exudative wounds. Not for use in mildly exudative or dry wounds. Dressing becomes hard if allowed to dry.	
		Pastes, powders, and beads interact with wound fluid to form a protective gel. The absorbent action draws microorganisms away from the wound, decreasing bacterial contamination and inflammation.	
	Remove retained starch-based dressings prior to reapplication.		

Care map for pressure ulcer management *(continued)*

Assessment	Plan	Rationale	Evaluation

CLOSED PRESSURE ULCER

Diagnosis: Impaired skin integrity	Care orders	Key rationale for care orders	Expected outcome
Large, bursalike cavity lined by chronic fibrosis extending to deep fascia or bone with drainage through a small sinus tract	Reduce individual risk with special emphasis on relief of pressure. Avoid pressure to affected area.	Risk assessment applies to every person with pressure ulcers.	
	Assess bony prominences for drainage from small sinus tracts.	The patient may be unaware of a closed pressure ulcer.	
	Consult physician if draining lesions are present.	Surgical intervention may be necessary.	
	Assess for signs of local infection in surrounding tissue: • Redness • Heat • Induration • Edema • Pain • Purulent drainage	Erythema, heat, induration, and pain may be evidence of tissue response to bacterial invasion.	
	Assess for signs of systemic infection: • Elevated temperature • Changes in WBC count • Confusion	Elevation in body temperature and an abnormal rise in WBC count may be signs of systemic infection. Body temperature should be monitored closely after surgical wound debridement because bacteria may enter the bloodstream at this time. Acute confusion may be an indication of sepsis.	
	Notify the physician if there are signs of local or systemic infection.		

pendices F through L for additional Harper Hospital care decision trees.) The topics include:

- skin care
- surgical wounds
- leg ulcers
- pressure ulcers
- debridement
- periwound skin care
- attachment of products without tape.

The care map on the following pages was developed for use at Harper Hospital. Institutions may use it as a guide for developing their own specific guidelines or standard care maps. The clinician who uses this map for guidance should base selections on each patient's risk factors, the characteristics of the pressure ulcer, and the environmental setting.

Many institutions now use standard care maps with daily checklists to decrease documentation time. These forms use a critical pathway format to track patient progress toward expected outcomes of care. The documentation forms give expected outcomes for patients with diagnoses of "risk for impaired skin integrity: pressure ulcers" and "impaired skin integrity: pressure ulcers." Documentation reflects daily progress toward outcomes. If the outcome is met, the clinician checks the box; if not, the clinician writes an explanation in the space provided and changes the care plan accordingly. This pathway is a precursor to a critical path that will give accompanying treatment and expected outcome timelines. (For an example of pressure ulcer care using the Harper Hospital documentation format, see Appendices N and O.)

Selected references

Ayello, E.A. "Assessment of pressure ulcer healing," *Advances in Wound Care* 10(5):10, 1997.

Baranoski, S., Salzberg, C.A., Staley, M.J., et al. "Obstacles and opportunities for the multidisciplinary wound care team. A resymposium on wound management," *Advances in Wound Care* 11(2):85-88, 1998.

Barnett, R.I., Shelton, F.E. "Measurement of support surface efficacy: pressure," *Advances in Wound Care* 10(7):21-29, 1997.

Barr, J.E., Cuzell, J. "Wound care clinical pathway: A conceptual model," *Ostomy/Wound Management* 42(7):18-26, 1996.

Fallon, R. "Critical paths for wound care," *Advances in Wound Care* 8(1):26-34, 1995.

Doan-Johnson, S. "The growing influence of wound care teams," *Advances in Wound Care* 11(2):54, 1998.

Gallagher, S.M. "Outcomes in clinical practice: Pressure ulcer prevalent incidence studies," *Ostomy/Wound Management* 43:28-32, 34-35, 38, 1997.

Hill, M., et al. "Managing skin care with the care map system," *Journal of Wound, Ostomy, and Continent Nursing* 24:26-27, 1997.

Salcido, R. "Will all pressure ulcers heal?" *Advances in Wound Care* 10(5):28-30, 1997.

Thomas, D.R. "Existing tools: Are they meeting the challenges of pressure ulcer healing?" *Advances in Wound Care* 10(5):86-90, 1997.

Chapter 9

Policy and procedure development

An institution-wide program for pressure ulcer management must begin with the development of policies that govern patient care. Administrators approve institutional policies, which determine the actions of its employees. A policy may include professional standards, patient care plans, procedures, and protocols that are implemented by the staff who work there. (See *Policy and procedure definitions,* page 144.)

The employees of an agency may be asked to assist in writing institutional protocols and procedures. Generally, the protocol format is standard and may include the title, purpose, desired patient outcome, personnel affected, steps of the procedure, and rationale, if necessary. Appropriate documentation is indicated, references are given, authors are credited, and approving signatures and titles are included.

The following section, pages 145 to 186, provides examples of pressure ulcer policies and procedures from Detroit Medical Center's Harper Hospital. Agencies may adapt the format to develop policies and procedures that are specific to their own institutions.

Policy and procedure definitions

Policy: statement governing a course of action

Procedure: steps required to complete a task

Protocol: actions prescribed to manage a problem

Standard: statement defining rules, conditions, or actions

Standard care plan: predetermined written plan for managing care

Standard of care: indicator that defines expected patient care

Standard of practice: indicator that defines expected nursing action

Standard precautions/isolation: Broad

1. Standard precautions apply to all healthcare workers who may be exposed to blood or other potentially infectious body fluids as a result of their job duties.

2. Gloves are worn when anticipating contact with blood, other body fluids, mucous membranes, or nonintact skin. Gloves must be changed after contact with each patient.

3. Handwashing is done immediately before and after gloving. Hands and other surfaces should be washed immediately and thoroughly if contaminated with blood or other body fluids.

4. Masks and protective eyewear are not routinely necessary but are used during procedures likely to generate droplets of blood or other body fluids, and to prevent exposure of the mucous membranes of the mouth, nose, and eyes.

5. Gowns are used during procedures likely to generate splashes of blood or other body fluids and to prevent soiling of clothes.

6. Sharp instruments (such as used needles) are not recapped, purposely bent or broken, removed from disposable syringes, or otherwise manipulated by hand. This includes needles used for blood cultures. Needles are not changed before placing specimens in the bottles. Disposable syringes, needles, sutures, scalpels, and similar items are placed in puncture-resistant sharps containers designed for this purpose and kept as close to the point of use as possible.

7. Blood and blood-contaminated body fluid specimens are handled as potentially infectious material and are bagged in clear plastic bags before being transported. Bags are not required for blood tubes transported on blood trays. Specimens are sent in a tube with a foam insert. See references at the end of this policy for more information.

8. Standard precaution equipment is located either in each patient room in the universal precaution bin, specified drawers in the intensive care units, or the medication room in the psychiatric units as well as the department treatment rooms and crash carts.

References:

OSHA Enforcement Policy and Procedures for Occupational Exposure to Tuberculosis, October, 1993.

OSHA Final Blood Borne Pathogen Rule, Federal Register, December, 1991.

Universal Precaution and Isolation Policy, Infection Control Manual.

Pneumatic Tube System Use, Administrative Policy and Procedure 1.14, October, 1993. Administrative Policy Manual.

Skin care

Policy:
Each patient has systematic skin assessment and care consisting of: inspection, cleaning, hydration, and protection.

Equipment:
Mild soap or detergent

Moisturizers

Barrier agent (such as aluminum paste)

Absorbent materials

Film dressing

Powder

Positioning products (cushions, wedge pillows, trapeze)

Procedure	Rationale/emphasis
A. Inspection	
1. Inspect skin during admission assessment.	
2. Evaluate skin integrity, color, temperature, texture, and turgor.	
3. Reassess the skin. Frequency of reassessment is determined by the patient's level of risk.	Ongoing assessment of the skin can be done during physical assessment, bathing, dressing changes, exercise routines, or other patient care activities.
	Risk factors include weight loss, inactivity, immobility, incontinence, and decreased LOC, malnutrition (decreased albumin), or both.
B. Cleansing	
1. Cleanse skin when needed.	The purpose of skin cleansing is to remove foreign materials, bacterial contaminants, and the residues of skin secretions.
2. Select mild soap or detergent for individual use.	The ideal soap or detergent will remove only the skin contaminants and will preserve the natural lipids and oils of the skin. Excessive cleansing or use of harsh cleansers leads to skin drying.
3. Minimize any force or friction during cleansing.	
4. Avoid chemical additives in soaps or detergents such as colorants, fragrances, and conditioners.	Chemical agents may lead to skin irritation or sensitization.
C. Hydration	
Apply topical moisturizing agents to dry skin after bathing and as needed.	Decreased skin hydration/dry skin is associated with fissuring and cracking of the skin.

Skin care *(continued)*

Procedure

D. Protection from excessive moisture

1. Avoid excessive moisture on skin (urine, stool, perspiration, wound drainage) by either of these methods:
   a. Urine or fecal pouch to manage incontinence
   b. Barrier agent to protect skin from excessive moisture

2. Place an absorbent material under the patient to absorb fluid. Avoid using plastic and paper protectors.

E. Protection from friction, shear, and pressure

1. Avoid elevating the head of the bed $>$ 30° for long periods if the patient can tolerate other positions.

2. Avoid massage over bony prominence and reddened or broken areas of skin.

3. Lift patient when repositioning. Avoid dragging skin across bed linens.

4. Use a film dressing or powder on areas of skin susceptible to friction forces.

5. Provide and teach patient to use overhead trapeze to assist in moving about in bed unless medically contraindicated.

6. Use positioning wedges or pillows.

7. Suspend patient's heels while in bed.

8. Use wheelchair/chair cushion when in sitting position.

9. Avoid using doughnuts and products shaped like doughnuts.

10. Teach patient to do small shifts in body weight at regular intervals.

Rationale/emphasis

Skin that is moist or wet is more susceptible to injury from friction, more easily abraded, more readily penetrated by irritating solutions, and promotes higher microbial growth.

Absorbent products wick moisture away from the skin. Such products are composed of at least two layers; the layer contacting the skin is usually permeable and dries quickly. The second layer is hydrophilic and highly absorbent.

Shear injury occurs when the head of the bed is raised. The tissues attached to the bone have a tendency to slide downward due to body weight while the surface tissues stick to the sheets and remain stationary.

Massage over bony prominence may cause maceration and tearing of underlying tissue.

Frictional trauma to the skin occurs when the skin, while under load, is moved across a coarse surface such as bed linen.

Material that can be placed on the skin to reduce its coefficient of friction will reduce the potential for friction injury.

Lifting prevents friction injury.

External support will assist position changes.

Because heels are the hardest area to bridge for pressure relief, care is needed to prevent pressure on heels while patient is in bed.

Ischial tuberosities are at increased risk for pressure when patient is in sitting position.

Products that circumscribe the pressure ulcer or bony prominence compromise the skin circulation around the area of concern.

Shifts in body weight provide intermittent pressure relief.

(continued)

Skin care *(continued)*

References:

Agency for Health Care Policy and Research. (1992). Clinical Practice Guidelines, Number 3, Publication No. 92-0047. *Pressure ulcers in adults: Prediction and prevention.* U.S. Department of Health and Human Services.

Leyden, J.J. (1984). Cornstarch, candida albicans, and diaper rash. *Pediatric Dermatology,* 1:(4), 322-325.

Leyden, J.J., Katz, S., Stewart, R., & Kligman, A.M. (1977). Urinary ammonia and ammonia producing microorganisms in infants with and without diaper dermatitis. *Archives Dermatology,* 113: (12), 1679-1680.

Maklebust, J., and Sieggreen, M. (1996). *Pressure ulcers: Guidelines for prevention and nursing management,* 2nd ed. Springhouse Corporation, Springhouse, Pa.

Shipes, E., and Stanley, I. (1981). Effects of a liquid copolymer skin barrier for preventing skin problems. *Ostomy/Wound Management,* 4: 19-23.

Shipes, E., and Stanley, I. (1983). A study of a liquid copolymer skin barrier for preventing and alleviating perineal irritations in incontinent patients. *Journal of Urological Nursing,* 2 (3): 32-34.

Zimmera, R.E., Lawson, K.D., and Calvert, C.J. (1986). The effects of wearing diapers on skin. *Pediatric Dermatology,* 3 (2): 95-101.

Wound culture: Aerobic and anaerobic

Policy:
1. A physician's order is required. Aerobic and anaerobic cultures must be ordered separately, although both can be ordered on the same specimen. Anaerobes are not ordered on a swab specimen.
2. If more than two organisms grow, they will be partially identified but not fully worked up, and no susceptibility testing will be performed. If additional workup is desired, please notify the laboratory within 72 hours.
3. Cultures are obtained before starting antibiotic therapy.
4. Tissue is the optimal specimen; swabs are not recommended. Swabs of dry wounds are not accepted by the microbiology laboratory. Swabs of sinus tracts provide inaccurate information and are not done.
5. Superficial wounds or abscesses and sinus tracts are not acceptable for anaerobic cultures. Anaerobic cultures may be obtained in tissue biopsy or needle aspiration specimens only.
6. Tissue biopsy and/or fine needle aspiration must be performed by a physician, physician assistant, or advanced practice nurse. Swab cultures may be done by RNs.

Equipment:
Aerobic specimen collector — Culturette II — and/or Anaerobic specimen collector

4″ × 4″ sponges

Clean gloves — two pair

Sterile gloves

Impervious bag

250 ml normal saline

Iodophor solution or 70% alcohol (for small wound openings)

Baxter irrigation tip

Sterile water

10-ml syringe with 22G needle or biopsy punch or #15 blade

Patient label

Procedure
A. Preparation
1. Wash hands and put on nonsterile gloves. Use no-touch technique to remove old dressings.
2. Discard soiled dressings in impervious bag.
3. Remove gloves and wash hands.
4. Put on sterile gloves and assess wound for origin of drainage.

Rationale/emphasis

To prevent further contamination of the wound.

To examine the wound bed for depth and any undermined areas.

(continued)

Wound culture: Aerobic and anaerobic *(continued)*

Procedure

5. Irrigate wound area with sterile normal saline solution.

6. Cleanse wound periphery, unless contraindicated, with sterile water or normal saline solution. An iodophor solution or 70% alcohol may be used around a small wound opening.

7. Dry skin around the wound gently but thoroughly with 4" × 4" sponge before performing culture.

8. Remove gloves.

B. Aerobic or anaerobic culture (Tissue biopsy — preferred specimen)

1. Prepare wound site as in Section A.

2. Put on nonsterile gloves.

3. Select site where tissue is viable and not covered with eschar or exudate.

4. Obtain a piece of tissue by punch biopsy or by using a #15 scalpel blade.

5. Obtain at least 5 mm of tissue in each direction.

6. Place the specimen in the sterile specimen container.

7. Attach patient label to the specimen collector. Label the specimen "tissue" and indicate the type and location of the wound.

8. Carry the specimen immediately to the lab or send via pneumatic tube to the microbiology laboratory in University Health Center.

Rationale/emphasis

To remove loose necrotic material and surface contaminants that colonize the wound and result in an inaccurate polymicrobial culture. Avoid the use of bacteriostatic solutions for wound irrigation, such as water or normal saline for injection, because they will inhibit recovery of pathogens.

Cleansing the wound periphery will prevent contamination of the swab when obtaining the specimen. Do not allow the antimicrobial solution to touch the wound surface being cultured because it will weaken or kill the offending pathogen.

Physicians, PAs, and APNs may obtain tissue biopsy for culture.

Areas of necrotic tissue are always colonized with multiple organisms.

Tissue biopsy is the preferred method to increase the chance of an accurate specimen collection.

The aerobic specimen collector may be used if an aerobic specimen only is ordered. The anaerobic specimen collector is used if an anaerobic culture or both aerobic and anaerobic cultures are ordered. The centers of larger tissue pieces can maintain their own anaerobiasis. However, the anaerobic collector is used if the tissue specimen is small.

To instruct the laboratory personnel to look for tissue and not to culture the swab.

Wound culture: Aerobic and anaerobic *(continued)*

Procedure

C. Anaerobic and/or anaerobic culture by aspiration

1. Prepare wound site as in Section A.

2. Put on nonsterile gloves.

3. Cleanse intact skin with antiseptic, such as povidone-iodine, and allow to dry.

4. Using a 22G needle and 10-ml syringe, insert the needle into area of tissue with suspected infection.

5. Create suction by withdrawing the plunger to the 10-ml mark. Keep the plunger retracted.

6. Move the needle backward and forward at different angles for two to four explorations. Do not depress the plunger.

7. Remove needle from the tissue. Retract the plunger to aspirate all tissue and fluid into barrel of syringe.

8. Expel any air from the syringe and needle.

9. Deposit aspirate into anaerobic specimen collector and label. Insert the swab and push down to activate the reducing agents. Both aerobic and anaerobic cultures can be performed on aspirate sent in the same anaerobic specimen collector.

10. Attach patient label to the specimen collector and indicate the type and location of the wound.

11. Transport specimen to the lab immediately: either hand carry or send via pneumatic tube to the microbiology lab at UHC.

D. Aerobic culture (swab)

1. Prepare wound site as in Section A.

2. If unable to get a tissue specimen and and a swab specimen is indicated, remove the swab from the aerobic specimen collector, being careful to touch only the top of the cap. Do not touch swab.

3. Select site where tissue is viable and not covered with eschar or exudate.

Rationale/emphasis

This method is used when obtaining tissue isn't feasible. Physicians, PAs, and APNs may obtain cultures by aspiration.

A complete seal and active reducing agent are necessary to prevent oxygen from killing pathogens.

Prevents death of pathogens or overgrowth of contaminants.

Staff RNs may obtain swab cultures.

(continued)

Wound culture: Aerobic and anaerobic *(continued)*

Procedure	Rationale/emphasis
4. Press the swab against the ulcer base. Move the swab back and forth over a 1-cm^2 area using sufficient force to cause fresh wound fluid to thoroughly wet the swab.	
5. Avoid contaminating the swab with organisms from the skin and adjacent tissues.	To decrease the chance of a contaminated culture.
6. Place the swab back into the specimen collector.	To preserve the pathogens by preventing specimen from drying out.
7. Attach patient label to the specimen collector. The label must indicate the type and location of the wound.	Specimens without appropriate labeling will not be accepted by the lab.
8. Transport specimen to the microbiology lab within 1 hour.	Prolonged time results in death of representative pathogens or allows other pathogens to multiply (microbial overgrowth).

References

Bergstrom, N., Bennett, M.A., and Carlson, C.E., et al. (1994). *Treatment of Pressure Ulcers.* Clinical Practice Guideline No. 15. Rockville, Md: U.S. Department of Health and Human Services. Public Health Service, Agency for Health Care Policy and Research. AHCPR Publication No. 95-0652.

Garner, J.S. (1988). CDC definitions for nosocomial infections. *American Journal of Infection Control,* 16(3):128-140.

Guevich, I. (1980). Appropriate collection of specimens for culture and sensitivity. *American Journal of Infection Control,* 8(4):113-119.

Levine, N.S., Lindberg, R.B., Mason, A.B., and Pruitt, B.A. (1976). The quantitative swab culture and smear: A quick simple method for determining the number of viable aerobic bacteria on an open wound. *Journal of Trauma,* 16:89-94.

Rousseau, P. (1989). Pressure ulcers in an aging society. *Wounds* 1(2):135-141.

Sapico, F.L., Witte, J.I., Canavati, H.N., et al. (1984). The infected foot of the diabetic patient: Quantitative microbiology and analysis of clinical features. *Reviews of Infectious Disease,* 6(51):5171-5176.

Sapico, F.L., Ginunas, V.J., Thornhill-Joynes, M., Canavati, H.N., et al. (1986). Quantitative microbiology of pressure sores in different stages of healing. *Diagnostic Microbiology and Infectious Disease,* 5(1):31-38.

Stotts, N.A. (1995). Determination of bacterial burden in wounds. NPUAP Proceedings. *Advances in Wound Care* 8(4):46-52.

Stotts, N.A. (1997). Associate Professor, Department of Physiologic Nursing, University of California-San Francisco (personal communication).

Resources

Fairfax, M.R., MD, PhD, Medical Director, Clinical Microbiology and Immunology Laboratories, December 1997.

Flanagan, E., MSA, BSN, RN, CIC, Manager, DMC Epidemiology, December 1997.

Pressure Ulcer Committee, Harper Hospital, 1995.

Wound irrigation

Equipment:

Clean gloves — two pair

Sterile normal saline 250 ml or sterile irrigant as ordered

Sterile gauze sponges

$4'' \times 4''$ gauze sponges and/or abdominal pads

Skin sealant (optional)

Irrigation cap

Paper tape

Impervious bag

Procedure	Rationale/emphasis
A. Preparation	
1. Label bottle of saline with date and time.	
2. Wash hands.	
3. Put on nonsterile gloves and remove old dressings and place in impervious bag.	
4. Remove gloves and wash hands.	
5. Measure wound and assess wound bed for presence of granulation tissue, necrosis, odor, and amount and color of drainage.	Wound assessment aids in selection of appropriate irrigation technique.
6. Open irrigation cap package. Save the bubble package to cover cap after procedure.	
7. Tightly secure irrigation cap to a 250-ml bottle of saline.	
8. Open sterile gauze dressing supplies, maintaining a sterile field.	
B. Irrigation	
1. Flush wound with prescribed irrigant. Hold tip 1 to 2 inches from wound:	Wound irrigation may dilute the bacterial count.
a. Gently irrigate clean granulating wounds.	Forceful irrigation may damage clean granulating wounds.
b. Forcefully irrigate necrotic wounds using full force to plunger of 30-ml syringe.	Forceful irrigation mechanically debrides loose necrotic tissue. Bacteria multiply and necrotic tissue easily accumulates in undermined areas of a wound or sinus tracts.
c. Flush away any wound drainage or residue from previous dressing.	

(continued)

Wound irrigation *(continued)*

Procedure	Rationale/emphasis
2. Put on nonsterile gloves.	
3. Dry surrounding skin with 4″ × 4″ gauze sponges.	
4. Apply prescribed dressing.	
5. Consult advanced practice nurse, ET nurse, or wound care specialist for alternative types of dressings that may be used in clean and necrotic wounds.	
6. Wash hands and discard impervious bag containing old dressings in soiled utility room.	
7. Replace the bubble package on top of the irrigation cap to protect it from dust and contamination. After a 24-hour period, discard bottle.	

References:

Brown, L., Shelton, H., Barnside, G., and Cohn, I., Jr. (1978). Evaluation of wound irrigation by pulsatile jet and conventional methods. *Annals of Surgery*, 187(2): 170-173.

Diekmann, C.M., Smith, J.M., and Wilk, J.R. (1985). A double life for a dental irrigation device. *American Journal of Nursing*, 85(10): 1157.

Green, V.A., Carlson, H.C., Briggs, R.L., and Stewart, J.L. (1971). A comparison of the efficacy of pulsed mechanical lavage with that of rubber bulb syringe irrigation in removal of debris from avulsive wounds. *Oral Surgical Oral Medical Pathology*. Jul; 32(1): 158-164.

Hamer, M.L., Robson, M.C., and Krizek, T.J., (1975). Quantitative bacterial analysis of comparative wound irrigations. *Annals of Surgery*, 181(6): 819-822.

Longmire, A.W., and Broon, L.A. (1987). Wound infection following high-pressure syringe and needle irrigation. *Americal Journal Emergency Medicine*, 5(2): 179-181.

Maklebust, J., and Sieggreen, M. (1996). *Pressure ulcers: Guidelines for prevention and nursing management*. 2nd ed. Springhouse Corporation, Springhouse, Pa., 110-111.

Rodeheaver, G.T., Pettry, D., Thacker, J.G., Edgerton, M.T., and Edlich, R.F. (1975). Wound cleansing by high pressure irrigation. *Surgical Gynecological Obstetrics*, 141(3): 357-362.

Rogness, H. (1985). High-pressure wound irrigation. *Journal of Enterostomal Therapy*, (12): 27-28.

Stotts, N.A. (1983). The most effective method of wound irrigation. *Focus Critical Care*, 10(5): 45-48.

Weller, K. (1991). In search of efficacy and efficiency. An alternative to conventional wound cleansing modalities. *Ostomy/Wound Management*, Nov-Dec; 37:23-28.

Dressings: Continuously moist saline

General information: Continuously moist saline gauze dressing: technique in which gauze moistened with normal saline is applied to the wound and remoistened with normal saline frequently enough so it will remain moist. The goal is to maintain a continuously moist environment.

Policy:
1. Physician order is not required.
2. When an order is written for pressure ulcer care or wound care, the practitioners will decide when to use a moist dressing. Consult an advanced practice nurse or wound care specialist for complex cases.

Equipment:
Sterile normal saline
Clean gloves
Impervious bag
Tape
4″ × 4″ gauze sponge or abdominal pads
Skin sealant (optional)

Procedure

A. Preparation
1. Wash hands.
2. Put on clean gloves.
3. Remove moist dressing and dispose of in impervious bag. If dressing is dry, soak with normal saline before removal.
4. Remove soiled gloves and wash hands.
5. Open dressings and normal saline.
6. Use normal saline to moisten enough gauze to fill the wound.
7. Put on nonsterile gloves.
8. Irrigate wound using a 250-ml bottle of normal saline and Baxter irrigating tip.
9. Apply moist gauze dressing:
   a. Squeeze excess saline from gauze sponges.
   b. Place layer of moist gauze against ulcer base. Tuck loosely into undermined areas or sinus tracts. Be sure there is a moist dressing next to all the tissue in the wound.

Rationale/emphasis

To prevent introduction of additional bacteria into wound and to comply with universal precautions.

Removal of dried dressing may damage granulating tissue. Granulating tissue is a gelatinous film that can easily be wiped or flushed away.

Irrigation dilutes the bacteria. Irrigation assists in debriding by washing loose necrotic tissue from wound.

(continued)

Dressings: Continuously moist saline *(continued)*

Procedure

    c. Fluff remaining gauze sponges and gently place into remainder of wound to fill dead space. Avoid overpacking the wound.

    d. Keep intact skin dry.

    e. May apply skin sealant to skin surrounding wound. Air dry.

10. Cover with a dry dressing and secure in place. Date, time, and initial dressing.

11. Maintain moist dressing by remoistening with saline.

12. Change dressing at least every 8 hours. If the dressing is dry when changed, the frequency of change must be increased.

13. Remove gloves, wash hands, and dispose of refuse in soiled utility room.

Rationale/emphasis

Overpacking increases pressure on tissue in wound bed causing additional tissue damage.

Moisture will macerate intact skin.

To prevent tissue maceration from damp dressing and skin stripping when tape is removed.

References

Bergstrom, N., Bennett, M.A., Carlson, C.E., et al. *Treatment of pressure ulcers.* Clinical Practice Guideline, No. 15. Rockville, Md: U.S. Department of Health and Human Services. Public Health Service, Agency for Health Care Policy and Research. AHCPR Publication No. 95-0652. December 1994.

Maklebust, J., and Sieggreen, M. (1996). *Pressure ulcers: Guidelines for prevention and nursing management,* 2nd ed. Springhouse, Pa.: Springhouse Corporation.

Panel for the Prediction and Prevention of Pressure Ulcers in Adults. (1992). *Pressure ulcers in adults: Prediction and prevention clinical practices guideline.* Number 3. AHRQ Publication No. 92-0047. Rockville, Md: Agency for Health Care Policy and Research, Public Health Service, U.S. Department of Health and Human Services.

Sieggreen, M. (1987). The healing of physical wounds. *Nursing Clinics of North America,* 22(2).

Xakellis, G.C., and Chrischilles, E.A. (1992). Hydrocolloid versus saline gauze dressings in treating pressure ulcers: A cost effectiveness analysis. *Archives of Physical Medicine Rehabilitation,* 73: 463-469.

Dressings: Moist-to-dry for debridement

General information: Moist-to-dry saline gauze: a dressing technique in which gauze moistened with normal saline is applied wet to the wound and removed once the gauze becomes dry and adheres to the wound bed. The goal is to debride the wound as the dressing is removed.

Policy:

When an order is written for pressure ulcer care or wound care, the practitioner will decide when to use a "moist-to-dry" dressing. Consult a wound care specialist for complex cases.

Equipment:

Sterile normal saline

Clean gloves — two pair

Impervious bag

Sterile 4″ × 4″ gauze sponges

Tape

Irrigation tray

Abdominal pad (optional)

Skin sealant (optional)

Procedure

1. Wash hands.
2. Put on nonsterile gloves.
3. Remove dry dressing from wound pulling away necrotic debris with dressing. Discard in impervious bag.
4. Remove gloves and wash hands.
5. Open normal saline and dressings.
6. Moisten sterile gauze with normal saline.
7. Put on nonsterile gloves.
8. Irrigate wound using a 250-ml bottle of normal saline and Baxter irrigation tip.
9. Apply moist dressing:
   a. Unfold moist gauze.
   b. Spread it in a single layer over open wound.
   c. Tuck moist gauze loosely into undermined areas or sinus tracts.
   d. Keep intact skin dry.

Rationale/emphasis

More frequent dressing changes may be necessary to facilitate a more rapid debridement when there is excess wound drainage.

Irrigation dilutes the bacteria. Irrigation assists in debriding by washing loose necrotic tissue from wound.

Gauze should be just moist enough to allow it to dry between dressing changes.

Moisture will macerate intact skin.

Dressings: Moist-to-dry for debridement *(continued)*

Procedure

10. Gently place fluffed gauze into remainder of wound.

11. May apply skin sealant to skin surrounding wound. Air dry. Secure dressing. Write date, time, and initial.

12. Remove gloves, wash hands, and discard impervious bag in soiled utility room.

13. Change dressing as needed. Dressing should be dry when removed.

Rationale/emphasis

The additional dressing assists with drying. Absorption of exudate into the gauze will aid in debriding the wound. May cover gauze with abdominal pad.

To prevent tissue maceration from damp dressing.

References

Alvarez, O.M., Mertz, P.M., and Eaglestein, W.H. (1983). The effect of occlusive dressings on collagen synthesis and re-epithelialization in superficial wounds. *Journal of Surgical Research,* 35(2): 142-148.

Bergstrom, N., Bennett, M.A., Carlson, C.E., et al. *Treatment of pressure ulcers. Clinical Practice Guideline,* No. 15. Rockville, MD: U.S. Department of Health and Human Services. Public Health Service, Agency for Health Care Policy and Research. AHCPR Publication No. 95-0652. December 1994.

Fowler, E., and Goupil, D.L. (1984). Comparison of the wet-to-dry dressing and a copolymer starch in the management of debrided pressure sores. *Journal of Enterostomal Therapy,* 11(1): 22-25.

Maklebust, J., and Sieggreen, M. (1996). Pressure ulcers: Guidelines for prevention and nursing management. 2nd ed. Springhouse Corporation, Springhouse, Pa.

Panel for the Prediction and Prevention of Pressure Ulcers in Adults. (1992). *Pressure ulcers in adults: Prediction and prevention,* Clinical practice guidelines, Number 3. AHCPR Publication No. 92-0047. Rockville, Md: Agency for Health Care Policy and Research, Public Health Service, U.S. Department of Health and Human Services.

Sieggreen, M. (1987). The healing of physical wounds. *Nursing Clinics of North America,* 22(2).

Dressings: Foam dressing to maintain a moist wound environment

Equipment:

Clean gloves — two pair
250-ml bottle sterile normal saline
Baxter irrigation cap
4″ × 4″ gauze sponges
Foam dressing
Paper tape
Impervious disposal bag

Procedure

A. Preparation

1. Wash hands and put on clean gloves.
2. Remove old dressing and discard in impervious bag.
3. Remove soiled gloves and discard.
4. Wash hands, apply second pair of clean gloves, and use 250 ml normal saline with Baxter irrigation tip to forcefully irrigate wound.

5. Dry skin surrounding the wound with a 4″ × 4″ sponge.
6. Assess wound bed and surrounding tissue for necrosis, erythema, odor, drainage, and size.

7. Select dressing size large enough to extend 1 inch beyond the wound margins on all sides.

B. Application

1. Assess wound depth to determine necessity of filling wound bed prior to application of foam covering.
2. If wound is superficial, cover wound with foam dressing positioning the dressing directly over the wound with the dressing extending 1 inch beyond wound bed on all sides.

Rationale/emphasis

Thorough cleansing or irrigation is needed to flush out cellular debris or loose necrotic tissue and reduce the bacterial count.

Normal saline does not damage granulation tissue.

To keep periulcer skin clean and dry.

Foam dressings can absorb exudate and facilitate removal of superficial necrotic tissue by autolysis in pressure ulcers or partial-and full-thickness wounds.

Absorbs wound exudate and maintains moist wound bed.

To avoid dead space in the wound.

To maintain moist wound environment.

(continued)

Dressings: Foam dressing to maintain a moist wound environment *(continued)*

Procedure

3. If wound is not flush with skin, select moist dressing material to fill wound crater prior to covering with foam.

4. Do not cover the foam dressing with occlusive films or tapes.

5. Adhere dressing with tape, roll gauze, or netting depending on periulcer skin condition.

6. Change dressing frequently enough to absorb exudate and keep wound bed moist.

7. Discontinue foam dressing if wound bed is sufficiently moist, wound exudate exceeds absorption capability, or frequency of dressing change needs to be decreased.

8. Remove gloves, wash hands, and discard impervious bag containing old dressings in soiled utility room.

Rationale/emphasis

To avoid dead space in wound.

Covering the foam can interfere with water vapor transmission and reduce dressing effectiveness.

Large necrotic or heavily draining wounds may require more frequent dressing changes due to exudate leakage. Wounds with a necrotic base may increase in size and depth during the initial phase of management as the necrotic debris is cleaned away.

References

Bergstrom, N., Bennett, M.A., Carlson, C.E., et al. Treatment of pressure ulcers. Clinical Practice Guideline, No. 15. Rockville, Md: U.S. Department of Health and Human Services, Agency for Health Care Policy and Research. AHCPR Publication No. 95-0652. December 1994.

Lyofoam dressing package insert, Acme United Corporation, 1995.

Wiseman, D.M., Rovee, S.T., and Alvarz, O.M. (1992). Wound dressings: design and use. In Cohen, I.K., Diegelmann, R.F., & Lindbald, W.J. (eds). *Wound Healing: Biochemical and Clinical Aspects.* Philadelphia: W.B. Saunders Co.

Dressings: Hydrogel-impregnated gauze dressing to maintain a moist wound environment

Equipment:

Clean gloves — two pair

250-ml bottle sterile normal saline

Baxter irrigation cap

Hydrogel-impregnated gauze dressing materials

4″ × 4″ gauze sponges or gauze rolls

Paper tape

Impervious disposal bag

Procedure

A. Preparation

1. Wash hands and put on clean gloves.

2. Remove old dressing and discard in impervious bag.

3. Remove soiled gloves and discard.

4. Wash hands, put on second pair of clean gloves, and use 250 ml normal saline with Baxter irrigation tip to forcefully irrigate wound.

5. Dry the area surrounding wound with a 4″ × 4″ sponge.

6. Assess wound bed and surrounding tissue for necrosis, erythema, odor, drainage, and size.

7. Select dressing size that will cover the wound bed.

B. Application

1. Assess wound depth to determine amount of hydrogel gauze dressing necessary to cover wound.

2. Place hydrogel dressing into wound, covering all exposed wound surface.

3. Cover with secondary dressing.

4. Adhere dressing with tape or roll gauze depending on periulcer skin condition.

Rationale/emphasis

Thorough cleansing and/or irrigation is needed to flush out cellular debris or loose necrotic tissue and reduce the bacterial count.

Normal saline does not damage granulation tissue.

To keep periulcer skin clean and dry.

Hydrogel dressings can facilitate removal of superficial necrotic tissue by autolysis in pressure ulcers or partial- and full-thickness wounds.

Maintains moist wound bed.

(continued)

Dressings: Hydrogel-impregnated gauze dressing to maintain a moist wound environment *(continued)*

Procedure

5. Change dressing every day and p.r.n. to keep wound bed moist.

6. Discontinue hydrogel dressing if wound bed is sufficiently moist or frequency of dressing change needs to be decreased.

7. Wash hands and discard impervious bag containing old dressings in soiled utility room.

Rationale/emphasis

Large necrotic or heavily draining wounds may require more frequent dressing changes due to exudate leakage. Wounds with a necrotic base may increase in size and depth during the initial phase of management as the necrotic debris is cleaned away.

References

Bergstrom, N., Bennett, M.A., Carlson, C.E., et al. *Treatment of pressure ulcers.* Clinical Practice Guideline, No. 15. Rockville, Md: U.S. Department of Health and Human Services, Agency for Health Care Policy and Research. AHCPR Publication No. 95-0652. December 1994.

Carrington Laboratories product insert, 1995.

Cuzzell, J. (1997). Choosing a wound dressing. *Geriatric Nurse* 18: 260-265.

Panel for the Prediction and Prevention of Pressure Ulcers in Adults. (1992). *Pressure ulcers in adults: Prediction and prevention.* Clinical practice guidelines, Number 3. AHRQ Publication No. 92-0047. Rockville, Md: Agency for Health Care Policy and Research, Public Health Service, U.S. Department of Health and Human Services.

Wiseman, D.M., Rovee, D.T., & Alvarez, O.M. (1992). Wound dressings: design and use. In Cohen, I.K., Dieglemann, R.F., & Lindbald, W.J. (eds). *Wound Healing: Biochemical and Clinical Aspects.* Philadelphia: W.B. Saunders Co.

Dressings: Hydrocolloid

Equipment:

Clean gloves — two pair

250-ml bottle sterile normal saline

Baxter irrigation tip

4″ × 4″ gauze sponges

Hydrocolloid dressing, 4″ × 4″ or 8″ × 8″

Skin sealant (optional)

Paper tape

Impervious disposal bag

Procedure

A. Preparation

1. Wash hands and put on clean gloves.

2. Remove old dressing by pressing down on the skin with one hand and lifting dressing edge toward the wound with the other hand.

3. Discard dressing and soiled gloves in impervious bag.

4. Set up normal saline irrigation bottle and tip.

5. Wash hands, put on second pair of clean gloves, and use 250 ml normal saline with Baxter irrigation tip to forcefully irrigate wound.

6. Dry the skin surrounding wound with a 4″ × 4″ sponge.

7. Assess wound bed and surrounding tissue for necrosis, erythema, odor, drainage, and size.

8. Select dressing size large enough to extend 1-½ inch beyond the wound margins on all sides.

B. Application

1. Remove backing from hydrocolloid wafer. Do not stretch wafer.

Rationale/emphasis

Liquefied wound drainage may appear purulent and odiferous. Both are normal reactions to the hydrocolloid dressing.

Thorough cleansing, irrigation, or both are needed to flush out cellular debris or loose necrotic tissue and reduce the bacterial count.

Normal saline does not damage granulation tissue.

Promotes adhesion and increases wear time of dressing.

Hydrocolloid dressings can absorb exudate and facilitate removal of superficial necrotic tissue by autolysis in pressure ulcers or partial- and full-thickness wounds.

Facilitates adhesion of the wafer and improves dressing wear time.

(continued)

Dressings: Hydrocolloid *(continued)*

Procedure

2. Apply wafer directly over wound surface in a rolling motion. The dressing may be cut if necessary to conform to different areas of the body.

3. Smooth the wafer firmly into place especially at the wound margins.

4. Picture-frame or tape edge of dressings, especially in sacral or perianal regions.

5. Leave dressing in place for 3 to 5 days. Change dressing frequently enough to avoid leakage.

6. Discontinue hydrocolloid dressings if wound exudate exceeds absorption capability or frequency of dressing change needs to be increased.

7. Remove gloves, wash hands, and discard impervious bag containing old dressings in soiled utility room.

Rationale/emphasis

Dressings on irregular surfaces are difficult to keep intact.

Wounds with a necrotic base may increase in size and depth during the initial phase of management as the necrotic debris is cleaned away.

References

Bergstrom, N., Bennett, M.A., Carlson, C.E., et al. *Treatment of pressure ulcers.* Clinical Practice Guideline, No. 15. Rockville, Md: U.S. Department of Health and Human Services. Public Health Service, Agency for Health Care Policy and Research. AHCPR Publication No. 95-0652. December 1994.

Colwell, J.C., Foreman, M.D., and Trotter, J.P. (1992). *A comparison of the efficacy and cost effectiveness of two methods of managing pressure ulcers.* Washington, D.C.: AHCPR.

Maklebust, J., and Sieggreen, M. (1996). *Pressure ulcers: Guidelines for prevention and nursing management.* 2nd ed. Springhouse Corporation, Springhouse, Pa.

Neill, K.M., Conforti, C., Kedas, A., and Burris, J.F. (1989). Pressure sore response to a new hydrocolloid dressing. *Wounds,* 1(3): 173-185.

Oleske, D.M., Smith, X.P., White, P., Pottage, J., and Donavan, M.L. (1986). A randomized clinical trial of two dressing methods for the treatment of low-grade pressure ulcers. *Journal Enterostomal Therapy,* 13(3): 90-98.

Panel for the Prediction and Prevention of Pressure Ulcers in Adults. (1992). *Pressure ulcers in adults: Prediction and prevention.* Clinical practice guidelines, Number 3. AHCPR Publication No. 92-0047. Rockville, Md: Agency for Health Care Policy and Research, Public Health Service, U.S. Department of Health and Human Services.

Shannon, M.L., and Miller, B. (1988). Evaluation of hydrocolloid dressings on healing of pressure ulcers in spinal cord injury patients. *Decubitus,* 1(1): 42-46.

Wiseman, D.M., Rovee, D.T., and Alvarez, O.M. (1992). Wound dressings: Design and use. In Cohen, I.K., Dieglemann, R.F., and Lindbald, W.J. (eds). *Wound healing: Biochemical and clinical aspects.* Philadelphia: W.B. Saunders Co.

Xakellis, G.C., and Chrischilles, E.A. (1992). Hydrocolloid versus saline gauze dressings in treating pressure ulcers: A cost-effectiveness analysis. *Archives of Physical Medicine Rehabilitation,* 73: 463-469.

Dressings: Polyurethane film

Equipment:
Polyurethane film dressing
    Small — 10 cm $\times$ 12 cm
    Large — 15 cm $\times$ 20 cm
Skin sealant
Clean gloves
250 ml sterile normal saline
Baxter irrigation tip
4" $\times$ 4" gauze sponge
Tape
Impervious bag
Syringe and 25G needle

Procedure	Rationale/emphasis
A. Preparation	
1. Wash hands.	
2. Put on nonsterile gloves and remove old dressing.	
3. Discard dressing and gloves in impervious bag.	
4. If skin is broken, put on sterile gloves and cleanse wound and surrounding skin gently with normal saline.	Normal saline will not damage tissue.
5. Dry intact surrounding skin with gauze. Clip hair if necessary.	Transparent film dressings will not stick to hair or a wet surface.
B. Application	
1. Select a dressing size that will cover at least 2 inches beyond the wound margin.	Dressing border on skin facilitates adhesion and improves wearing time of the dressing. Large wounds may be covered with overlapping pieces of film dressing.
2. Apply a skin sealant to the surrounding skin as needed. Air dry.	Protects skin from maceration from wound drainage and prolongs seal or dressing.
3. Remove and discard center cutout window.	
4. Peel printed paper backing from the paper frame of dressing exposing adhesive surface.	
5. View the wound site through the window and center dressing over the site.	

(continued)

Dressings: Polyurethane film *(continued)*

Procedure	Rationale/emphasis
6. Press in place, firmly smoothing from center to edges of dressing.	Pulling or stretching the film dressing across wound area causes excessive tension on skin, tissue shearing, and patient discomfort.
7. Slowly remove the paper frame from the dressing and firmly smooth the dressing edges. Smooth entire dressing using firm pressure.	
8. Wipe edges of film dressing with skin sealant.	
9. Put a piece of tape on the dressing, if needed, and record date and initials on tape.	
10. Inspect wound and integrity of film dressing every day and p.r.n.	
11. If excessive exudate forms under the dressing compromising the seal, use sterile technique to aspirate exudate with a 25G needle. Patch the puncture site with a small piece of film dressing.	It's normal for the wound to form a layer of fluid under the dressing.
12. Dispose of needle in sharps container.	
13. Change dressing if:	Film dressings may be left on for 2 to 3 days.
a. Leakage occurs.	
b. Edges roll up or dressing naturally sloughs off.	
c. Excessive granulation tissue forms in the wound bed.	Excess tissue may extend above and beyond wound margins.
14. Remove film dressings by stretching and releasing edges slowly in direction of hair growth. For fragile skin, use warm water soaks to release dressing from skin.	
15. Discontinue use of dressings if clinical signs of wound infection are present.	Drainage under film dressing will appear purulent and have a foul odor. This is a result of bacteria and white blood cell interaction. Wound culture and/or tissue biopsy may be indicated if there are clinical signs of infection (erythema, increased size of wound, pain, swelling, fever, and excessive purulent drainage).

References

Ahmed, M. (1982). Op-Site for decubitus care. *American Journal of Nursing,* 82(1): 61-64.

Alvarez, O., Rozent, J., and Wiseman, D. (1989). Moist environment for healing: Matching the dressing to the wound. *Wounds,* 1(1): 35-51.

Dressings: Polyurethane film *(continued)*

Bergstrom, N., Bennett, M.A., Carlson, C.E., et al. *Treatment of Pressure Ulcers.* Clinical Practice Guideline, No. 15. Rockville, Md: U.S. Department of Health and Human Services, Agency for Health Care Policy and Research. AHCPR Publication No. 95-0652. December 1994.

Brady, S.M. (1987). Management of pressure sores with OCC/SIU dressings in a select population. *Nursing Management*, 18:41.

Maklebust, J., and Sieggreen, M. (1996). *Pressure ulcers: Guidelines for prevention and nursing management,* 2nd ed. Springhouse Corporation, Springhouse, Pa.

Sebern, M.D. (1986). Pressure ulcer management in home health care: Efficiency and cost effectiveness of moisture vapor permeable dressings. *Archives of Medicine Rehabilitation,* 67(10):729.

Dressings: Alginate

Equipment:

Clean gloves

Sterile normal saline

4″ × 4″ gauze sponge and/or abdominal pads

Impervious bag

Paper tape

Barrier agent

Gauze wrap (optional)

250 ml normal saline

Irrigation cap

Procedure

A. Preparation

1. Wash hands. Put on clean gloves and remove old dressing.

2. Discard soiled dressing and gloves in impervious bag.

3. Throughout the procedure, assess wound and surrounding tissue for erythema, degree of necrotic tissue, odor, amount of drainage, and size.

4. Wash hands. Put on clean gloves. Use "no touch" technique to irrigate wound with normal saline.

5. Leave wound bed moist. Dry intact skin with 4″ × 4″ gauze sponge.

6. Apply a barrier agent to intact skin around the wound and allow to dry.

B. Application

1. Apply alginate to the moist wound surface.

2. Pat down to conform to the wound surface.

3. Cover alginate:

   a. For a moderately draining wound, use a secondary absorbent dressing or semiocclusive film dressing.

Rationale/emphasis

Alginate is used for moderately to heavily draining wounds. It turns into a gel as it absorbs drainage.

Alginate dressings are not effective for ulcers with dry eschar or clean granulation wound beds. Alginate dressings are not debriding agents; as much necrotic tissue as possible should be debrided prior to application.

To keep absorbent dressing off healthy skin.

Hydrophilic absorptive dressings must have room for expansion in the wound bed because they absorb drainage and odor.

Absorption dressings should be applied to a moist wound surface. Do not overfill or pack the wound bed.

Do not use alginate in deep fistulae, sinus tracts, or body cavities, where complete removal is not assured.

Dressings: Alginate *(continued)*

Procedure	Rationale/emphasis
b. For a heavily draining wound, use a thick absorbent dressing such as layers of gauze or an ABD pad.	
4. Secure alginate and cover dressing over bony prominence with stretch gauze wrap. Where stretch gauze would not be indicated, such as over a hip wound, secure in place with tape along the edges.	

C. Dressing change

Procedure	Rationale/emphasis
1. Wash hands and put on clean gloves.	
2. Gently remove outer dressings down to the gel.	The frequency of dressing changes will depend on the volume of exudate. The dressing should be changed when the secondary dressing becomes moist. A heavily draining wound may require one or two changes daily for the first 3 to 5 days.
3. Remove nongelled alginate and discard.	As the wound begins to heal and drainage decreases, dressing changes may be made less frequently— every 2 to 4 days or as directed by a nurse specialist.
4. Irrigate the wound with normal saline to rinse away the remaining gel. Should the gel be too thick to rinse, the bulk of the gel should be wiped from the wound. Any remaining gel should then be rinsed away.	Retained foreign bodies have been associated with impaired wound healing.
5. Remove gloves, wash hands, and apply clean gloves.	
6. Redress the wound.	
7. Discontinue treatment when the wound has a healthy granulation base and is no longer draining.	
8. Collaborate with physician or wound specialist to select another primary dressing that will continue to maintain a moist wound environment.	

References

Attwood, A.I. (1989). Calcium alginate dressing accelerates split skin graft donor site healing. *British Journal of Plastic Surgery,* 42(4): 373-379.

Maklebust, J., and Sieggreen, M. (1996). *Pressure ulcers: Guidelines for prevention and nursing management,* 2nd ed. Springhouse Corporation, Springhouse, Pa.

Motta, G.J. (1991). Calcium alginate topical wound dressings, a new dimension in the cost-effective treatment for exudating dermal wounds and pressure sores. *Ostomy/Wound Management,* 25: 52-56.

Enzymatic agent to debride necrotic tissue

Equipment:

Clean gloves

Sterile tongue blade

4″ × 4″ gauze sponge and/or abdominal pads

250 ml bottle sterile normal saline

Collagenase (Santyl)

Baxter irrigation tip

Tape

Impervious bag

Skin sealant (optional)

Polysporin powder

Procedure

A. Preparation

Procedure	Rationale/emphasis
1. Wash hands.	
2. Put on clean gloves.	To protect against nosocomial infections.
3. Remove old dressing.	
4. Discard gloves and dressing in impervious bag.	
5. Wash hands.	
6. Open tongue blade or sponge and squeeze enzymatic debriding ointment onto tongue blade or sponge.	Amount of ointment used depends on size of necrotic area.
7. Open normal saline, apply Baxter irrigation tip. Set bubble cap aside.	
8. Put on clean gloves.	
9. Irrigate wound by squeezing bottle of saline with full force.	Forceful irrigation mechanically debrides loose necrotic tissue. The wound must be cleansed of antiseptics or heavy metal antibacterials, which may denature the enzyme.
10. Dry intact surrounding skin.	To prevent maceration of skin.
11. Measure wound. Assess wound and surrounding tissue for erythema, degree of necrotic tissue, odor, and drainage.	Surgical debridement and/or crosshatching of dry, hard, necrotic tissue may be necessary. Debriding agents cannot penetrate dry, hard, necrotic tissue (eschar). Crosshatching refers to using a scalpel to cut through the depth of the eschar allowing the enzymatic agent to penetrate.

Enzymatic agent to debride necrotic tissue *(continued)*

Procedure

12. Apply skin sealant to skin surrounding wound. Air dry.

B. Application

1. Apply polysporin powder to surface of wound. This may be applied by sprinkling into the wound directly or onto a 4″ × 4″ and touching to the wound surface.

2. Apply Santyl to necrotic tissue staying within the lesion area.

3. Cover wound with dry 4″ × 4″ or ABD dressing.

4. Change dressing at least once a day.

5. Remove gloves and discard in impervious bag.

6. Secure dressing. Date and initial.

Rationale/emphasis

To prevent tissue maceration and skin stripping when tape is removed.

A topical antibiotic is applied to the wound prior to application of the enzymatic agent to decrease the risk of bacteria entering healthy tissue as the enzymes debride.

To prevent a transient erythema in surrounding intact skin areas.

More frequent dressing changes may be necessary due to excessive drainage.

References

Bergstrom, N., Bennett, M.A., Carlson, C.E., et al. *Treatment of pressure ulcers.* Clinical Practice Guideline, No. 15. Rockville, Md: U.S. Department of Health and Human Services, Agency for Health Care Policy and Research. AHCPR Publication No. 95-0652. December 1994.

Cuzzeli, J.Z. (1985). Wound care forum: Artful solutions to chronic problems. *American Journal of Nursing,* 85(2): 162-166.

Lee, L.K., and Ambrus, J.L. (1975). Collagenase therapy for decubitus ulcers. *Geriatrics* 30(5), 91-93, 97-98.

Maklebust, J., and Sieggreen, M. (1996). *Pressure ulcers: Guidelines for prevention and nursing management.* 2nd ed. Springhouse Corporation, Springhouse, Pa., 134-136.

Low-air-loss therapy for pressure or pain

Policy:
1. Check maximum weight allowed as specified by manufacturer.
2. If patient is transferred or discharged or therapy is discontinued, call company to remove bed.

Equipment:
Low-air-loss bed and user manual

Sheet

Optional: Full-length drawsheet, trapeze bar, air sacs with different configuration, head and foot boards

Procedure	Rationale/emphasis
A. Setup	
1. Verify that user manual is available with bed.	User manual is available with bed.
2. Validate determination of need and physician's order for low-air-loss bed.	To order bed.
3. Order bed; complete a charge slip and send to procurement.	
4. Plug bed in.	
5. Have company representative position bed.	
6. Adjust temperature, usually to about 93° F.	A temperature of about 93° F (33.8° C) is usually satisfactory.
7. Note operation of hand control.	
8. Note operation of air supply control panel.	
B. Maintenance	
1. If drainage accumulates, wash air sac with soap and water.	
2. Call company for bed replacement if drainage is excessive. Company will either clean or replace the bed.	Company will either clean the bed or replace it.
3. When bed is discontinued, cover with company-supplied plastic shroud before removing from the room.	

References

Ferrell, B.A., Keeler, E., Sui, A.L., Ahn, S.H., and Osterweil, D. Cost effectiveness of low-air-loss beds for treatment of pressure ulcers. *Journal of Gerontology,* 1995; 50A (3): M141-6.

Jeneid, P. (1976) Static and dynamic support systems — Pressure differences on the body. In Kenedi, R.M., Cowden, J. M., and Scales, J.T., eds. *Bed sore biomechanics.* London: Macmillan.

Low-air-loss therapy for pressure or pain *(continued)*

Maklebust, J., Mondoux, L., and Sieggreen, M. (1986). Pressure relief characteristics of various support surfaces used in prevention and treatment of pressure ulcers. *Journal of Enterostomal Therapy* 14(3): 85-89.

Scales, J.T. (1976). Air support systems for the prevention of bed sores. In: Kenedi, R.M., Cowden, J.M., and Scales, J.T., eds. *Bed sore biomechanics.* London: Macmillan.

Thomas, C. (1989). Specialty beds: Decision making made easy. *Ostomy/Wound Management* 23: 51-59. Summer, 1989

Wyllie, F.J., McLean, N.R., and McGregor, J.C. (1984). The problem of pressure sores in a regional plastic surgery unit. *Journal of the Royle College of Surgeons Edinburgh*, 29: 38-43.

Stewart, T. Support systems. In L.C. Parish, J.A. Witowski, and Crissey (eds.) *The decubitus ulcer in clinical practice.* New York: Springer-Verlag, 1997.

Sof-Care mattress overlay

Policy:

1. A hand check of the Sof-Care mattress is performed.

2. Sof-Care is a single-patient-use item and may be sent home with the patient upon discharge with the Sof-Care instruction booklet.

3. Adapters for home inflation are available in the nursing office.

4. The cushion must be deflated before initiating chest compressions during CPR.

Equipment:

Sof-Care mattress overlay
Sof-Care monitor

Procedure	Rationale/emphasis
A. Setup	
1. Detach sign from patient booklet and position it in a visible location.	To save instruction booklet.
2. Unroll cushion, positioning air valve at the foot of the bed.	Cushion is marked "Foot End" on end of strap.
3. Mount the pump on the foot panel of the bed and plug unit in.	
4. Unscrew cap from Sof-Care cushion.	
5. Pull tab to remove check valve and place on retaining ring on side of monitor.	Failure to remove the check valve may delay therapy.
6. Install cap attached to monitor tubing and tighten. Ensure that air supply tubing is not kinked or twisted.	
7. Push power switch to ON. Set control knob to arrow.	
8. Allow the monitor to inflate the cushion.	Patient may be on or off the bed cushion during inflation. Inflation will take about 30 minutes.
9. Position corner straps around bed mattress.	May be done before or after inflation.
10. Cover cushion loosely with a sheet.	An incontinent pad, bath blanket, or draw sheet may be used. Do not use foam or sheepskin.
11. Confirm operation of the system by using the hand check procedure. Slide hand underneath the cushion under bony prominence.	Patient should be elevated just off the hand. If a bony prominence is not felt, the monitor and cushion are functioning properly.
12. If a bony prominence is felt, check to see that: • Monitor is plugged in • Monitor is turned on	

Sof-Care mattress overlay *(continued)*

Procedure

- Control is set at arrow
- Air tubing is not kinked
- Monitor air tubing is attached to cushion.

13. If system is set up properly, turn the monitor to high and ensure the bed cushion is fully inflated.

14. If a bony prominence is felt, an alternative pressure-reducing therapy is indicated.

B. Cleaning monitor

1. Unplug monitor from wall.
2. Clean outside of monitor with mild detergent and damp cloth.
3. Wipe dry with a clean cloth before operating.

C. Cleaning bed cushion

1. Clean with a mild detergent and damp cloth.
2. Wipe dry.

D. Deflation

1. Remove valve screw cap.
2. For a slow or partial deflation: Insert sturdy pen point or any other blunt probing device into one of the four holes in the valve disc. Air will escape slowly

For a fast or complete deflation: Insert finger into ring check valve and pull firmly so that the check valve is removed from the valve body. The cushion may also be slashed to accomplish rapid deflation. In either case, the patient will "bottom" in 3 to 4 seconds. Note: Before initiating CPR, the cushion must be deflated.

3. Gently begin rolling cushion from the head to the foot end as marked. Air will escape through the valve body.
4. If the valve disc was removed, reinsert into valve body. The rubber flap on the valve disc must be inside when reassembled with the holes on the disc facing up. Valve disc will snap into place when properly positioned.

Rationale/emphasis

If the cushion doesn't inflate, it should be replaced.

Patient's weight may exceed the pressure-reducing capabilities of the system. Patients weighing more than 300 lbs (136 kg) may have an increased risk of bottoming out.

Do not allow fluids to get inside the monitor. *Do not autoclave.*

Don't use alcohol or alcohol-based agents. It is not necessary to deflate before cleaning.

(continued)

Sof-Care mattress overlay *(continued)*

Procedure

E. Discontinue

1. Turn switch on monitor to OFF.
2. Remove valve screw cap from cushion.
3. Gently roll from head to foot of bed.

F. For use after discharge

1. Offer the Sof-Care bed cushion to the patient if continued short-term use is anticipated at home, and hospital protocol allows.

2. Train the patient and family in the home inflation procedure and use of the hand check. Give them the instruction booklet.

3. Home inflation can be achieved through use of a bicycle pump or canister-type vacuum cleaner, CP300 or CP500.

4. The Sof-Care bed cushion is a single-patient-use product.

Rationale/emphasis

Air will escape through valve body.

Cushion can be gently rolled while inflated and secured with corner straps or deflated for transport.

The home inflation procedure and hand check procedure are described in the instruction booklet. This booklet should be given to the patient's family upon discharge.

This procedure is described in the instruction booklet that accompanies each Sof-Care bed cushion. A bicycle pump adapter is available to assist with inflation at home. Consult discharge planner or Gaymar at 800-828-7431 or 716-662-2551.

References

The use of Gaymar Sof-Care bed cushion and monitor. Orchard Park, NY: Gaymar Industries, Inc.

Maklebust, J.M., Brunkhorst, L., Cracchiolo-Caraway, A., Ducharme, M.A., Dundon, R., Panfilli, R., and Sieggreen, M. (1986). Pressure relief characteristics of various support surfaces used in the prevention and treatment of pressure ulcers. *Journal of Enterostomal Therapy* 14(3): 85-89.

Maklebust, J., and Sieggreen, M. (1996). *Pressure ulcers: Guidelines for prevention and nursing management,* 2nd ed. Springhouse Corporation, Springhouse, Pa.

Maklebust, J., Sieggreen, M., and Mondoux, L. (1988). "Pressure relief capabilities of the Sof-Care bed cushion and the Clinitron bed. *Ostomy/Wound Management,* 21: 32-41.

Panel for the Prediction and Prevention of Pressure Ulcers in Adults. (1992). *Pressure ulcers in adults: Prediction and prevention. Clinical Practice Guideline No. 3.* AHCPR Pub. 92-0047. Rockville, Md: U.S. Department of Health and Human Services, Agency for Health Care Policy and Research.

Warner, D.J. (1992). A clinical comparison of two pressure reducing surfaces in the management of pressure ulcers. *Decubitus,* 5(3): 52-64.

Air-fluidized therapy for pressure/pain relief

Policy:
Check manufacturer's specific weight limit.

Equipment:
Air-fluidized bed
Foam wedge
User manual
Optional: Lift

Procedure	Rationale/emphasis
A. Setup	User manual accompanies bed.
1. Validate determination of need and physician's order for air-fluidized bed.	
2. Send completed charge slip to procurement.	
3. Position bed at least 18 inches from wall.	To allow movement around bed.
4. Explain and demonstrate operation of bed to patient. Explain reasons for use and how it will feel to patient.	
5. Place bed sheet over filter sheet and secure with elastic cord attached to bed.	To prevent billowing of bed sheets.
6. Turn bed on and off using hand or control.	To ascertain proper functioning.
B. Patient care measures	
1. Transfer patient to bed with airflow off.	
2. Place pillow under head.	Protects ears from airflow.
3. Turn bed for continuous flotation.	
4. Set temperature selector at 86° to 95° F (30° to 35° C). Adjust for patient's comfort or set to increase or decrease the body temperature.	Heat is lost through evaporation by circulating airflow.
5. Check temperature dial each shift for correct temperature setting.	
6. Avoid external heat sources such as hyperthermia blanket or heating pad.	Avoids overheating bed.
7. Position the patient.	
8. Monitor the following while patient is on the bed:	
	Studies show that even on air-fluidized therapy, heels may be at risk for tissue damage.

(continued)

Air-fluidized therapy for pressure/pain relief *(continued)*

Procedure	Rationale/emphasis
• Tissue integrity	Dehydration is a risk because of an insensible water loss due to warm, dry airflow.
• Intake and output	
• Vital signs every 8 hours	A decrease in blood pressure or heart rate may occur because of the relaxing effect of air-fluidized therapy.
• Weight daily	Air-fluidized therapy may increase sedative effect.
• Effect of narcotics, barbiturates, or sedatives.	May damage filtering system or coating on beads.

9. Avoid use of petroleum, betadine, or silver-based ointments. If used, keep wound covered with dressings.

10. Avoid convoluted foam, sheepskin, gel pads, linen savers, and other devices. — Interfere with airflow.

C. Maintenance

1. The company representative will service the bed as needed.

2. Transfer the patient from the bed to a stretcher during maintenance procedures. — Company representative is responsible for the bed only.

3. Supply company representative with plastic bags to cover floor around bed. Bag micro spheres and sheet. — Microspheres are contaminated.

References

Allman, R.M., Walker, J.M., Hart, M.K., Laprade, C.A., Noel, L.B., and Smith, C.R. (1987). Air-fluidized beds or conventional therapy for pressure sores. *Annals of Internal Medicine,* 107:641-648.

Coker, K. (1979). The intermittent air-fluidized bed and the neurologically impaired patient. *Journal of Neurosurgical Nursing* 11(1): 31-33.

Greer, D.M., Morris, E.J., Walsh, N.E., Glenn, A.M., and Keppler, J. (1988). Cost-effectiveness and efficacy of air-fluidized therapy in the treatment of pressure ulcers. *Journal of Enterostomal Therapy* 15(6): 247-251

Jackson, B.S., Chagares, R., and Freeman, K. (1988). The effects of a therapeutic bed on pressure ulcers: An experimental study. *Journal of Enterostomal Therapy* 15(6): 220-226.

Maklebust, J.M., Brunkhorst, L., Cracchiolo-Caraway, A., Ducharme, M.A., Dundon, R., Panfilli, R., and Sieggreen, M. (1986). Pressure relief characteristics of various support surfaces used in the prevention and treatment of pressure ulcers. *Journal of Enterostomal Therapy* 14(3): 85-89.

Maklebust, J., Sieggreen, M., and Mondoux, L. (1988). Pressure relief capabilities of the Sof-Care bed cushion and the Clinitron bed. *Ostomy/Wound Management,* 21: 32-41.

Parish, L., and Witkowski, J. (1980). Clinitron therapy and the decubitus ulcer: Preliminary dermatologic studies. *Dermatology* 19: 517-518.

Scheidt, A., and Lewis, D. (1983). Bacteriologic contamination tn an air-fluidized bed. *Journal of Trauma* 3: 241-242.

Dressings: Absorptive for wounds with excessive drainage and odor

Equipment:

Nonsterile gloves — two pair

Sterile normal saline

Sterile tongue blade

4″ × 4″ sterile sponge or abdominal pads

Impervious bag

Paper tape

Skin sealant (Bard Protective Barrier Film Wipe)

Sterile container for paste

Absorptive dressing product

Procedure

A. Preparation

1. Wash hands. Put on gloves and remove old dressing.

2. Discard soiled dressing and gloves in impervious bag.

3. Wash hands. Put on a second pair of gloves. Use sterile technique to irrigate wound with normal saline.

4. Leave wound bed moist. Wipe intact surrounding skin dry with 4″ × 4″ sponge.

5. Assess wound and surrounding tissue for erythema, degree of necrotic tissue, odor, amount of drainage, and size.

6. Apply a skin sealant to intact skin around wound. Air dry.

B. Application

1. Debrisan:

   a. Pour beads 1 cm thick into the wound. Add a thin layer of sterile petrolatum around the wound margin to aid in bead containment.

Rationale/emphasis

To protect wound surface from contamination.

Forceful irrigation removes loose debris and necrotic tissue.

Absorptive dressings are hydrophilic and adhere better to wet wound surfaces.

Absorptive dressings are not effective for ulcers with dry eschar or clean, granulating wound beds. Absorptive dressings are not debriding agents. As much necrotic tissue as possible should be debrided before application.

To keep absorbent dressing off healthy skin.

Hydrophilic absorptive dressings must have room for expansion in the wound bed because they absorb drainage and odor. Absorptive dressings should be applied to a moist wound surface. Do not overfill or pack the wound bed.

Thickness of 1 cm is required to achieve desired hydrophilic suction effect of the dextranomer beads.

(continued)

Dressings: Absorptive for wounds with excessive drainage and odor *(continued)*

Procedure

    b. Use a paste mixture 1 cm thick, instead of beads, in irregular or hard-to-reach wound areas. Mix 3 parts beads with 1 part glycerin in a sterile container.

    c. Cover beads or paste with a dry 4" $\times$ 4" sponge or abdominal pad. Tape all 4 sides "picture frame" method. Write date, time, and initials.

    d. Change and reapply beads or paste every 12 hours or more frequently, if necessary.

    e. Use sterile technique to irrigate all beads or paste from the wound.

2. Bard Absorptive Dressing:

    a. Using a sterile tongue blade or gloved finger, fill the wound to a depth of approximately 1 cm.

    b. Cover with a dry 4" $\times$ 4" sponge or abdominal pad. Tape edges "picture frame" method. Date and initial.

    c. Change dressing daily or more frequently if necessary.

    d. Dressings can be easily removed with a gauze or sterile gloved finger followed by forceful wound irrigation.

3. Hollister Wound Exudate Absorber:

    a. Pour the granular powder 1 cm thick directly into the wound bed.

    b. Use a paste mixture 1 cm thick, instead of the powder, when it is difficult to reach wound areas. Use the Hollister tub container for mixing, blending the absorber with enough glycerin to create a paste consistency.

    c. Cover powder or paste with a dry 4" $\times$ 4" sponge or abdominal pad. Tape edges "picture frame" method. Date and initial.

Rationale/emphasis

Do not use beads or paste in deep fistulae, sinus tracts, or body cavities, where complete removal is not assured.

Helps contain beads and paste in the wound, preventing leakage. Bard Protective Barrier Skin Wipes applied to healthy skin may promote good tape adhesion and skin protection.

When beads or paste become saturated, a color change will be noted, indicating that they should be removed.

Retained dextranomer beads and paste have been associated with impaired wound healing.

Bard Absorptive Dressing can hold 30 times its dry weight in wound exudate.

Antibiotics or other topical medications such as enzymatic debriding agents should be applied before dressing the wound.

Frequency of dressing change depends on amount of drainage.

Dressings: Absorptive for wounds with
excessive drainage and odor *(continued)*

Procedure	Rationale/emphasis
d. Change dressing daily or more frequently if necessary.	Frequency of dressing change depends on amount of drainage.
e. Using sterile technique, rinse any powder or paste remaining in the wound when the dressing is removed with water and normal saline solution.	
4. Discontinue treatment when the wound has a healthy granulation base and is no longer draining.	
5. Select another primary dressing that will continue to maintain a moist wound environment to optimize rate of healing such as a moist dressing, polyurethane, or hydroactive Duo-DERM.	

References

Cuzell, J.Z. (1985). Wound care forum: Artful solutions to chronic problems. *American Journal of Nursing* 85(2): 162-166.

Freeman, B., Carwell, G., and McGraw, J. (1981). The quantitative study of the use of dextranomer in the management of infected wounds. *Surgery, Gynecology and Obstetrics* 153: 81-86.

Jeter, K.F., Chapman, R.M., Tintle, T., and Davis, A. (1986). Comprehensive wound management with a starch-based copolymer dressing. *Journal of Enterostomal Therapy* 13(6): 217-225.

Miksta, J.A. (1986). Industry responseto patient safety concerns. *Journal of Enterostomal Therapy* 13(5): 180-181.

Montgomery, B.A. (1985). Product ingredients: Important ramifications. *Journal of Enterostomal Therapy* 12(6): 203-204.

Thermal wound therapy

Policy:

1. Physician order is required.

2. Wound care specialist, advanced practice nurse, or ET nurse should be consulted to assist with complex wound care management.

3. Special order: Send special order form to Procurement.

Equipment:

Normal saline for irrigation

Baxter tip

Wound cover

Warming card

Temperature control unit

Protective barrier wipes

Procedure

1. Explain procedure to patient.

2. Select a wound cover size to match the wound.

3. Position patient to access ulcer.

4. Irrigate ulcer with normal saline. Use Baxter irrigation tip.

5. Cleanse surrounding skin with soap and water to remove oils and debris. Dry.

6. Apply barrier to intact skin.

7. Apply wound cover over wound so that wound can be seen. Don't wrinkle wound cover edges. Avoid stretching skin or wound cover.

8. Plug the warming card into the temperature control unit. Insert the warming card into the wound cover pocket.

9. Select AC or battery for power delivery. Change battery daily if it is used.

10. Press the ON button to begin therapy.

11. Provide warming therapy for 1 hour.

12. Turn off the temperature control unit. Remove warming card.

13. Leave wound cover in place.

Rationale/emphasis

Cleanse ulcer before treatment.

To facilitate adhesive.

To protect from adhesive.

To ensure power for treatment

Thermal wound therapy *(continued)*

Procedure

Replace wound cover when:

1. leakage occurs.
2. wound cover is loose from skin.
3. wound requires assessment.
4. drainage is copious.

Cleaning and disinfecting equipment

1. Clean and disinfect the temperature control unit and AC adapter between patient uses.
2. Don't immerse the devices.

3. Don't use solvents.
4. Don't autoclave.
5. Disconnect the AC adapter from the wall outlet. Disconnect the temperature control unit from the AC adapter.
6. Use a damp cloth to remove dirt and debris.
7. Dry with a dry cloth.
8. If the unit requires disinfecting, wipe all surfaces with a low-level disinfecting solution. Dampen another cloth with water. Wipe all surfaces, and dry with another cloth.
9. The *warming card* is a single-patient-use item. If it's soiled, it may be cleaned with a slightly damp cloth moistened with clean water. Dry with a separate cloth.
10. Don't store the temperature control unit or the AC adapter in a wet or damp place. Place warming card in the patient storage bag and the temperature control unit in the carrying pouch. Store both in a cool dry place.
11. Customer Service: (800)733-7775 or (952)947-1200
12. Document:
    a. frequency and duration of therapy
    b. date and time of wound cover changes

Rationale/emphasis

Moisture may seep inside and damage the electrical components.
Damage to the unit may result.
Damage to the unit may result.

(continued)

Thermal wound therapy *(continued)*

Procedure   **Rationale/emphasis**

   c. size and condition of wound and periwound
      tissue

   d. patient response to treatment.

References

Hess, C.T. *Nurse's clinical guide: Wound care*, 2nd ed. Springhouse, PA. Springhouse Corporation.

Vacuum-assisted closure

Policy:
1. Physician order is required.
2. Wound care specialist, advance practice nurse, or ET nurse should be consulted to assist with complex wound care management.
3. Special order: Send special order request to Procurement.
4. Therapy is used for patients with copious draining wounds of large volume.

Equipment:
Normal saline
Baxter tip
Reticulated foam
Evacuation tubing
Air-permeable drape
Collection canister
Vacuum unit

Procedure

1. Explain procedure to patient.
2. Thoroughly cleanse wound using normal saline for irrigation and the Baxter tip.
3. Position patient to allow maximum exposure of the wound.
4. Cut the foam to the shape and measurement of the ulcer. More than one piece of foam may be used if the initial piece is cut too small.
5. Place the foam in the wound cavity.
6. Place the fenestrated tube into the center of the foam.
7. Use a protective barrier on the skin adjacent to the ulcer to protect the ulcer from the adhesive.
8. Open the transparent dressing and place over the foam, enclosing the foam and the tubing together.
9. Connect the fenestrated tube to the tube connected to the evacuation canister.
10. Change dressing every 48 hours.

Rationale/emphasis

Seal allows pressure to system.

(continued)

Vacuum-assisted closure *(continued)*

Procedure

11. Document procedures.
    a. frequency and duration of therapy
    b. size and condition of wound and periwound tissue
    c. patient response to treatment

Rationale/emphasis

References

KCI product information

Chapter 10
Continuum of care

Planning for care across different service settings is becoming increasingly important. Many patients receive care from different people in various settings as medical or social conditions change. The Joint Commission for Accreditation of Health Care Organizations (JCAHO) states that each health care organization must view the care it provides as part of a continuum that provides access to an integrated system of settings, services, and care levels as the need occurs. Within this continuum of care, each organization defines, shapes, and sequences over time the following processes and activities to maximize coordination of care:

■ appropriate level of care based on patient's needs
■ coordination among health care professionals
■ referral, transfer, or discharge to another level of care, health care professional, or setting
■ exchange of patient care and clinical information.

Essential components of an effective continuum of care include the following:

■ **Integration of payment sources.** Patients may have insurance only for services that are provided in an acute-care setting, such as a hospital, but some services required may be more appropriately provided in a less expensive setting. Integrating the payment resources by appointing an individual to establish which services the patient needs and determine the best way to meet those needs in a cost-effective way will result in better management of existing finances.

■ **Shared data.** Establishing a communication system across settings may include sharing procedures and forms. A shared database should reduce the time needed for data collection. Use of a common language across services improves communication and facilitates continuity of care.

■ **Management.** Determining how the patient and system converge should be the responsibility of one person who recognizes the patient's needs and preferences and knows the available services. Which discipline is best suited to provide this service has not yet been determined. The patient and system must somehow interface in a way that is beneficial to both.

■ **Multidisciplinary team.** Providing effective, comprehensive, integrated, ongoing services requires effective multidisciplinary teamwork. For example, comprehensive wound management teams provide optimal care for the wounded patient. Each team includes physicians, nurses, pharmacists, dieticians, physical therapists, and social workers and operates as a unit of care.

A continuum of health services can be a progression from wellness to illness and return to wellness or it may be described in terms of type of service, such as preventive care, primary outpatient care, inpatient care, restorative care, or supportive care.

■ Preventive care for patients at risk for pressure ulcers includes education of patient and caregivers, referrals to community resources, and provision of equipment and supplies for prevention.

■ Primary care requires a knowledgeable provider who periodically performs comprehensive assessments of health status and risk factors.

■ Patients with advanced pressure ulcers that can't be managed at home require inpatient care; for example, patients with sepsis, or those requiring reconstructive operations to repair deep pressure ulcers, should be eligible for inpatient services.

■ A recovering patient can receive restorative care in a long-term care facility, a rehabilitative agency, or at home. Restorative care may include physical therapy, occupational therapy, or wound management.

■ Supportive care may include sitters for caregiver respite, day care, assisted living arrangements, and hospice care.

Patients who require long-term or chronic care may use all the services in a system at one time or another. Anticipatory management addresses the chronic care needs of people with pressure ulcers. When initiated at the preventive end of the continuum, care is financially, socially, and personally more economical.

For many years, ill or injured people remained in acute-care hospitals until wounds and diseases were under control or cured. A hospitalized patient was discharged by order of the physician when medically stable. Today, patients are discharged in the midst of workups, sometimes before a definitive diagnosis is made and well before they can safely care for themselves. The physician is only one of a number of people who plan and determine readiness for discharge. Factors that should influence the discharge date include medical stabilization and availability of:

■ appropriate living arrangements
■ community resources

▩ financial resources

▩ ability to direct the activities of caregivers or assistants.

Discharge planning emerged along with new reimbursement mechanisms, high-tech medical care, and regulations in the health care delivery system. In 1982, Medicare's new Prospective Payment System (PPS) forced hospitals to reduce costs and length of stay in the acute-care setting. Since its inception, planning for early discharge became a hospital priority, length of stay in the acute-care setting dropped, and utilization of services was shifted to the community. Continuity of care became even more imperative as early discharge became the norm.

Realizing that emphasis on controlling hospital costs might impinge on the quality of patient care, legislators amended the Social Security Act to require that hospitals have a discharge planning program. The JCAHO issued special guidelines to its member hospitals to recognize discharge planning as part of high-quality services.

The American Hospital Association's General Council published guidelines on discharge planning that contain the definition, purpose, principles, essential elements, and need for quality assurance. The elements of a discharge planning program are as follows:

▩ early identification of patients likely to need complex posthospital care

▩ patient and family education

▩ patient and family assessment and counseling

▩ discharge plan development

▩ discharge plan coordination and implementation

▩ postdischarge follow-up to determine outcomes.

Discharge planning has become a multidisciplinary task. Patient and family participation increases the chance of successful outcomes.

Hospital care

Planning for hospital discharge begins when the physician and patient or family agree on the need for hospitalization. Admitting clinicians should begin planning for discharge at the initial interview and record information about anticipated discharge needs. Ongoing information regarding discharge plans, equipment ordered, or intended disposition should all be listed in the discharge planning section of the medical record. Anticipated discharge disposition is recorded as well as consults requested, current living arrangements, support systems, barriers to self care, and other significant discharge data. New consults and additions to or changes in the plan are added as they occur. (See *Discharge planning assessment,* pages 190 and 191.)

As the patient's condition or needs change, information such as wound care treatment and supplies is updated in the progress notes. A simple statement on the discharge form (such as "see progress notes 9/15, mattress or-

Discharge planning assessment

Detroit Medical Center
Harper
Hospital

DISCHARGE PLANNING ASSESSMENT

Patient lives with _____ ☐ Alone

Legal guardian: ☐ No ☐ Yes   Name/Phone #: _____

Emergency contact (name/phone#) : _____

Responsible for the care of someone else: ☐ No ☐ Yes Relation(s): _____

Services pre-hospitalization: ☐ None ☐ Home care   Reason _____

    If yes, Agency _____   Last visit _____

    Equipment in home _____   Name of company _____

    ☐ Meal service   ☐ Chore service/Housekeeper

Mobility: ☐ No problems ☐ Need assistance _____ ☐ Assistive devices/type _____

Self care: ☐ No problems ☐ Need assistance/type _____
(Feed self, bathe, take own meds , energy for required activities, home maintenance, shopping)

Environment: ☐ No problems ☐ Architectural barriers in home ☐ Bathroom not on 1st level
    ☐ Bed not on 1st level ☐ Stairs in home ☐ Stairs to enter home ☐ Other: _____

Transportation needs: ☐ No problems ☐ Transport to appointments ☐ Clinic/MD appointments
    ☐ ROC ☐ Van service   ☐ Other _____

Financial: ☐ No problems ☐ Unable to obtain medications ☐ Assist with insurance ☐ Other: _____

Caregivers (name/relation): _____

Discharge plan at time of admission	(complete this section on admission)		Additional Self-Care Assessment
	Disposition:	Referral made to:	
☐	Home - Independently or with adequate support	☐ None at this time	_____
☐	Dependent on response to treatment	☐ None at this time	_____
☐	Home - With skilled Home Care	☐ Home Care Coordinator	_____
☐	Home with Medical Equipment	Name _____	_____
☐	Home - Hospice Care	Reason for referral: _____	_____
		See HCC notes for detailed plan.	_____
☐	Home with other community support	☐ Social Worker	_____
☐	Nursing home	Name: _____	_____
☐	Hospice - Inpatient	Reason for referral: _____	_____
☐	Hospice - Nursing home		_____
☐	Ventilator hospital		_____
☐	Adult foster care		_____
☐	Shelter		_____
☐	Psych hospital	See SW notes for detailed plan.	_____
☐	Rehabilitation facility		_____
☐	Other hospital		**Date/Signature:** _____

Discharge planning assessment *(continued)*

Discharge Plan Revisions

Additional discharge related consults placed to:
(Check all that apply)

Date/Signature   Date/Signature

Complex Nursing Issues
☐ Case Manager

Special teaching needs _____   ☐ Physical therapy _____
☐ Diabetes Educator _____   ☐ Occupational therapy _____
☐ Enterostomal Therapist _____   ☐ Speech therapy _____
☐ Pharmacist _____   ☐ Pulmonary Rehab/Home 0$_2$ _____
☐ IVDT _____   ☐ Home Care Coordinator _____
☐ TPN Team _____   ☐ Social Worker _____
☐ Advanced Practive Nurse _____   ☐ Dietitian _____
☐ Other _____   ☐ Other _____

Ongoing Revisions to Discharge/Disposition

Date	Disposition Plan	Signature

dered for home delivery") will make discharge information elsewhere in the record available to all caregivers. Many facilities have developed discharge planning tools to assist clinicians in obtaining important information for home care. To facilitate documentation, some use a discharge criteria checklist for patients with pressure ulcers. Areas of instruction for patients with pressure ulcers include wound care, insurance coverage, pressure ulcer prevention techniques, and where to obtain specific medical equipment and supplies. Development of a discharge criteria checklist may facilitate communication of vital information to the receiving health care provider. Much of the essential information for discharge planning can be obtained at group conferences or multidisciplinary rounds.

An effective discharge plan requires that the clinician be able to identify the patient's functional status, evaluating exactly what the patient is able to do and what support staff can contribute to meeting the patient's activities of daily living in the home setting. Then follows an attempt to foresee problems the patient may encounter in different levels of care. Finally, to ease the transition from one health care setting to another, the discharge planner facilitates completion of a continuing patient care form for home care or an interagency transfer summary for transfer to another health care facility, including as much information as possible for the professional caregiver in the new setting. (See *Interagency transfer summary*.) To implement the plan of care, the community health nurse or physical therapist assesses the patient's home for safety and comfort and makes appropriate requests for assistive devices as necessary.

Many health care agencies have developed criteria for screening patients who are at risk for problems after discharge. Patients at risk for pressure ulcers generally fall into this category. With the advent of prospective payment, patients are discharged from the hospital sicker and more dependent than ever before; this patient population is at greatest risk for developing pressure ulcers. Patients who are discharged from the hospital with pressure ulcers must have consistent observation and treatment at home to prevent further tissue breakdown.

One way to monitor patients as they move from a controlled inpatient setting into the home is to contact them after discharge. Geriatric patients with newly diagnosed incontinence, pressure ulcers, and cognitive impairment are at risk for functional decline or death during or following hospitalization. Although expensive, postdischarge home assessment and follow-up intervention for geriatric patients can be effective and can have long-term benefits.

Patients with pressure ulcers may be discharged to a subacute, long-term care, or rehabilitation facility or they may be sent home with instructions to rely on community support resources. Patients who are terminally ill may be discharged and sent home with hospice services. It is essential that health care staff in every agency be educated regarding pressure ulcer prevention.

Interagency transfer summary

DMC Wayne State University
The Detroit Medical Center
Interagency Transfer Summary

Brown, Janella
04592036
10/1/11
Feldspar, Jasper MD

1. Patient's last name	2. First name	3. Middle	4. Sex	5. Date of transfer	6. Religion
Brown	*Janella*	*B*	M ☒F	*01-27-00*	*B*

7. Address (Street number, city, state, zip)
4291 West Detroit 48203

8. Date of birth
10-1-11

9. Transfer to:	10. Transfer from:
Name *Rehab Inst* Address *John R*	Name *Harper Hospital* Address:

11. Contact person
Name *Ella Brown*   Address: *4291 West*   Phone number: *(313) 491-7342*   Relationship *Mother*

12. Patient lives
Alone ☐   with spouse ☐   with family ☐   Other ☒   Please specify:

13. Insurance information:	14. Physician at time of transfer
BCBSM x 42 411590192 6P11166	Name: *J. Feldspar* Phone number: *(313) 145-4009*

15. Allergies:	16. Previous hospitalizations and/or extended care facilities:
NKA	*MVA Paralysis 1996 - Rehab 8 weeks*

P H Y S I C I A N   I N F O R M A T I O N

17. Diagnosis (es) at time of transfer
Primary: *Sacral Pressure Ulcer, Infected*
Other conditions: *Paraplegia*

18. Surgical procedures and dates
Debridement, Sacral Pressure Ulcer

19. Physician orders on transfer: *1. See ulcer care - next page, 2. Maximize function*
  A. Diet: *Regular - Supplement with Ensure Cl CAN TID?*
  B. Medications: Name/dose/route/frequency

  Vicodin ES 1-2 tabs
  Pepcid
  Metamucil
  Cipro
  MVI
  Ascorbic Acid

  C. Therapies: *Physical Therapy, Occupational Therapy*

  D. Other:

  E. Weight bearing: *Non AMB*

  Full _____ Partial _____ None _____ On _____ Leg

20. Labs:
			Mode of transport: *W/C*
CBC	date *1/26/00*	result *WBC.9 / Hgl 10 / Hct 38*	
Urinalysis	date *1/26/00*	result *neg*	
Serology	date _____	result _____	Ambulance _____
Other	date _____	result _____	
Chest x-ray*	date *1/08/00*	result *neg*	Car _____
	(* Report to be sent with patient)		

21. Patient* family aware of disease process   ☒ Yes   ☐ No

Physician signature   Date:
  J. Feldspar MD   *1-21-00*

(continued)

Interagency transfer summary *(continued)*

DMC Wayne State University
The Detroit Medical Center
Interagency Transfer Summary

Brown, Janella
0459 2036
10-1-11
Feldspar, Jasper MD

N U R S I N G

E V A L U A T I O N

22. Vital signs: Blood pressure _118/76_ Pulse _72_   Temperature _98_   Height _5'4"_   Weight _110_

23. Speech: normal ☒   impaired ☐   unable to speak ☐   speaks no English ☐
                                                                         understands no English ☐

24. Hearing: normal ☒   impaired ☐   deaf ☐   hearing aid ☐

25. Sight: normal ☒   impaired ☐   blind ☐   glasses ☐

26. Mental status: oriented ☒   confused ☐   agitated ☐   other ☐

27. Feeding: independent ☒ needs help ☐   cannot feed self ☐   dentures ☐   tube ☐

28. Dressing: independent ☐ needs help ☒   cannot dress self ☐

29. Bathing: independent ☐ needs help ☒   bedbath with help ☐   bedbath ☐

30. Elimination: independent ☒   help to bathroom ☐   bedpan or urinal ☐   last bowel movement
    offer supplies incontinent: urine ☐   stool ☐   Foley ☐   ostomy ☐   *1-21-00*

31. Ambulatory status: independent ☐   chair ☒   help with ambulation ☐   bedbound ☐
                       assistance: one ☐   two ☐   three ☐
                       equipment _____

32. Dressing and bandages   Or, check none ☐

33. Skin integrity: normal ☐   pressure sore ☒   Stage I   ☒ *heels*
                                                        Stage II ☐
                      Other ☐   Stage III ☐
                      Special Skin   Stage IV ☒ *Sacrum 8 x 8 cm, 4 cm deep*
                      Products: _Moist saline gauze_   *granulating tissue necrosis*
                                change 9 - 8 hr, rinse with saline

34. Unresolved nursing diagnosis (es) and plan:
    1. Tissue integrity - continue above dressing change
    *   - keep off ulcer*
    *   - patient to return to hospital for rotation flap when infection cleared*

35. Special needs: *1. Pressure reducing bed cushion*
                    2. pressure reducing chair cushion

Signature and title   Date:
    Susan Wilfse RN   *1-21-00*

36. Special hospital services: social work, dietary, physical therapy, pharmacy and patient education.
    SW: check family situation for care giver assistance
    CMS: Arrange for home health supplies and equipment

Registered nurses, licensed practical nurses, home health aides, and other caregivers must be included in the education process.

Subacute care

Subacute care facilities evolved from the need for health care that is more intensive than that provided by nursing homes or home care. The duration of stay is expected to be short. Patients with open pressure ulcers requiring complex dressing changes, and those in a lengthy postoperative phase after pressure ulcer reconstruction, will spend part of their recovery in a subacute care facility. Patients admitted to subacute care facilities without pressure ulcers, but requiring high-technology care and equipment, are at risk for pressure ulcers while they are in the facility. Policies and procedures must be in place in the facility for pressure ulcer prevention and treatment (see chapter 9).

Long-term care

Residents of long-term care facilities and nursing homes frequently are at high risk for pressure ulcers. The Omnibus Budget Reconciliation Act (OBRA) of 1991 established that all residents of long-term care facilities must be assessed with a standardized assessment tool, the Minimum Data Set (MDS). This tool contains "triggers"; that is, components of the assessment considered to be potential problems that may require development of a care plan. Triggers in the MDS associated with pressure ulcers and risk for pressure ulcers include presence of a pressure ulcer and the following 12 risk factors: impaired transfer or bed mobility; bedfast, hemiplegia, quadriplegia; urinary or bowel incontinence; peripheral vascular disease; diabetes mellitus; hip fracture; weight loss; history of pressure ulcers; impaired tactile sensory perception; medications such as antipsychotics and tranquilizers; restraints used daily; and no adequate skin care program.

Most skilled nursing facilities now receive prospective payment under a Medicare Part A qualifying stay. Medicare's Skilled Nursing Facility (SNF) Prospective Payment System (PPS) follows the intent of the Balanced Budget Act of 1997, which mandates that other SNF PPSs work on a per diem payment system modified by case mix adjustments. Medicare pays nursing facilities a fixed amount of money each day, based on the documented needs of the patient. Prospective payment means that nursing facilities must be aware of their exact costs for various clinical conditions, services, and supplies. Clinicians need to determine how to reduce costs by finding the lowest priced products that achieve the desired clinical outcome. For pressure ulcers, this means demonstrating evidence of healing or prevention. Staff education becomes more important than ever because knowledgeable staff members can assist administrators with smart purchasing by reporting products that offer the best value.

Admitting patients with existing pressure ulcers generates tremendous anxiety among caregivers in long-term care facilities. Patients with pressure ulcers often are denied admission or readmission to skilled or long-term care facilities because their wound cultures show growth of multiple organisms. Some nursing homes require two negative wound cultures as criteria for admission. The problem stems from lack of knowledge about colonization versus infection in chronic wounds. All chronic wounds will grow organisms when cultured, just as organisms will grow from a skin surface culture. Wound culture isn't a valid criterion for denial for admission to a health care facility. If discharge planners are informed that a negative wound culture is required for placement in a given institution, the hospital epidemiologist should be consulted to assist the agency in interpreting the regulations. Skilled nursing facilities should do all they can to provide the best possible wound care prevention and treatment and create a win-win situation for patients who need wound and skin care.

Home care

Home care agencies have registered nurses, licensed practical nurses, physical therapists, social workers, dieticians, and home health aides who participate in the care of patients with pressure ulcers. Each of these providers must be educated about pressure ulcer prevention and treatment. As patients make the transition from the hospital environment to home care, professionals perform periodic assessments to update patient information and to verify the continued accuracy of the treatment plan.

A home care agency admission assessment form can be a useful tool. Because this tool includes a body diagram, information about pressure ulcer location and characteristics can be communicated easily to caregivers. Specific instructions for pressure ulcer care are written on the Home Health Aide Care Plan. This includes required procedures, the duration and frequency of treatments, activity allowed, and body positioning to avoid pressure. (See *Home health aide care plan.*) Routine pressure ulcer documentation by home care providers includes weekly information on wound measurements, ulcer stage, location, appearance, and drainage.

Providing home care for a patient with a pressure ulcer often is complicated and overwhelming for the caregiver. The professional nurse's time in the home is intermittent, and the family caregiver's skills are limited. The lay person finds most medication regimens, treatments, diet, and wound care management plans to be complex. Family members who usually are adept at routine care may be overwhelmed by the task of preventing and treating pressure ulcers on their own. Even treatments that professionals think of as easy can be frightening for patients at home without professional

Home health aide care plan

RENAISSANCE HOME HEALTH CARE

HOME HEALTH AIDE CARE PLAN

Patient				Age	Sex	Pt. No.		Today's date		Times Weekly (Range)

Patient address			Apt. #	Team	Insurance □ Care □ Caid	□ BC □ HMO □ Other	Therapy only □	Diagnosis	

City		Zip	Phone	Directions (cross streets)

		VITAL SIGNS	
PERSONAL CARE	Encourage participation ADL/bathing	X	TEMPERATURE NOTIFY:
	Assist bath	X	PULSE NOTIFY:
	Complete bed bath	X	RESPIRATIONS NOTIFY:
	Progress to:	X	DATE OF LAST BM Report if no BM x days
	Assist bath as tolerated	X	Maintain Clean, Safe Environment
	Tub/shower as tolerated		DIET □ Regular □ _____

PLEASE NOTE: □ Speech impaired □ Disoriented   □ Blind

□ Hard of hearing □ Unconscious □ Incontinence □ Amputation

□ Contractures □ Hemiplegia □ Quadriplegia □ Paraplegia

LIMITATIONS

PERSONAL CARE (cont.)
- Skin care
- Shave client
- Shampoo ___ Weekly and PRN
  ___ Bi-monthly and PRN
- Comb hair
- Oral hygiene
- Nail care
- Linen change ___ Weekly and PRN
  ___ Other (specify) _____

PRECAUTIONS
- Safe Disposal of contaminated materials
- No smoking with oxygen in use
- Seizures
- Lock wheelchair with transfers
- Side rails up
- Total hip precautions
- Other (specify) _____

ACTIVITY
- Ambulation with assistance of _____
- Transfer bed/ chair with assistance of _____
- Complete bed rest
- ROM to _____

REPORT TO RN:

SIGNS AND SYMPTOMS
- Dizziness, headache, blurred vision, fainting
- Report foley plugged, leaking, blood in urine, cloudy, burning or strong odor to urine.
- Report redness, warmth, change in wound drainage or foul odor
- Change in LOC/Change in gait
- Excessive thirst, urination, and hunger
- Abru t onset of excessive sweating, faintness, trembling and confusion
- Severe SOB, unrelieved chest pain, swelling lower extrem.
- Weight gain/loss greater than _____ #'s
- OTHER:_____

OTHER DUTIES
- **Catheter Care:** Dsg change/cleanse with _____
- Irrigate with _____ every _____
- Change bag every _____
- **Wound/Decubitus care** (specify) _____
- Frequency for HHA: q. _____ .
- Oxygen at _____ Liters/min per _____
- Weigh: q. _____ .
- Other (specify)_____

RN SIGNATURE:	PRIMARY YES □ NO □	REVISION YES □ NO □	AIDE ASSIGNED:	FIRST HHA VISIT:	SUPERVISORY VISIT DUE:

supervision. The age and physical condition of the caregiver plays an important role in determining whether a specific treatment protocol will work. During the patient's first few days at home, it isn't unusual for the patient or caregiver to perform wound care once or twice a day, with a nurse visiting daily for another dressing change. When the nurse believes that the caregiver is comfortable with the technique, the number of visits to the home can be reduced. Teaching the family home care of pressure ulcers can be broken down into three steps:

■ explain the cause
■ assess each ulcer and select the appropriate treatment plan
■ explain the treatment plan to the family member.

See Chapter 11 for more detailed patient and family education regarding home care of the patient with pressure ulcers.

Hospice care

Pressure ulcers in hospice patients greatly complicate care, increase costs, and seriously threaten quality of remaining life. Recommended daytime care strategies are directed toward increasing patient comfort. Needless pain and suffering associated with pressure ulceration can be avoided by teaching hospice staff the essentials of pressure ulcer prevention. If and when pressure ulcer care becomes burdensome to the patient, the patient and family may choose to eliminate turning or painful dressing changes in favor of comfort-only measures. The plan of care always follows the patient and family preferences, as long as it is well documented.

Cost considerations

Home health care is growing rapidly, primarily because of the pressures on hospitals to discharge patients early. Recuperation with home-based nursing care is an essential link between the hospital and a return to daily living. Unfortunately, the current climate suggests that only direct physical care is reimbursable; nurses need to pursue changes in reimbursement mechanisms for home health care.

Immobile patients are at high risk for pressure ulcers and require a pressure-relieving sleep surface at home. Often the choice of a pressure-relieving device will be determined by the family's financial situation and not by what's best for the patient. If a pressure-relieving surface isn't sent home from the acute-care setting, the patient who is at risk for pressure ulcers may not be able to obtain one after discharge, despite the fact that it is much less expensive to treat a patient in the home setting than in the hospital. Currently, Medicare selectively reimburses for prevention and treatment of pressure sores under the Part B home care benefit. Nurses need to continue to track such cases and submit the findings to fiscal intermediaries. Home care nursing agencies are lobbying for legislative changes to ensure quality nursing care. All nurses need to support changes in Medicare reimbursement for interventions that affect pressure ulcer management.

The PPS is contributing to a growing access problem for hospital patients who require and would be more appropriately provided care in a skilled nursing facility or at home. PPS often results in denial of access to the frailest Medicare patients. Because many patients' needs have daily costs in excess of the allowable rates, many SNFs turn away medically complex patients. Home health care agencies also refuse care to many patients because the cost of care is too high.

Summary

Health care cost containment policies have been the major impetus for the increasing importance of discharge planning. Health care cost containment will remain a major concern for the foreseeable future because of the following:

- the Balanced Budget Act
- the aging of the population
- medical technology prolonging life without cure
- the shift of care from inpatient to outpatient
- recognition that resources are limited
- uneven distribution of health care professionals
- the attempt to provide access to care while also trying to guarantee quality of life.

Planning for the appropriate level of care is increasing in importance as more third-party payers adopt prospective payment. Clinicians must shift their thinking about patient care from the episodic acute incident to an ongoing continuum. Responsibility for planning expands as patients become part of a system that offers lifetime health and illness care and insurance companies assume responsibility for "covered lives." Pressure ulcers are chronic problems that demand lifetime surveillance as part of a management program. Planning for appropriate level of care takes on a global dimension as it shifts from discharge planning to ongoing planning. Discharge from one facility to another or from a facility to the home isn't discharge from the system. It is merely a transition along the continuum of care.

Selected references

Andrews, G. "HCFA calls town meeting on skilled nursing facilities," *WOCN News*, Issue 2:6, 1999.

Berquist, S., and Frantz, R.A. "Pressure ulcers in community-based older adults receiving home health care," *Advances in Wound Care* 12(7):339-351, 1999.

Buckbinder, D., et al. "Building a wound care healing team. Part I," *ECPN* 62:17-18, 1999.

Erwin-Toth, P." Cost-effective pressure ulcer management in extended care," *Ostomy/Wound Management* 41(7A Suppl):64S-69S, 1995.

Fenner, S.P. "Developing and implementing a wound care program in long term care," *JWOCN* 26(5):25-60, 1999.

Fontaine, K. "The transition from hospital to home health nursing," *CME Resources*, ANCC, 1999.

Joint Commission for Accreditation of Health Care Organizations. 1995 *Comprehensive accreditation manual for hospitals*. Oakbrook Terrace: JCAHO, 1994.

Knapp, M.T. "Nurses' basic guide to understanding the Medicare PPS," *Nursing Management* 30(5):14-15, 1999.

Krafitz, R.L., et al. "Geriatric home assessment after hospital discharge," *Journal of the American Geriatric Society* 42(12):1229-1234, 1994.

Micheletti, J.A., and Shalala, T.J. "Understanding and operationalizing subacute services," *Nursing Management* (Continuing Care Edition) 26(6):49-56, 1995.

Motta, G.J. "Can SNF under PPS afford to use support surfaces?" *ECPN* 61:5, 1999.

Xakellis, G., and Frantz, R.A. "Cost effectiveness of an intensive pressure ulcer prevention protocol in long term care," *Advances in Wound Care* 11:22-29, 1998.

Zulkowski, K. "MDS and items not contained in the pressure ulcer RAP associated with pressure ulcer prevalence in the newly institutionalized elderly," *Ostomy/Wound Management* 45(1):24-33, 1999.

Chapter 11
Education

As patients move from inpatient settings of hospitals and long-term care facilities into their homes, responsibility for care moves to family members and to patients themselves. This shift away from professional care dramatically increases the need for patients and caregivers to have the requisite knowledge and skills. Educating patients leads to improved risk-related behavior, less postoperative pain and distress, decreased length of stay, and fewer hospital readmissions.

Identifying educational needs of family members or caregivers for patients with pressure ulcers is a difficult process. The few studies available suggest that family members who serve as caregivers have little idea about how to obtain knowledge about pressure ulcers; many have never heard of pressure ulcers and have no information on risk factors or preventive measures. Yet, when patients are hospitalized for sepsis or other complications of pressure ulcers, professionals may blame the family for providing poor care. Elderly caregivers, often wives caring for husbands, tend to be frail themselves; these women have difficulty providing the physical, emotional, and financial care their husbands need. Social support systems may be limited or nonexistent, and the caregivers often lack basic caregiving knowledge. Many neglect their own health to provide the care they believe their husbands need. Because many insurance plans don't cover home-care services, and Medicare reimbursement doesn't cover most home health care supplies, the cost of dressings, equipment, and nutritional supplements creates a financial burden for these families.

Education empowers patients and caregivers. Health care professionals in hospitals, long-term care facilities, outpatient clinics, and offices have a responsibility to educate patients and families about pressure ulcer risk factors. The optimal time for teaching each person is an individual matter. Patient education is more effective when given in more than one session and enhanced with follow-up because presenting large amounts of new educational content in a single session hinders the patient's ability to process information. Patient education should focus on promoting the acquisition of knowledge and skills and on supporting decision making.

Adult learning

Patients and families enter the health care environment with a variety of beliefs and a wide range of educational experiences and abilities. Their interpretations of current situations reflect their own past experiences. The educator may be well qualified to teach a patient how to perform a procedure or modify risk factors, but the patient who doesn't value this knowledge won't learn. Established principles of adult learning help the educator provide health education for adult patients and families. In general, the following points hold true about adult learners:

■ They need to know *why* they should learn something.
■ They need to be self-directed.
■ They have a greater variety and different quality of experiences than youth.
■ They're ready to learn information or practices that allow them to function more effectively and satisfyingly.
■ enter a learning experience with a task-centered, problem-centered, or life-centered orientation to learning.
■ They're stimulated to learn by extrinsic and intrinsic motivators.

These principles should be applied as formal or informal education is developed.

Assessing needs

Health care professionals collect comprehensive data to determine a patient's current and past health status, functional status, and coping patterns. This database must include assessment of patient and family learning needs and identification of available resources for patient and caregiver education. Assessment of patients with pressure ulcers includes identifying of caregivers and patient and family characteristics that may inhibit or enhance learning. Interpersonal and intrapersonal patient and caregiver characteristics may influence both the teaching-learning process and the outcome.

Pressure ulcer prevention information should be directed toward the person who will use it — the patient himself or his chosen primary caregiver. Some patients can obtain information and either carry out the functions or direct someone else to perform the skills. Others may be cognitively impaired, unable to retain information, or physically unable to perform the tasks necessary for self-care. For any number of reasons, a capable patient may wish to have someone else assume the primary provider role.

The teacher must be familiar with how different cultures vary in their expectations of the health care system. Some patients may use "healing remedies" that are in fact detrimental to healing. Others may be uncomfortable having another person perform skin inspection, particularly around the pelvic girdle, an area that often is vulnerable to pressure ulceration. Health care professionals must develop culturally sensitive strategies to teach pressure ulcer prevention and treatment.

Before teaching, the educator must perform a comprehensive pressure ulcer history and risk assessment to identify current practices that increase the risk for pressure ulcers. Only then can a decision be made regarding what educational content should be stressed.

Establishing goals and objectives

The clinician and the patient or caregiver must set goals and objectives together. The goals identify what needs to be accomplished and guide the teaching-learning process. The objectives are the behaviors expected at completion of the process. They are stated in behavioral terms so that they can be measured. For example, one goal may be to have the patient's pressure ulcer heal. Objectives related to this goal may include a patient demonstration of a dressing change or preparation of a menu with a balanced nutrition plan for wound healing.

Combining the expertise of clinicians with the patient's and caregiver's desires improves the chances for realistic goal setting. A patient may have many risk factors and may require several goals to reduce the risks or to promote healing. Risks are commonly embedded in lifestyles or routines, and patients may have priorities that are in conflict with risk factor management. For example, a young, insensate, wheelchair-bound person may need a reminder to perform wheelchair pushups or shift body weight during long classes at school. One mother found a watch with an alarm to remind her wheelchair-bound daughter to shift her weight on schedule. However, because the alarm brought attention to her handicap, the young girl chose not to use it. A watch with a vibrating alarm turned out to be an acceptable alternative.

Facing a large number of goals may be an overwhelming experience for both patient and caregiver. Dividing long-term goals into short-term goals can make a plan more manageable. Whenever possible, family members should participate in goal setting and caregiving. Sharing the care relieves the burden and reduces caregiver strain. Matching tasks to the skills of different family members creates a sense of teamwork and mutual responsibility. If it's acceptable to the patient and family, children can participate in care by moisturizing skin and providing oral fluids, and adolescents can run errands. Participation in the team helps all members of the family understand frustrations when they occur.

When the number of goals seems overwhelming, setting subjective goals also may help. Indeed, a subjective goal may be more important to the caregiver than an objective goal. For example, the objective goal of decreasing the size of the pressure ulcer provides the patient or caregiver with the subjective goal of experiencing a sense of relief as the frequency of dressing changes decreases.

Clinicians should continually reassess the situation in terms of goals or expected outcomes. As the patient's risk factors change, the goals may require adjustment or revision. Revisions indicate that caregivers are responding to the needs of the patient and not just working with a routine plan that has lost its benefit.

Strategies and methods

An effective educator uses a variety of teaching strategies to reach the desired educational outcome. Matching the clinician's teaching style with the patient's preferred learning style increases the chance that learning will take place. Most learners require multisensory stimulation. Even when a caregiver must master a certain task, more than one learning strategy may exist. The teacher may request a repeat demonstration if the essential component of a lesson is mastering a required skill. Teaching may include written instruction and diagrams as well as demonstration. One family videotaped the physical therapist as she taught the patient safe transfer techniques. The patient could then view the video to reinforce learning.

The demonstration-practice method of instruction is effective for teaching prevention and care skills, such as positioning, use of equipment, and dressing change procedures. Demonstration is accompanied by instructions and written outcome criteria, often in the form of a checklist. All instructions should be written in clear, simple terminology so that family members may refer to them. The checklist can serve as a reminder to the patient when a procedure is performed at home without supervision. Demonstration-practice has three components:

■ telling the patient how to do the procedure
■ demonstrating the procedure
■ asking the patient to duplicate the demonstration, including all the items on the written checklist

When referring a hospitalized patient for continuing care, the discharging clinician should document the following:

■ patient education covered during the hospital stay
■ patient's and family's level of understanding
■ patient's ability to provide self-care.

Clinicians can use their own experience in caring for many patients with the same type of health care problem as a basis for developing teaching-outcome checklists. Such checklists may be modified to fit the desired objectives, goals, and needs of each patient. (See *Dressing change and wound care: Teaching outcome checklist.*)

Dressing change and wound care: Teaching outcome checklist

Detroit Medical Center
Harper Hospital

Performance Criteria: Dressing Change/Wound Care		Initiated by Nurse	Verbalized or Demonstrated by Patient
1. Patient verbalizes need/rationale and frequency for dressing changes.	1.	_____	_____
2. Selects the correct amount and type of dressing supplies.	2.	_____	_____
3. Discusses technique of dressing changes (e.g., clean, sterile).	3.	_____	
4. Demonstrates steps of dressing change/wound care:			
a. Washes hands and prepares new dressings	4. a.	_____	_____
b. Removes old dressing	b.	_____	_____
c. Rewashes hands	c.	_____	_____
d. Changes dressing per correct procedure	d.	_____	_____

☐ dry ☐ soaks

☐ wet and dry ☐ other (specify)

☐ packing _____

☐ other (specify) _____

e. Disposes of old dressing properly	e.	_____	_____
5. Verbalizes confidence in changing dressing	5.	_____	_____
6. States intended method of changing dressing at home:			
a. Sitting	6. a.	_____	_____
b. Standing	b.	_____	_____
c. Use of mirror	c.	_____	_____
7. States where to obtain dressing supplies/needed resources.	7.	_____	_____
8. States signs and symptoms to report to physician:			
a. Color of tissue in wound	8. a.	_____	_____
b. Color of drainage from wound	b.	_____	_____
c. Color of tissue surrounding wound	c.	_____	_____
d. Chills, fever, pain, swelling, tenderness of wound	d.	_____	_____
9. States date of and intention to keep follow-up appointment with physician.	9.	_____	_____

COMMENTS _____

_____

Initials	Signature/Title	Initials	Signature/Title	Initials	Signature/Title

SMOG readability formula and conversion table

Use the formula and conversion table below to determine whether the reading material you are using is appropriate for your patient's educational level.

1. For a test sample of 30 sentences, count off 10 consecutive sentences near the beginning, in the middle, and near the end of the text. If the entire text has fewer than 30 sentences, use all.

2. Count the number of words containing three or more syllables, including repetitions of the same words.

3. Find the approximate grade level on the table below.

Total number of polysyllabic words	Approximate grade level
0 to 2	4
3 to 6	5
7 to 12	6
13 to 20	7
21 to 30	8
31 to 42	9
43 to 56	10
57 to 72	11
73 to 90	12
91 to 110	13
111 to 132	14
133 to 156	15
157 to 182	16
183 to 210	17
211 to 240	18

Adapted from U.S. Department of Health and Human Services. *Pretesting in health communications*. NH Pub. 84–1493. Washington, DC: US Government Printing Office. Table developed by Harold C. McGraw, Office of Education Research, Baltimore County Schools, Towson, Md.

Reading levels

The reading level of printed educational material should match the learner's reading ability. If the reading level is too high, less educated patients won't understand the written information. If the level is too low, more educated patients will lose interest. A readability formula, such as the simplified measure of gobbledygook (SMOG), is a useful tool for determining whether written material is appropriate for a specific patient or caregiver. (See *SMOG readability formula and conversion table*.)

What patients need to know

All patients with pressure ulcers and those who are at risk for pressure ulcers need to know basic information about prevention and treatment. The consumer guides of the Agency for Healthcare Research and Quality (AHRQ) *Preventing Pressure Ulcers: A Patient's Guide* and *Treating Pressure Sores* are available from the U.S. Department of Health and Human Services for patient and caregiver education. These guides describe how pressure ulcers form, how to identify risk factors, steps to prevent pressure ulcers, and how to treat them if they do occur. They also address skin care, pressure reduction, nutrition, mobility and activity, positioning, ulcer treatment, complications, and what to report to a health care provider. Pharmaceutical companies, medical equipment manufacturers, and wound care companies also provide educational material that can be adapted for individual use. The following sections highlight essential information for patients and caregivers.

Prevention and treatment

A program for pressure ulcer education should address both prevention and treatment (see Chapters 6 and 7). Patients must be taught that healed pressure ulcers are at high risk for ulceration. The scar resulting from granulation and re-epithelialization of soft tissue ulceration has only 80% of the tensile strength of normal body tissue. Lifelong surveillance of this tissue is necessary.

Everyone who comes into contact with a patient with pressure ulcers needs to know that unrelieved pressure is the main cause of pressure ulcers. Visual signs make a description of the consequence of prolonged pressure easier to understand, For example, give a simple explanation about compression of blood vessels and the need for tissue oxygenation and nutrition. Demonstrate the effect of pressure against soft tissue by pressing the fingers tightly around a clear drinking glass. With enough pressure, the finger pads become pale from compression of the blood vessels. Reactive hyperemia is apparent on the finger pads when the pressure is relieved. Patients can see the effect of pressure through the clear glass.

Skin care

The first step in the program is teaching the appropriate skin care. This includes accurate inspection, careful cleansing, and avoiding friction.

Inspection

■ Inspect and care for the skin at least twice daily. In addition, inspect areas over bony prominences after each position change. (See *How to perform a skin check,* page 208.)

How to perform a skin check

An effective skin check includes the following steps:

- Check all surface areas at least twice daily. Convenient times may be on waking and at bedtime.
- Check pressure points at every change in position.
- Check previously reddened areas every 15 minutes to 1 hour as indicated by the care plan.
- Remove the patient's clothing, and position the patient so that areas to be checked are accessible. The patient's position will depend on the previous activity or position and the current care plan.
- Identify the areas to be inspected.
- Examine the skin for signs of pressure (redness, loss of skin, changes in color or temperature), moisture or dryness, and presence of rashes.
- Check for temperature changes by placing the back of the hand against the skin surface. Compare findings with the temperature of other skin surface areas. This method will detect even a 5° difference in temperature.
- If you note a reddened area, reassess it in 15 minutes. If the reddened area has not changed, do not position the patient with pressure on this area. Continue to monitor until the condition resolves. Report the finding to the professional health care provider.
- If you note a rash , cleanse the area with plain water and pat dry. Report findings to the professional health care provider. Apply topical lotions, powders, or ointments only under the direction of the health care provider.

■ Pressure points may vary when joints become contracted, after flap operations for repair of pressure ulcers, and as soft tissue redistributes on the body after weight changes.

■ Every person has unique pressure points. It's helpful to create a diagram of the patient's body with identified pressure points to be used as a check sheet for inspection.

■ Inspection of the entire skin surface is essential.

■ Pay special attention to areas that remain reddened after position changes. Make sure that reddened areas are completely free from pressure after a position change. Use pillows, rolled towels, or foam wedges to relieve pressure.

■ Never massage over bony prominences or reddened areas. Massage may rupture capillaries and damage the tissue under the skin.

Cleansing

■ Clean skin only when it's soiled. Warm water is safer than hot water for bathing or showering, particularly over skin areas that are insensate. If the patient prefers daily bathing, take measures to prevent dry skin, such as applying moisturizing creams or oils.

■ Urine, stool, and perspiration irritate skin and increase pressure ulcer risk. A program for incontinence management will reduce the risk for skin breakdown. The cause of incontinence should be investigated and treated. *Managing Urinary Incontinence: A Patient's Guide* can be ordered from AHRQ Publications.

▪ Fecal incontinence is especially detrimental to skin. Use of a skin barrier will help protect the skin. Incontinence pads that wick moisture away from the skin will help keep the skin dry. Incontinence pads are readily available and can be used if urinary or fecal incontinence is minimal.

▪ Cleanse and dry the perianal and pelvic areas after each soiling and prior to use of an incontinence product. For more information about continence products and services, contact Help for Incontinent People, P.O. Box 544, Union, SC 29397.

Friction

▪ Avoid friction against the skin during repositioning by lifting, rather than dragging, the body across a bed or chair surface. Friction can rub away the skin surface.

▪ An overbed trapeze allows the patient to help lift the body during repositioning. Caregivers should use lift sheets to prevent friction when repositioning.

▪ Wearing clothing, such as long-sleeved pajamas and socks, or using a thin film of cornstarch on the skin will also reduce friction.

Pressure reduction

Removing pressure is the most important part of prevention and treatment of pressure ulcers. The family needs to know how to relieve pressure in the home setting. People who are confined to bed need a special mattress or mattress overlay made of foam, air, gel, or water. The patient and caregiver should understand that the clinician will help with selection of the best product. Insurance companies with case management services may identify preferred products. (See chapter 6 for more information on pressure-reduction devices and proper positioning.) However, the family must be taught that a pressure-reducing device doesn't substitute for proper positioning and frequent repositioning. A pictorial diagram of the recommended positioning schedule can remind the caregiver to routinely turn the patient.

The teaching plan should include the following points:

▪ Good body positioning in bed begins with good body alignment. Pillows and foam wedges maintain correct body alignment and support the patient's position.

▪ The head of the bed should be raised as little as necessary and for as short a time as possible. Maintaining the head with less than 30 degrees elevation will avoid a shearing effect of the bony skeleton sliding inside the soft tissue of the pelvis.

▪ Using a foot board on a hospital bed will help prevent the patient from slipping while in a sitting position.

Teaching caregivers the 30-degree laterally inclined position

Assessment addresses the skin's functional integrity. The chart below shows how to assess important skin factors by function along with normal and abnormal assessment findings.

- Show the family or caregiver a picture of the 30-degree angle, side-lying position. Explain that there's no pressure on the hip bone (trochanter of the femur) or tailbone (sacrum).
- Demonstrate the positioning technique by first moving the patient into the 30-degree angle, side-lying position, then placing a pillow or wedge behind the patient to maintain the position.
- When the patient is properly positioned, have the caregiver slide a hand, palm upward, under the patient's hip.
- Call caregiver's attention to how the weight of the patient's body rests on the fleshy part of the buttocks, not on the hipbone.
- Return the patient to a back-lying position. Have the caregiver correctly position the patient while you provide verbal coaching. When the patient is positioned, have the caregiver repeat the hand check to confirm that positioning is correct.

▪ The 30-degree, lateral, side-lying position eliminates direct pressure on the greater trochanter of the femur and places the weight of the pelvis on the soft tissue of the buttocks. (See *Teaching caregivers the 30-degree laterally inclined position.*)

▪ A support surface can be assessed for effectiveness in reducing pressure by a "hand check" procedure. (See chapter 6.) If support is inadequate, the health care provider may recommend a different support surface.

▪ The patient's heels require extra protection. Devices that suspend the heels are preferred, but pillows placed under the ankle and calf are an inexpensive alternative. If a piece of paper can slide between the heel and the surface of the bed, the device is effective.

▪ Avoid placing pillows or other support devices behind the knee, as this may cause undue pressure to the popliteal area.

Wheelchair positioning

Correct posture for chair sitting is shown in Chapter 6. Instruct the patient to keep thighs horizontal to the chair seat.

▪ A patient who uses a wheelchair should never sit directly on a pressure ulcer.

▪ The feet should rest comfortably on the foot rest and the arms horizontally on the arm rests.

▪ The wheelchair-bound patient needs a pressure-reducing chair cushion. Such cushions are available in foam, gel, or air. The health care provider will help the patient and caregiver select appropriate products. Don't use doughnut-type cushions because they cause rather than relieve pressure as well as reduce blood flow to the tissue surrounding the ulcer.

■ Using a chair cushion doesn't eliminate the need for frequent moving and repositioning or shifting of body weight.

■ A person who is confined to a chair should change position at least every hour and make small shifts in body weight at 15-minute intervals. A person with sufficient upper body strength should also do wheelchair pushups.

Teaching pressure-reduction activities

These activities provide regular relief of pressure over bony prominences. Develop an individualized schedule for pressure relief activities that is compatible with the patient's daily routine. Be sure to consider the following:

■ *Frequency of activity.* Determine the patient's tissue tolerance and capacity to tolerate position changes and shifts in body weight. Initially, inspect skin every 15 minutes for redness at the pressure points. Extend evaluation time by 15-minute intervals until the maximum time is established.

■ *Length of pressure relief.* Relieve the pressure for at least 10 seconds every 15 minutes while the patient is sitting.

■ *Assistance.* When the patient is unable or unwilling to carry out the recommended measures for pressure ulcer prevention, a caregiver must perform the activities. Use of assistive devices may increase the patient's independence. The physical therapist and occupational therapist will make suggestions about appropriate devices. Whenever possible, the patient should direct the care that others provide.

■ *Effectiveness.* Absence of tissue breakdown and skin redness is the goal of pressure relief. The first sign of tissue injury — redness — requires a revision in the plan to provide complete pressure relief until the tissue is healed. Shorten the time between pressure-relief activities. Determine whether the patient is following the plan as established. Does the patient have any problems in carrying out the activity? Are the risks and benefits of the activity clear to the patient? Can the procedure be simplified in any way to improve compliance? Are there any incentives that can be used for this patient to encourage desired behavior? (See *Teaching pressure relief in the wheelchair,* page 212.)

Nutrition

Malnutrition may reflect an underlying disease process or social or economic problems. Some people simply don't know what constitutes a balanced diet. Patients need to be taught that skin breaks down more easily and wounds won't heal with inadequate nutrition. Nutritional deficiencies predispose patients to wound infections, wound dehiscence, sepsis, and other complications. Good nutrition is essential for healing wounds, preventing infections, and maintaining a general sense of well-being. Designing a patient's personal nutrition plan is as important as any other part of goal setting.

Teaching pressure relief in the wheelchair

Establish the goal for sitting tolerance with the patient. For most patients, resumption of life activities requires tolerance of several hours.

- Inform the patient of frequency for pressure relief. Teach pushups or leans if the patient has the upper body strength and coordination to perform these activities.
- Gradually increase sitting time by 30 minutes.
- Maintain increased time for 2 days before increasing sitting time again.
- Examine skin over ischia, posterior trochanters, and sacral-coccygeal bony prominences for hyperemia whenever the patient returns to bed.
- Remind the patient to perform pressure-relief activities every 30 minutes.

Periodic nutritional assessment helps clinicians recognize early signs of malnutrition, correct problems, and minimize the loss of patient strength. Patients and caregivers must report weight loss, poor appetite, or gastrointestinal disturbances that interfere with eating.

Any decrease in oral fluid intake increases the elderly person's risk for dehydration. Without water, nutrients can't reach the wound. Fluid also helps cushion the cells and organs. The National Research Council recommends 1 ml of water per calorie intake or 30 ml per kilogram of body weight per day. For example, a 110-pound person should drink approximately six to eight cups of fluid every day. (See *Tips for increasing fluid intake.*)

Diet education for patients and their families should include information about types of foods that contain nutrients necessary for wound healing. Protein, vitamins, and minerals are needed for new tissue growth, and calories are needed for energy. High-protein, high-calorie supplements may be necessary. Families should bring in any favorite foods that might stimulate the patient's appetite, and they should learn to read labels on food products. Grocery stores may carry less expensive supplements with the same nutritional value as brand-name products.

Patients who can't or won't consume adequate oral intake may require enteral feedings. The National Center for Nutrition and Dietetics of the American Dietetic Association and its Foundation recommends using the Food Guide Pyramid as a guide to nutritional well-being. (See *Using the Food Guide Pyramid,* page 214.)

Comprehensive self-care education includes teaching patients and their caregivers to perform their own nutritional assessments. (See *Self-assessment of nutritional health,* page 215, and *Warning signs of nutritional deficiencies,* page 216.) Patients and caregivers need to report any problems to their clinician, who may consult with a dietitian for assistance with menu selection, food substitution, and dietary instruction.

Tips for increasing fluid intake

- Offer large amounts of fluids with medications.
- Add flavoring, such as lemon or lime juice, to water.
- Mix ginger ale or other carbonated soft drinks with fruit juice.
- Offer popsicles, soup, and jello between meals.
- Provide ice cream or frozen yogurt cones.
- Serve hot or cold cereal with extra milk.
- Remind all visitors to offer fluids at periodic intervals.

Adapted with permission from Kobriger, A. "The healing power of water," *Contemporary Long Term Care* (18)6:68-69, 1995.

Treatment

A treatment plan is developed by a team that includes the patient, the patient's caregiver(s), physicians, nurses, dieticians, physical and occupational therapists, social workers, and pharmacists. Case managers working for insurance companies may also participate as part of the team. According to the AHRQ Consumer Guide for Pressure Ulcer Treatment, the patient and caregiver need to do the following:

- know their roles in the treatment program
- learn how to perform care
- know what to report to the clinician
- know how to tell if the treatment is working
- help change the treatment plan when needed
- know what questions to ask
- get understandable answers.

Patients can participate in their care more effectively if they understand the reason for the plan. They should be aware that clinicians will ask about general health, other illnesses, medications, and available support of family and friends. The team bases the plan on information obtained from the history and physical examination and the goals of the patient. It will include pressure reduction, pressure ulcer care, and promotion of healing.

Pressure ulcer care

Care of pressure ulcers includes cleansing, debridement, and dressing application. Only experienced clinicians should perform debridement. Patients or caregivers expected to perform dressing changes should be taught proper handwashing technique, how to perform the dressing changes, how to store and care for the dressings, and how to dispose of the soiled dressings.

(Text continues on page 217.)

Using the Food Guide Pyramid

Fats, oils, sweets
Use sparingly

Milk, yogurt, cheese
2–3 servings daily

Meat, poultry, fish, dry beans, eggs, nuts
2–3 servings daily

Vegetables
3–5 servings daily

Fruits
2–4 servings daily

Bread, cereal, rice, pasta
6–11 servings daily

What counts as a serving?

Bread, cereal, rice, pasta
- 1 slice of bread, $\frac{1}{2}$ bagel or hamburger bun
- 1 ounce of ready-to-eat cereal
- $\frac{1}{2}$ cp of cooked cereal, rice, or pasta

Vegetables
- 1 cup of raw, leafy vegetables
- $\frac{1}{2}$ cup of other vegetables, chopped raw or cooked
- $\frac{3}{4}$ cup of vegetable juice

Fruits
- 1 medium apple, banana, or orange
- $\frac{1}{2}$ cup of chopped canned or cooked fruit
- $\frac{3}{4}$ cup of fruit juice

Milk, yogurt, cheese
- 1 cup of milk or yogurt
- $1\frac{1}{2}$ ounces of natural cheese
- 2 ounces of processed cheese

Meat, poultry, fish, dry beans, eggs, nuts
- 2 to 3 ounces of cooked lean meat, poultry, or fish
- $\frac{1}{2}$ cup of cooked dry beans, 1 egg, or 2 tablespoons of peanut butter (counts as 1 ounce of lean meat)

Pyramid source: U.S. Department of Agriculture, U.S. Department of Health and Human Services. Serving information source: *Nutrition and your health*, 3rd ed. U.S. Department of Agriculture, U.S. Department of Health and Human Services, 1990.

Self-assessment of nutritional health

The warning signs of poor nutritional health are often overlooked. Use this checklist to find out if you or someone you know is at nutritional risk. Read the statements below. Circle the number in the yes column for those that apply to you or someone you know. For each yes answer, circle the number in the box. Total your nutritional score.

	YES
I have an illness or condition that made me change the kind or amount of food I eat.	2
I eat fewer than 2 meals per day.	3
I eat few fruits or vegetables, or milk products.	2
I have 3 or more drinks of beer, liquor, or wine almost every day.	2
I have tooth or mouth problems that make it hard for me to eat.	2
I don't always have enough money to buy the food I need.	4
I eat alone most of the time.	1
I take 3 or more different prescribed or over-the-counter drugs a day.	1
Without wanting to, I have lost or gained 10 pounds in the last 6 months.	2
I am not always physically able to shop, cook, or feed myself.	2
TOTAL	

If your nutritional score is:

0 to 2 ....Good! Recheck your nutritional score in 6 months.

3 to 5 ....You are at moderate nutritional risk. See what can be done to improve your eating habits and lifestyle. Your office on aging, senior nutrition program, senior citizens center, or health department can help. Recheck your nutritional score in 3 months.

6 or more ....You are at high nutritional risk. Bring this checklist the next time you see your doctor, dietitian or other qualified health or social service professional. Talk with them about any problems you may have. Ask for help to improve your nutritional health.

Remember that warning signs suggest risk but do not represent diagnosis of any condition.

Source. Nutrition Screening Initiative, a project of the American Academy of Family Physicians, the American Dietetic Association, and the National Council On the Aging, Inc., funded in part by Ross Products, a division of Abbott Laboratories.

Warning signs of nutritional deficiencies

The self-assessment of nutritional health is based on the warning signs described below. If you have one or more of these warning signs, you may be at risk for nutritional deficiency.

Disease

Any disease, illness, or chronic condition that causes you to change the way you eat or makes it difficult for you to eat puts your nutritional health at risk. Four out of five adults have chronic diseases that are affected by diet. Confusion or memory loss that keeps getting worse is estimated to affect one out of five older adults. This can make it difficult to remember what, when, or if you've eaten. Feeling sad or depressed, which happens to about one in eight older adults, can cause big changes in appetite, digestion, energy level, weight, and well-being.

Eating poorly

Eating too little or too much can lead to poor health. Eating the same foods day after day or not eating fruit, vegetables, or milk products daily will also cause poor nutritional health. One in five adults skips meals daily. Only 13% of adults eat the minimum amount of fruit and vegetables needed. One in four older adults drinks too much alcohol. Many health problems become worse if you drink more than one or two alcoholic beverages per day.

Tooth loss or mouth pain

A healthy mouth, teeth, and gums are needed to eat. Missing, loose, or rotten teeth or dentures that don't fit well or cause mouth sores make it eating difficult.

Economic hardship

As many as 40% of older Americans have an income under $6,000 per year. Having less — or choosing to spend less — than $25 to $30 per week for food makes it very difficult to get the foods you need to stay healthy.

Reduced social contact

One-third of all older people live alone. Being with people daily has a positive effect on morale, well-being, and eating.

Multiple medicines

Many older Americans must take medicines for health problems, and almost half take multiple medicines daily. Growing old may change the way the body responds to drugs. The more medicines you take, the greater the chance for side effects such as increased or decreased appetite, change in taste, constipation, weakness, drowsiness, diarrhea, and nausea. Vitamins or minerals, when taken in large doses, act like drugs and can be harmful. Alert your doctor to everything you take.

Involuntary weight loss or gain

Losing or gaining a lot of weight when you're not trying to do so is an important warning sign that you mustn't ignore. Being overweight or underweight increases your chances for poor health.

Needs assistance for self-care

Although most older people are able to eat, one of every five has trouble walking, shopping, or buying and cooking food. The difficulty increases with age.

Elder years above age 80

Most older people lead full and productive lives, but as age increases, the risk of frailty and health problems increases. Checking your nutritional health regularly makes good sense.

Source: Nutrition Screening Initiative, a project of the American Academy of Family Physicians, the American Dietetic Association, and the National Council on Aging, Inc., funded in part by Ross Products, a division of Abbot Laboratories.

Recipe for normal saline

Here's how to make normal saline solution to use in cleansing pressure ulcers.

- Boil mixing utensils and a storage container to ensure that they're clean.
- For the saline, use 1 gallon of distilled water or boil 1 gallon of tap water for 5 minutes. *Don't use well water or seawater.*
- Add 8 teaspoons of table salt to the distilled or boiled water.
- Mix the solution well until the salt is completely dissolved.
- Cool to room temperature before using.

You can store this solution at room temperature in a tightly covered glass or plastic container for up to 1 week.

Cleansing

Cleansing provides an optimum environment for wound healing by removing exudate, loose necrotic tissue, dressing residue, residual topical agents, and metabolic wastes. Although many commercial wound-cleansing agents are available, the safest agent to use is normal saline. Normal saline can be purchased or made in the home. (See *Recipe for normal saline.*)

Professionals who teach patients about cleansing should assess the resources available in the home. If the water supply is unsafe for drinking, it may be unsafe for use in the wound. Bottled distilled water can be purchased to create the saline solution.

Pressure ulcers should be cleansed at each dressing change. The AHRQ Treatment Guidelines recommend the use of irrigation pressures from 4 to 15 psi for safe and effective cleansing. A soft plastic 250-ml bottle of normal saline fitted with an irrigation cap provides approximately 4 to 5 psi when squeezed with full force (see Chapter 7 for use of this irrigation device). Patients and caregivers can use, clean, and refill these containers at home. (See *Teaching about pressure ulcer characteristics,* page 218, and *Teaching about prevention and care,* page 219.)

When to call the clinician

Caregivers should notify a health care professional if any of the following problems occurs:

- bleeding that doesn't stop with pressure
- foul, odorous drainage
- increased redness or warmth of the skin surrounding the ulcer
- a fever over 101°F, especially if accompanied by chills
- generalized decrease in activity or alertness.

Health care providers should discuss the rationale for treatment decisions with patients so that they will be able to make informed decisions about new treatment options.

Teaching about pressure ulcer characteristics

Teach patients and caregivers to report characteristics of pressure ulcers systematically. Using common terminology will facilitate communication between the patient and practitioner and ensure that ulcer changes are correctly identified.

Size

Measure the ulcer by using these steps:
- Use a ruler or measuring tape to measure across the ulcer at the two widest points. (Take two measurements.)
- If no ruler is available, place a piece of paper or string across the ulcer and mark the two widest measurements by using a pencil or marker. Then measure the marks on the paper or string.

Depth

Measure the ulcer's depth by gently inserting a gloved finger into the wound and rotating the finger to touch all sides of the wound bed. Note on the gloved finger how far it extends into the wound. Remove the finger from the wound, and measure the depth it was inserted.

Color of the wound bed

- A *red* color, often referred to as having a "beefy red" appearance, usually means there is a good blood supply. When new tissue is growing to fill in the wound, new blood vessels form to feed this new granulation tissue.
- A *yellow*, *cream*, or *light green* color of stringy tissue in the ulcer is usually fibrous tissue that needs to be removed. If allowed to dry, it will become a dark black, hard crust.
- *Black* hard tissue is dead and may require removal by the health care provider before healing can occur.

Location

If pressure ulcers exist in more than one area, assess the same characteristics for each ulcer.

Drainage

Report the thickness, color, and odor of any drainage.

Swelling

Feel the surrounding tissue with the back of the hand to check for an increase in firmness or temperature, and examine the area visually for redness and swelling.

Evaluating learning

Learning should be reflected by the achievement of goals and objectives. Changes in behavior will indicate that the patient or caregiver has acquired knowledge about prevention and the necessary skills to use that knowledge.

Teaching about prevention and care

Include the following points when educating patients and caregivers about pressure ulcer prevention and care.

What are pressure ulcers?

Pressure ulcers, also called bed sores, pressure sores, and decubitus ulcers, are red areas or sores on the skin. The sores can occur over any bony part of the body such as heels, hips, or back. There may be drainage or odor from these sores if they're deep.

What causes them?

Pressure ulcers are caused by lying in one position too long. The skin and body need a blood supply to get oxygen and food. Prolonged pressure on a bony portion of the body blocks the blood supply, causing a red area to appear. If the pressure isn't relieved by changing the body position, an ulcer or sore may form. Pressure ulcers can form in less than 2 hours.

Who gets them?

People who are immobilized due to sickness or injury are at risk for pressure ulcers.

What can be done to prevent pressure ulcers?

Pressure ulcers are prevented by moving, turning, or lifting the patient in the bed or wheelchair.
DO move or turn every 2 hours.
DO make small turns between the 2-hour positional changes.
DO use padding on the bed or chair.
DO use a trapeze to lift, if possible.
DO look at the skin three times a day for any red areas or other skin changes. Use a mirror to look at the back of the legs. Ask for help if needed.
DO keep skin clean and dry.
DO keep bed sheets smooth.
DO use an extra sheet to help turn, lift, or change position to help prevent sheet burns.
DO eat the right kinds of food and drink plenty of fluids. Ask the health care provider about special foods and vitamins.
DO ask the provider about the use of lotions or medicines.
DO tell the provider about changes, including increased drainage from existing sores.
DON'T sit on a rubber or plastic air ring.
DON'T rub any sore areas.
DON'T use heat on any pressure ulcer.
DON'T sit in a chair longer than 2 hours without shifting weight.

The patient's response to a request to evaluate the teaching method will also provide useful information.

Patients and caregivers should be able to verbalize the information and perform the procedures. Evaluation is ongoing. If conditions change, the plan may have to be altered. For example, a type of dressing that was effective may no longer be available or affordable or a patient may develop a medical problem that necessitates changing the plan.

Summary

Recognizing the need for health care education is the mutual responsibility of the learner and the educator. Through experience, educators identify essential information and necessary skills for care of patients with pressure ulcers. Using a variety of educational techniques and methods increases the effectiveness of the learning experience. The patient and caregiver together must set realistic goals.

The learner is responsible for incorporating newly acquired knowledge and skills into useful behavior. The AHRQ Pressure Ulcer Prevention and Treatment guides provide a basis for patients and professionals to build individualized educational programs.

In addition to learning about pressure relief, patients and families need to know how to reduce the risk factors. Adequate nutrition, management of incontinence, good body hygiene, skin care maintenance, and relief of pressure are topics that need to be reviewed on every nursing visit.

The purpose of education is to facilitate the patient's understanding of the pressure ulcer problem, encourage participation in decision making, maximize skills, and promote a healthful lifestyle. Educating patients about risk factors, pressure ulcer prevention, and pressure ulcer management gives them the power to manage their own care and to oversee the care others provide for them.

Selected references

AHCPR Patient Care Guidelines. Treating Pressure Sores. Publication No. 92-0047. Rockville, Md.: Agency for Health Care Policy and Research. Public Health Service, U.S. Department of Health and Human Services, 1994.

Ayello, E.A., et al. "Educational assessment and teaching of older clients with pressure ulcers," *Clinics in Geriatric Medicine* 13:484-496, 1997.

Beitz, J.M., et al. "Perceived need for education vs. actual knowledge of pressure ulcer care in a hospital nursing staff," *Med Surg Nurse* 7:283-301, 1998

Brylinsky, C.M. "Nutrition and wound healing: An overview," *Ostomy/Wound Management* 41(10):14-16, 1995.

Maklebust, J. "Preventing pressure ulcers in home care patients," *Home Healthcare Nurse* 17(4):229-238, 1999.

Maklebust, J." Treating pressure ulcers in the home," *Home Healthcare Nurse* 17(5):307-316, 1999.

Parsons, Y. "Healing more than wounds," *Contemporary Long Term Care* 18(6):57-76, 1995.

Warner, D., and Konnerth, K. "A patient teaching protocol for pressure ulcer prevention and management," *Ostomy/Wound Management* 39(2):34-44, 1993.

Chapter 12

Performance improvement

To reduce the large human and financial costs of pressure ulcers, medical researchers and health care providers have moved vigorously to identify many areas where prevention and treatment can be improved. During the 1990s many facilities changed their quality improvement (QI) efforts from traditional, reactive quality assurance (QA) programs to proactive continuous quality improvement (CQI) programs. CQI goes beyond QA to include surveillance of not only the 10% of care that falls below accepted norms but also of the acceptable 90%. The result is improved quality of care.

The basis of CQI is that the quality of care reflects the quality of the process; when the process is improved, outcomes improve. When selecting opportunities for CQI, clinicians should give priority to high-volume, high-risk, problem-prone areas. Pressure ulcers are one such area. The *Clinical Practice Guideline for Treatment of Pressure Ulcers* issued by the Agency for Healthcare Research and Quality (AHRQ) directs clinicians to gain administrative support for including pressure ulcer management as a major aspect of care. AHRQ has also issued a *Clinical Practice Guideline for Prediction and Prevention of Pressure Ulcers in Adults*. More about AHRQ's efforts will be found in Chapter 13, "Meeting future needs." Today, the focus has changed to patient outcome and improving the process to attain predefined outcomes. The process is now called performance improvement (PI). This chapter outlines methods of identifying quality improvement needs and monitoring progress, utilizing Harper Hospital's CQI experience.

The pressure ulcer PI committee

Pressure ulcer management is most efficient when a pressure ulcer or skin care PI committee of interested and knowledgeable people has been organized to develop policies and procedures. Depending on the nature of the health care provided, the committee may include nurses, doctors, dieticians, physical therapists, social workers, discharge planners, PI specialists, and infection control practitioners. Staff nurses should be included to promote communication with bedside caregivers. The committee chair must have strong administrative support.

The pressure ulcer PI committee develops, implements, and evaluates education and quality improvement programs. Most pressure ulcer PI programs have the following components:

▪ *measurement* to determine the size and severity of the problem, including local prevalence and incidence
▪ *risk assessment* to identify the at-risk population
▪ *policies and procedures* to specify standards of care and treatment protocols
▪ *monitoring* to evaluate the clinical and operational processes and outcomes associated with pressure ulcer management.

A word about this last point. Operational processes produce a service or a product for an internal or external customer. For example, a PI project might focus on improving operational processes to obtain goods from pharmacy or central supply. Clinical processes focus on medical or therapeutic processes that improve a person's health, such as pressure ulcer management. Specific aspects of clinical processes might be related to staff competence in patient care or value analysis of dressing products or support surfaces. All processes are directed toward producing specific clinical outcomes for the patient.

Any effort to improve clinical or operational processes will fail without support from clinical departments as well as nonclinical departments such as data management, utilization management, purchasing, pharmacy, and central supply.

Improving the cost and quality equation

Pressure ulcers affect the cost of care, reimbursement, and the patient's quality of life. Assessing local prevalence rates and patient risk profiles, standardizing therapy protocols, and increasing staff awareness will have a positive effect on the balance between cost and quality patient outcomes if the team or committee has the authority to affect clinical and financial decisions. Practice standards can be modified through overall clinical evaluation.

Pressure ulcer prevalence has been measured in acute, long-term, and home care settings. In 1995, the Health Care Financing Administration (HCFA) mandated use of the Outcome and Assessment Information Set (OASIS) in all certified home health agencies. These data are already providing a basis for performance improvement and relating costs to clinical outcomes. (See Appendix T.)

Pressure ulcer audit instruction sheet

These steps should be followed for each patient on your unit. The data collection tool must be completed by the staff nurse caring for the patient.

1. Stamp pressure ulcer data collection tool with addressograph plate.
2. Carefully read instructions on data collection form.
3. Assess each patient's entire body for pressure ulcers.
   (Don't include venous stasis ulcers, tape burns, skin lesions not caused by pressure, or skin irritation from incontinence)
4. If a pressure ulcer *is* present:
   a. Assess each ulcer for stage. (Nonblanchable erythema is considered Stage I and should be recorded.)
   b. Measure each ulcer's length and width in centimeters (using Measuring Grid).
   c. Indicate where each ulcer was acquired (e.g., home, hospital).
   d. Complete Side 2 of audit form in its entirety.
   e. Date and sign the audit sheet.
5. If *no* pressure ulcer is present, check the "No Pressure Ulcer" box.
   a. Complete Side 2 of the data collection form in its entirety.
   b. Date and sign the data collection.
6. Place the form in the designated area on your unit for APN, CNS, or ET nurse to validate.

NOTE: **DO assess ALL patients on your unit on the day shift.**
DON'T include afternoon admissions.
DO include patients being discharged.
DO include patients going to the OR (assess them before they leave the unit).

At Harper Hospital in the Detroit Medical Center, the Pressure Ulcer PI Committee measures pressure ulcer prevalence twice each year. All nursing units receive pressure ulcer measuring grids, audit instruction sheets, and data collection forms. (See *Pressure ulcer audit instruction sheet,* above, and *Pressure ulcer data collection form,* pages 224 to 226.) Every clinician inspects the skin of each assigned patient on that day, and another clinician validates every pressure ulcer found. The clinician records:
■ depth, length, and width of each ulcer
■ relevant risk factors
■ use of nutritional consultations
■ patient use of pressure ulcer prevention products.

(Text continues on page 226.)

Pressure ulcer data collection form

1. <u>Do you think the patient is at risk for pressure ulcers?</u>   YES ❑   NO ❑
2. Instructions:
   A. Read Pressure Ulcer Audit Instructions posted on unit.
   B. Inspect entire body from head to toe.
   C. Assess skin condition at each body site on numbered figure.
   D. Use stage key to determine stage of pressure ulcer and record after appropriate number at right.
   E. Measure and record the size of each pressure ulcer in cm.
   F. Indicate where each ulcer was acquired.
   G. Complete <u>both sides</u> of audit sheet.

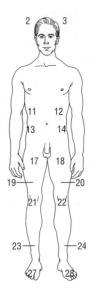 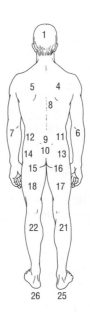

Stage Key

Stage 0	No redness or breakdown
Stage 1	Nonblanchable erythema of intact skin
Stage 2	Break in skin such as blisters or abrasions
Stage 3	Break in skin exposing subcutaneous tissue
Stage 4	Break in skin tissue extending through tissue and subcutaneous layers, exposing muscle or bone
Stage 9	Nonstageable (wound bed can't be observed)

Pressure ulcer data collection form *(continued)*

	Size Stage	Harper (in cm)	Indicate Where Each Ulcer Was Acquired				
			Another Hospital	Nursing Hospital	Home	Home	Unknown
1) Back of head							
2) Right ear	_____	_____	_____	_____	_____	_____	_____
3) Left ear	_____	_____	_____	_____	_____	_____	_____
4) Right scapula	_____	_____	_____	_____	_____	_____	_____
5) Left scapula	_____	_____	_____	_____	_____	_____	_____
6) Right elbow	_____	_____	_____	_____	_____	_____	_____
7) Left elbow	_____	_____	_____	_____	_____	_____	_____
8) Vertebrae (upper-mid)	_____	_____	_____	_____	_____	_____	_____
9) Sacrum	_____	_____	_____	_____	_____	_____	_____
10) Coccyx	_____	_____	_____	_____	_____	_____	_____
11) Right iliac crest	_____	_____	_____	_____	_____	_____	_____
12) Left iliac crest	_____	_____	_____	_____	_____	_____	_____
13) Right trochanter (hip)	_____	_____	_____	_____	_____	_____	_____
14) Left trochanter (hip)	_____	_____	_____	_____	_____	_____	_____
15) Right ischial tuberosity	_____	_____	_____	_____	_____	_____	_____
16) Left ischial tuberosity	_____	_____	_____	_____	_____	_____	_____
17) Right thigh (front/back)	_____	_____	_____	_____	_____	_____	_____
18) Left thigh (front/back)	_____	_____	_____	_____	_____	_____	_____
19) Right knee	_____	_____	_____	_____	_____	_____	_____
20) Left knee	_____	_____	_____	_____	_____	_____	_____
21) Right lower leg (front/back)	_____	_____	_____	_____	_____	_____	_____
22) Left lower leg (front/back)	_____	_____	_____	_____	_____	_____	_____
23) Right ankle (inner/outer)	_____	_____	_____	_____	_____	_____	_____
24) Left ankle (inner/outer)	_____	_____	_____	_____	_____	_____	_____
25) Right heel	_____	_____	_____	_____	_____	_____	_____
26) Left heel	_____	_____	_____	_____	_____	_____	_____
27) Right toe(s)	_____	_____	_____	_____	_____	_____	_____
28) Left toe(s)	_____	_____	_____	_____	_____	_____	_____
29) Other (specify)	_____	_____	_____	_____	_____	_____	_____
30) NO PRESSURE ULCER	▢						

(continued)

Pressure ulcer data collection form *(continued)*

31. Is the patient using a pressure-relieving device? Yes ❑ No ❑
    If yes:
    A. Vascular boot ❑
    B. Sof-Care bed cushion ❑
       On manual check, is the Sof-Care adequately inflated? Yes ❑ No ❑
    C. Special bed (specify type): _____
    D. Other (specify): _____

32. Is there a **completed pink nutrition assessment form**
    in the medical record? Yes ❑ No ❑

33. The following list contains factors that increase the risk for developing pressure ulcers. Circle all that apply to
    your patient.
    1) Decreased mental status
    2) Impaired mobility
    3) Malnutrition
    4) Fecal incontinence
    5) Urinary incontinence
    6) Diabetes
    7) Vascular disease
    8) Spinal cord injury
    9) Multiple sclerosis
    10) Metastatic CA

Date: _____

Signature: _____

Title: _____

Validating Nurse: _____

Harper Hospital also assesses the medical records of patients with pressure ulcers to determine the accuracy of pressure ulcer documentation. (See *Pressure ulcer medical record data sheet.*) Initially, after pressure ulcer is reported, members of the pressure ulcer PI committee review the charts of patients with pressure ulcers. The goal is to ensure that documentation includes the following:

■ onset of the ulcer (preadmission or unit-specific origin)
■ description of the ulcer
■ treatment plan, including pressure relief and local wound care
■ evidence that care was delivered according to the plan of care.

Pressure ulcer medical record data sheet

Date: _____

Time: _____

Demographic data _____

	YES	NO	N/A	COMMENTS
IF ULCER WAS ACQUIRED OUTSIDE OF HOSPITAL:				
1. Is it documented on the admission data base? (include date)				
2. Is there a plan of care including pressure reduction? (indicate date written)				
3. Is there evidence that interventions were carried out? (shift assessment, progress notes, etc.)				
4. Was a pressure-reduction device applied? (indicate date)				
IF ULCER WAS ACQUIRED AT HOSPITAL:				
1. Was there a risk for impaired skin/tissue integrity plan of care prior to the ulcer formation, including preventive measures?				
2. Was a pressure-reduction device applied?				
3. Indicate date and nursing unit where pressure ulcer was first identified.				
4 Is there an impaired tissue integrity plan of care including pressure reduction and local wound care? (indicate date written)				
5. Is there evidence that the interventions were carried out? (shift assessment, progress notes, etc.)				

Signature of Validator: _____

Committee members analyze the data, which are distributed to managers in tabular format. (See *Pressure ulcer report form*, pages 228 and 229.)

When reporting data, it is important to include as much information as possible so that others will know exactly what the data mean. A useful re-

Pressure ulcer report form

Service / Census	Number of Patients with Ulcers	Total Number of Pressure Ulcers	Stages				
			1	2	3	4	9*
Oncology /							
Medicine /							
Surgery /							
Cardiology / Critical Care /							
TOTALS							

*nonstageable

TOTALS = Prevalence Rate (All pressure ulcer patients in hospital on day of data collection)
Percentage of Ulcers Acquired at Harper Hospital =

port should include the number of ulcers in each stage and the definition of each stage. For example, many reports do not indicate whether non-blanchable reddened areas are counted as Stage I ulcers.

Calculating prevalence

The difference between prevalence and incidence is essential in any useful study. Prevalence reflects the total number of patients with pressure ulcers on any given day, regardless of where the ulcers were acquired. Data are reported as percentage of patients with pressure ulcers among the patient population included in data collection. The formula for calculating a pressure ulcer prevalence rate is given below.

Harper Hospital Acquired Ulcers	Other Hospital Acquired Ulcers	Nursing Home Acquired Ulcers	Home Acquired Ulcers	Source of Ulcers Unknown

National acute care prevalence rate $=$ 5% to 11%
National acute care incidence rate $=$ 1% to 5%

$$\text{PU Prevalence Rate} = \frac{\text{Number of patients with pressure ulcers on data collection day}}{\text{Number of patients in facility included in data collection}} \times 100$$

Calculating incidence

Incidence reflects the number of patients who acquire pressure ulcers while in the care of a given facility. This can be determined only by assessing patients for pressure ulcers on admission and monitoring those without to see if they develop pressure ulcers during their admission. Data are reported as percentages of patients developing pressure ulcers among patients admitted during a specified period. Incidence can be calculated for an individual nursing unit or an entire facility.

$$\text{PU Incidence Rate} = \frac{\text{Total number of patients developing pressure ulcers per period}}{\text{Total number of patients admitted per period}} \times 100$$

A more accurate approach may be to identify at-risk patients and then calculate the percentage of those patients who develop pressure ulcers within a specified time period, as follows:

$$\text{PU Incidence Rate} = \frac{\text{Number of at-risk patients developing pressure ulcers per period}}{\text{Number of at-risk patients admitted per period}} \times 100$$

Showing prevalence or incidence in bar graphs or pie charts categorized by stage presents a clinically useful picture. (See *Pressure ulcer prevalence trends*.) Graphing prevalence or incidence trends also provides visual reinforcement. (See *Pressure ulcer prevalence by stage*, page 232.)

Each facility should identify intended improvements by comparing local findings to national as well as local baseline data. This means identifying established standards so that the committee can evaluate treatment and make necessary changes. Improvements may include changing policies and procedures, educating or redistributing staff, altering use of equipment and supplies, or correcting communication processes. If introducing a PI program reduces the incidence of pressure ulcers, a facility usually can further improve outcomes by continuing to improve operational and clinical processes.

Improving outcomes with risk assessment

Identifying the percentage of at-risk patients helps health care providers plan allocation of human and material resources to lower the risk and improve outcomes. Incorporating risk assessment scales into a daily clinical flow sheet is an important way to detect changes in patients' risk status. The pressure ulcer risk assessment scale must be simple enough that caregivers will complete it. (See *Braden Scale*, Appendix B.) In today's climate of restructured health care delivery and patient-focused care, the number of clinicians working at the bedside is dwindling. It is important for clinicians to delegate col-

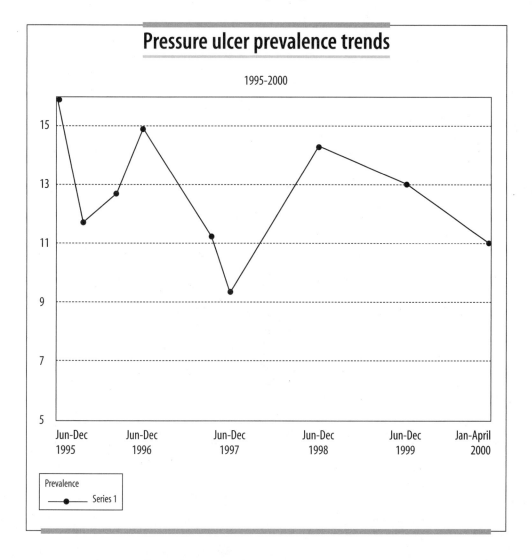

Pressure ulcer prevalence trends

1995-2000

lection of specific patient data and then have adequate time to interpret its significance.

Research shows that the risk of pressure ulcer development seems to be highest in older adults receiving care at home or in a long-term care facility if they:

■ are confined to a wheelchair

■ need assistance with activities of daily living (ADLs) such as dressing or bowel or bladder incontinence

■ have a Braden Scale mobility subscore of "very limited"

■ have an adult child as primary caregiver

■ are malnourished

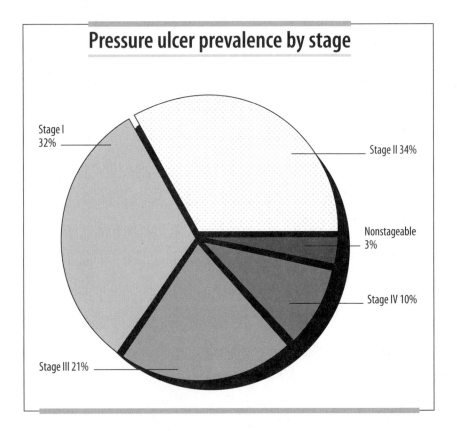

Pressure ulcer prevalence by stage

Stage I 32%

Stage II 34%

Nonstageable 3%

Stage IV 10%

Stage III 21%

- have a recent fracture
- use oxygen.

Similar factors emerged in long-term care settings where inability to perform ADLs was strongly associated with prevalence of pressure ulcers. It has been suggested that ADL items from the Minimum Data Set be included in the pressure ulcer Resident Assessment Protocol.

Harper Hospital examined the relationship between risk factors and pressure ulceration by retrospectively analyzing pressure ulcer data collected from five hospitalwide prevalence measurements. Pooled data showed a pressure ulcer prevalence rate of 12.3%. Immobility was the most frequently reported risk factor, but it was not associated with the greatest odds of acquiring a pressure ulcer; the widespread use of pressure-reducing surfaces for immobile patients may have compensated for the risk of impaired mobility. The most significant risk factor was fecal incontinence, which carried a 22-fold greater risk than that of fecal continence. Fecally incontinent patients also had more pressure ulcers per patient than continent patients.

Analysis of these data led to new measures to protect the patients' skin from caustic fecal enzymes. Skin and wound care flowcharts were developed, and the process was computerized so that nurses could independently or-

Standards of care for prevention and treatment of pressure ulcers

Standard for pressure ulcer prevention

- All patients with mobility or activity deficits will have a formal risk assessment tool administered to determine pressure ulcer risk.
- All patients at risk will have a systematic skin assessment at least once daily.
- Skin exposure to pressure, friction, shear, and moisture will be minimized.
- At-risk patients will be repositioned according to their tissue tolerance.
- At-risk patients will be placed on pressure-reducing surfaces.
- At-risk patients' nutritional status will be assessed for adequacy.
- At-risk patients and caregivers will be taught pressure ulcer prevention techniques.
- Pressure ulcer prevention interventions and patient/family instruction will be documented.

Standard for pressure ulcer treatment

- Patients with pressure ulcers will have prevention standards instituted.
- Pressure ulcers will be assessed for stage, size, condition, etiology, duration, and previous treatment.
- Condition of skin surrounding pressure ulcers will be assessed.
- Pressure ulcers with necrotic tissue will be assessed for need of debridement.
- Pressure ulcers will be cleansed with physiologic solutions.
- Pressure ulcers will be protected with appropriate dressings.
- Pressure ulcers will be reassessed with each dressing change for improvement or deterioration.
- Pressure ulcer treatment and patient outcomes will be documented.
- Patients and families will be educated about pressure ulcer treatment.

der appropriate products from pharmacy or central supply. A similar process can be used to reduce the impact of any pressure ulcer risk factor. Frequently, staff at the bedside are best at developing patient-related protocols and desired outcomes. Not only do they claim ownership of protocols that they design but, if they believe it makes a difference, they will work to make the process successful.

Standards of care

The pressure ulcer guidelines from the AHRQ represent the best scientific information available for pressure ulcer prevention and treatment. Before releasing the guidelines, the AHRQ tested them at Harper Hospital and other pilot sites. At Harper, the Pressure Ulcer PI Committee incorporated guideline recommendations into the Harper Hospital Pressure Ulcer Standards of Care. (See *Standards of care for prevention and treatment of pressure ulcers.*)

These standards are generic, allowing individualized patient care. Protocols, policies, procedures, and patient documentation records elaborate more specific clinical and operational processes of care. (See Chapter 9 for Harper Hospital protocols, policies, procedures, and documentation formats.)

Improving management processes

To adequately improve pressure ulcer management, clinical education must be ongoing. Documentation is critical to ensure reimbursement. In addition, pressure ulcer products must be analyzed, including support surfaces and dressings.

Clinician education

The AHRQ Pressure Ulcer Guidelines include content recommendations for educating caregivers. Extensive educational resources exist for disseminating information to staff, patients, and families. For example, the National Pressure Ulcer Advisory Panel (NPUAP) has developed slide sets to augment the AHRQ Pressure Ulcer Guidelines. The slides contain clinical photographs of patients being cared for in various settings. To facilitate in-service training, a companion script accompanies each slide set. (For information on how to obtain a set of slides, call NPUAP at 703-464-4849, or check their Website, www.npuap.org.)

The research findings embodied in the AHRQ guidelines will affect clinical practice in many ways. For example, the venerable nursing practice of massaging a patient's skin over bony prominences to increase circulation has actually been found to damage soft tissue. Another example is the proper way to position and reposition patients. For many years, nurses were taught to turn bedbound patients from one side to another every 2 hours. Now, research-based evidence shows that patients should not be placed on the greater trochanter of the femur but instead in a 30-degree laterally inclined position to avoid pressure over the bony prominence of the hip. This position needs to be demonstrated to bedside caregivers.

The AHRQ Pressure Ulcer Treatment Guideline specifies accurate wound assessment, appropriate wound irrigation pressure, and correct techniques for culturing wounds. It also differentiates colonization from infection and indicates toxicities of various topical treatments. Recommended infection control practices support use of clean, no-touch technique rather than sterile technique for pressure ulcer care. All of these recommendations need to be transferred to the caregiver level. It is a formidable task to educate all caregivers, but the guideline itself provides a good start by giving a rationale for each guideline recommendation.

Agencies can begin by inservicing nursing personnel taking direct care of patients; nurses can be messengers for the other disciplines as well. Research shows that teaching and hands-on practice are more effective than demonstration alone and that education of caregivers can reduce the incidence and severity of pressure ulcers in hospitalized patients.

It is helpful if bedside caregivers first are taught the relevant knowledge and then precepted clinically to determine competency in pressure ulcer prevention and management. Pressure ulcer treatment options should focus on a person's normal lifestyle. Clinical competency tools are available for preceptor documentation of pressure ulcer prevention and management. (See *Clinical competency tool*, pages 236 and 237.) Studies of changes in nurses' behavior after continuing education show that support from colleagues and superiors is the most important determinant of ongoing behavioral change in nursing practice.

Documentation

Regulatory issues and reimbursement mechanisms have an enormous impact on the quality of care, the introduction of new technology, use of products and services, patient access to care, and outcome of care delivered. One of the single most important factors in favorable coverage of services and supplies for Medicare and Medicaid patients is complete, accurate, and descriptive documentation. This emphasis on documentation also holds true in cases of litigation against agencies and caregivers of patients who acquire pressure ulcers. Each type of patient care setting has its own specific format for documentation. Examples of such documentation are included in Appendices L through R.

Value analysis of pressure ulcer products

Performance improvement goes beyond caregiver education and patient care to include measuring and analyzing the value of products used in pressure ulcer management programs, such as support surfaces (various pads or special beds), dressings, topical solutions, and medical exam gloves.

Support surfaces

Pressure-reducing equipment options range from inexpensive, 1-inch, convoluted foam products to expensive, sophisticated specialty beds. (See Chapter 6, "Prevention.") It helps to have a basic understanding of the principles of pressure relief when evaluating various support surfaces on the market; the cost of a pressure-relieving device does not necessarily reflect its usefulness. The magnitude of pressure at the support surface/tissue interface must be considered when choosing products for pressure relief.

Before using tissue interface pressures quoted in the literature or advertising materials to screen devices for pressure relief, the PI committee must be sure that the data are really comparable. Data collected by different investigators using different measuring devices are not usually comparable. The best way to report interface pressure data is to use both absolute values and percentages of the interface pressure generated on a control surface,

Clinical competency tool

Clinician Signature: _____

Title/Department: _____

Intervention	Initial & Date—(Clinician)		Initial & Date—(Preceptor)
	Verbalized Knowledge	**Demonstrate Skill**	
1. Identifies clients at risk for loss of skin integrity	_____	_____	_____
2. Completes risk assessment tool	_____	_____	_____
3. Completes a thorough skin assessment	_____	_____	_____
4. Develops and implements plan of care to maintain and improve skin integrity			
- cleansing and remoisturizing	_____	_____	_____
- positioning (bed and chair)	_____	_____	_____
- support surface	_____	_____	_____
- nutritional support	_____	_____	_____
- management of incontinence	_____	_____	_____
- encourage mobility	_____	_____	_____
- minimize shear and friction	_____	_____	_____
- pain control	_____	_____	_____
- appropriate transfer	_____	_____	_____
5. Initiates appropriate referrals to consults			
- nurse	_____	_____	_____
- dietician	_____	_____	_____
- pharmacy	_____	_____	_____
- physical therapy	_____	_____	_____
- enterostomal therapist	_____	_____	_____
- pharmacist	_____	_____	_____
- infection control	_____	_____	_____
6. Appropriately stages and identifies characteristics of a wound			
- stage	_____	_____	_____
- size	_____	_____	_____
- undermining/tunneling	_____	_____	_____
- eschar	_____	_____	_____
- slough	_____	_____	_____
- drainage	_____	_____	_____
- hyperplasia	_____	_____	_____
- granulation	_____	_____	_____
- epithelialization	_____	_____	_____
- erythema	_____	_____	_____
- location	_____	_____	_____
- surrounding tissue	_____	_____	_____
- depth	_____	_____	_____
7. Identifies characteristics of wound healing physiology	_____	_____	_____
8. Differentiates clean, contaminated, and infected wounds	_____	_____	_____
9. Demonstrates and discusses selective versus nonselective debridement			
- surgical	_____	_____	_____
- autolytic	_____	_____	_____
- chemical	_____	_____	_____
- mechanical	_____	_____	_____

(continued)

Clinical competency tool *(continued)*

Intervention	Initial & Date—(Clinician)		Initial & Date—(Preceptor)
	Verbalized Knowledge	**Demonstrate Skill**	
10. Identifies the goal of moist wound therapy in wounds that are:			
- granular, draining	_____	_____	_____
- granular, nondraining	_____	_____	_____
- necrotic, draining	_____	_____	_____
- necrotic, nondraining	_____	_____	_____
11. Selects and appropriately implements use of moist wound therapy dressings and cleansers			
- surfactant	_____	_____	_____
- saline	_____	_____	_____
- transparent film	_____	_____	_____
- hydrocolloid	_____	_____	_____
- foam	_____	_____	_____
- skin protectant	_____	_____	_____
- hydrogel/gels	_____	_____	_____
- absorptive fillers	_____	_____	_____
- alginates	_____	_____	_____
12. Demonstrates the use of devices to control incontinence	_____	_____	_____
- intermittent catheterization	_____	_____	_____
- indwelling catheterization	_____	_____	_____
- external catheter	_____	_____	_____
- external pouches	_____	_____	_____
13. Selects adjunctive topical treatments (antimicrobial, antibacterial)	_____	_____	_____
14. Appropriately obtains and interprets wound cultures	_____	_____	_____
15. Demonstrates ability to assess the effectiveness of current wound therapy and initiates changed therapies as needed	_____	_____	_____
16. Implements interventions that prevent recurrence of breakdown	_____	_____	_____
17. Documents the prevention and management of pressure ulcers	_____	_____	_____
18. Reports findings to the appropriate resource	_____	_____	_____
- physician	_____	_____	_____
- supervisor	_____	_____	_____
- infection control	_____	_____	_____
- quality improvement	_____	_____	_____
- utilization review	_____	_____	_____
- social service	_____	_____	_____
- case management	_____	_____	_____
- PT/OT/ST	_____	_____	_____
- enterostomal therapist	_____	_____	_____
19. Participates in the development of protocols	_____	_____	_____

Preceptor's Signature: _____ Date of Completion: _____

Used with permission. ©Mary Cardy Weaver. "A tool to document the competence of clinicians to prevent and manage pressure ulcers," *Decubitus* 5(6): 47-48, Nov. 1992.

Measuring the value of dressings

Characteristics	Rating (Circle Score)					Subtotal
	Acceptable ⟶ Unacceptable					
Wear time/meltdown	5	4	3	2	1	
Skin protection	5	4	3	2	1	
Ease of application	5	4	3	2	1	
Ease of cutting	5	4	3	2	1	
Ease of molding	5	4	3	2	1	
Ease of removal	5	4	3	2	1	
Patient comfort	5	4	3	2	1	

such as a standard hospital mattress or unpadded chair. The absolute value of an interface pressure measurement can be compared with average capillary closing pressure (32 mm Hg) to decide about the adequacy of pressure relief. The interface pressure measurement data expressed as a percentage of interface pressure obtained on a standard mattress reflect the relative amount of pressure relief obtained. Biomedical engineers recommend that a standard format be developed for reporting research data on tissue interface pressure measurements.

Dressings

Dressings and topical solutions must be chosen as carefully as support surfaces. Today's clinicians need a thorough knowledge of current research on wound healing and the effects of dressings and topical solutions on human tissue. Measurement criteria for value analysis of dressings include several parameters related to ease of use. (See *Measuring the value of dressings.*) When evaluating marketing information for wound dressings, clinicians should ask company representatives for bona fide controlled clinical trials on dressings used for pressure ulcers. A research template gives the information needed to make inferences from published studies. (See *Template for pressure ulcer dressing study data.*)

Medical exam gloves

The skin offers the body protection against infection. Medical exam gloves provide an additional layer of protection for both patients and caregivers, but they cannot offer total protection against infection. Good handwashing techniques and practices, along with the use of gloves, offer the best protection.

Template for pressure ulcer dressing study data

Category	Descriptions and Examples
Authors' Names, Places of Employment, Date	
Study Time Frame	
Research Design	Examples: Case series, randomized controlled trial
Setting	Examples: Hospital, long-term care, home
Inclusion/Exclusion Criteria	
Method of Pressure Ulcer Risk Assessment	
Study Protocol	Example: Pressure Ulcer Risk Assessment Scale
	Examples: randomization process; use of ulcers or patients as unit of analysis; how multiple ulcers on one patient were handled in study design; cleansing protocol, cleansing materials (for example, saline, hydrogen peroxide); dressing protocol for experimental group, dressing protocol for control group, person changing dressing, frequency of dressing change, criteria for dressing change; use of adjunctive therapies, such as pressure reduction, turning regimens, or nutritional interventions.
Outcome Variables and Measurement	Primary outcome variables (usually a measure of healing
	Examples: Time to healing; percentage healed within a specified period of time; change in ulcer surface area, depth, or volume; methods of healing measurement (for example, tracings of ulcer perimeter and measurement length and width); frequency of measurement.
	Secondary outcome variables
	Examples: Patient or caregiver subjective assessments; level of ulcer pain; occurrence of ulcer complications; time needed to change dressings; monetary costs associated with dressings (cost may be primary outcome variable in some studies); cost measurement methods and frequency of measurement.
Study Endpoints	
Identified End of Treatment for Individual Subjects Specified Apriori	Examples: All ulcers treated for 14 days or complete ulcer healing with prespecified maximum length of treatment time for ulcers not healed.
Statistical Methods	Examples: Type of statistical tests; use of power analysis to detect whether sample size can show significant differences between or among treatments being studied.

(continued)

Template for pressure ulcer dressing study data *(continued)*

Category	Descriptions and Examples
Results	Subjects' demographics, including age, gender, pressure ulcer risk levels and score
	Medical diagnoses of subjects
	Baseline ulcer characteristics: etiology, size, stage, location, appearance (for example, exudate, odor, necrosis, periulcer skin condition), ulcer duration, prior treatment.
	Outcome results: unit of analysis (subjects or pressure ulcers); number of subjects enrolled; number of subjects who reached study endpoint; number of subject dropouts; reason for dropped status (for example, withdrew, died, discharged from care prior to study endpoint, had ulcer complications); number of subjects in data analysis; results of major outcome variables (for example, time to healing, percentage healed) analyzed by appropriate statistical tests; operational definition of "improved" if used to describe major outcome variables; results of secondary outcome variables; presence or absence of complications; analysis of costs if appropriate.
Summary/Conclusion	Discussion of author's opinion and possible rationales for study findings; comparison of study results with findings from other published research on the topic; identified study weaknesses; implications for clinical practice or healthcare policy; suggestions for further research in the area.

Used with permission from Xakellis, G., and Maklebust, J. "Template for pressure ulcer research," *Advances in Wound Care* 8(1): 46-48, January/February 1995.

Medical exam gloves may be made of latex, vinyl, or other substances. They are either sterile or nonsterile, powdered or powder-free. Latex and vinyl gloves can be used for protection against blood and body fluids. Tests have shown that they can be an effective barrier against HIV and hepatitis. Latex gloves can be used for protection only if the person is not allergic to latex. Vinyl gloves cannot be used when handling chemotherapeutic agents, and they do not stretch and fit as well as latex gloves. In simulations designed to approximate clinical use, latex gloves were more watertight and less permeable to bacteria than vinyl gloves. The relative risk of bacterial transmission was not studied.

Many gloves are prelubricated with cornstarch to make it easier to put them on. When cornstarch powder is used on latex gloves, the cornstarch absorbs allergens from the latex, which may cause an allergic reaction in latex-sensitive individuals. Sterile gloves must be used for sterile procedures, and nonsterile (or clean) gloves may be worn when sterile technique is not necessary.

Using benchmarks

Benchmarking is a search for industry best practices. A benchmark can be a source of best practice or a desired result or outcome. Many agencies do comparative benchmarking to identify improvement opportunities. However, benchmarking data from one department to another or from one organization to another is useful only if data are collected and reported in such a way that allows meaningful comparisons. Like the nursing process, the benchmarking process has sequential steps. In the nursing process, the phase that follows data analysis is diagnosis. In benchmarking, the phase that follows data analysis is discovery, which then leads to opportunities for CQI.

In 1995, the Sun Health Alliance of Hospitals, in the Southern United States, began benchmarking the prevention and treatment of pressure ulcers. Within their alliance, they searched for hospitals with the best overall pressure ulcer program or with the best components of a pressure ulcer program. Examples of program components were ease of use, content, staff education, patient education, policies and procedures, documentation, and so forth. Each of these components was rated by representatives of different disciplines at several other hospitals. They combined all the best-rated components into a new and better program for superior outcomes, which represents the industry's best practice.

Efficiency is the key to success in the best practice health care environment. The effort requires correlating clinical with financial data, documenting outcomes, and analyzing problems. In today's health care market, procedures and regulatory standards must be followed, and care must be provided with fewer resources in less time as it yields better outcomes.

Unit-based continuous performance improvement

Once a pressure ulcer program is established, the clinical staff needs a method to evaluate its effectiveness. Unit-based PI programs can identify potential or actual practice-related strengths and problems. Managers should include staff nurses and bedside caregivers in unit PI activities to evaluate policies, procedures, and patient outcomes.

Unit-based assessment of all patients can determine the prevalence and incidence of pressure ulcers. Tools for data collection may be found in the literature or developed by the nurses on the unit. Harper Hospital has developed a pressure ulcer PI report form. (See *Performance improvement report*, page 242.) Nursing units keep the PI forms in a unit log so they can trend information on any patients with pressure ulcers. If problems surface on more than one unit, they can be discussed and solved in the hospitalwide pressure ulcer committee.

Clinicians may tackle other unit-based projects. Before data collection, unit committee members identify problem-prone areas and then aim for im-

Performance improvement report

Initiate This Form for <u>ALL PRESSURE ULCERS</u>

Fill in the boxes below. Use the numbered figure and staging scale provided.

Ulcers on Admission

Location by No.	Stage
___	___
___	___
___	___
___	___
___	___
___	___

NONE _____

Ulcers Acquired at Harper

Location by No.	Stage	Date Discovered
___	___	___
___	___	___
___	___	___
___	___	___
___	___	___
___	___	___

Circle all the patient's current pressure ulcer risk factors.

Decreased activity:	Bedbound	Chairbound
Impaired mobility:	Repositions self	Requires turning
Poor nutritional status		
Incontinent of urine:	Foley catheter	Condom catheter
Incontinent of stool:	Fecal collector	
Decreased mental status		
Decreased sensation		

Chronic Disease, Specify _____

Other _____

Circle all devices in use at this time.

None	Vascular boot
Sof-Care mattress	Sheepskin pad
Convoluted foam mattress	Heel protectors
Acucair mattress	Chair cushion
Clinitron bed	Other _____

Has a "High-Risk for Impaired Skin Integrity" or "Impaired Tissue Integrity" problem been identified in the chart?

Yes ☐   No ☐

Name of person completing this form: _____

Nursing Unit:_____   Date: _____

PLEASE SUBMIT TO ADMINISTRATIVE MANAGER ON UNIT

Stage(s)

I) Nonblanchable erythema, intact skin

II) Skin loss through epidermis

III) Skin loss exposing subcutaneous fat

IV) Full thickness loss to muscle/bone.

E) Eschar — Not able to stage

Specify right or left when applicable

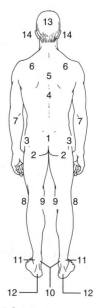

1. Sacrum
2. Ischial tuberosity
3. Trochanter
4. Lumbar vertebrae
5. Thoracic vertebrae
6. Scapula
7. Elbow (olecranon)
8. Lateral knee
9. Medial knee
10. Medial malleolus (inner ankle)
11. Lateral malleolus (outer ankle)
12. Heel
13. Occipital
14. Ear

proving operational and clinical processes to improve outcomes. Caregivers on the unit collect the desired data — this serves as both an educational process and a form of peer review. Unit committee members analyze and summarize the data. The final summary should include both staff feedback and an action plan to improve any problematic clinical or operational processes. This process also will determine the next project that the unit wishes to undertake. Staff nurses or physical therapists may suggest new procedure trials or new products to improve outcomes in problem-prone areas.

Some of the most beneficial outcomes of unit-based PI occur when members of the unit staff rotate turns on the PI committee. Participation in PI helps clinicians develop insight and perspective into standards of care. Involved clinicians accept the professional responsibility for monitoring and evaluating their own practices.

When the AHRQ pressure ulcer guidelines were first released, Harper staff on the pressure ulcer committee held a "pressure ulcer awareness day" to disseminate the information hospitalwide. Dieticians had posters and displays of nutrition information, physical therapists had positioning demonstrations and articles about hydrotherapy and debridement, and nurses presented prevention and treatment strategies. The results of Harper-based research on pressure ulcers were highlighted on poster boards. Every nursing unit was given a set of the AHRQ pressure ulcer guidelines and educational material from the National Pressure Ulcer Advisory Panel. A video monitor continuously played an educational tape on pressure ulcer care. To stimulate interest, attendees participated in a drawing for subscriptions to wound care journals. The all-day event was such a big success that many nurses asked it be held twice yearly.

As new scientific information is generated, guidelines must be revised and updated to reflect new research findings, emerging technologies, and innovative approaches. Pressure ulcer PI committees can help keep pace by educating health care practitioners. It is important for practitioners to learn how to read clinical research papers so they can interpret findings and apply them to practice. (See *How to read a clinical quantitative research paper*, pages 244 to 246.)

Summary

Ongoing systematic improvement of the quality of patient care will become increasingly important in today's health care market. Health care providers in every health care facility need to be aware of the potential for pressure ulcer development. If information in the AHRQ guidelines is widely disseminated and incorporated into practice, the pressure ulcer incidence rate and associated pressure ulcer costs will come down. Clinicians have a responsibility and an opportunity to help reduce the number of patients who suffer from pressure ulceration. We can begin now to effect changes in practice by starting multidisciplinary skin care teams in our own agencies.

(Text continues on page 246.)

How to read a clinical quantitative research paper

The practice of wound care is rich in experience, but many claims lack a rigorous scientific basis. The wound care community is now charged with producing evidence-based practice to improve standards for prediction, prevention, and care. This involves keeping abreast of current literature. A clinician who wishes to understand and interpret clinical research papers must know which basic elements constitute a sound paper, which factors are affected by the trial design, and how to interpret the statistical results.

A clinical research paper contains an abstract, an introduction, sections describing methods and results, a discussion or summary, and references.

Abstract

The abstract functions as the "road map" to the study. In 100 words or less, it describes:
- the purpose of the clinical trial (the specific treatment the trial will assess)
- the methods that were used
- critical results
- a brief statement of the researchers' conclusions.
  The abstract may also tell readers why the trial was necessary and how the results will be useful.

Introduction

The purpose of a clinical trial is to assess the efficacy of a specific treatment. The paper's Introduction includes:
- a review of the literature on the treatment under investigation, including prior research and discussions of current treatment methods
- an explanation of how prior research warrants the current trial's usefulness and potential clinical significance of its findings
- a statement of purpose that clearly defines the goal of the clinical trial being presented.

Methods

The methods section explains the trial protocol — how the data were collected and analyzed. The protocol may include:
- patient characteristics
- experimental design
- controls used to ensure reliable results
- statistical methods used to analyze the data.
  This section should include sufficient information for the reader to determine the reliability and validity of the study. *Reliability* describes the consistency of the study results — how well the results can be reproduced under similar circumstances. *Validity* describes whether the study proves what it was intended to prove.
  The methods section generally contains three parts:
- *Patient characteristics* — A listing of the inclusion and exclusion criteria (such as symptoms, age, gender) helps the reader determine whether the researchers have selected an appropriate study population.
- *Design* — The structure of the study includes its duration, the size of the study population, the number of groups in the study population, the method of data collection, and the types of statistical methods used to analyze the results. An experimental design is determined by the objectives of the study, the variables that must be measured to answer the questions dictated by the objectives, the characteristics of the study population, and the possible error or bias problems anticipated in data collection and analysis.
- *Statistical methods* — The information on how the data were analyzed helps the reader assess the authors' conclusions.

How to read a clinical quantitative research paper *(continued)*

Methods terminology

- *Conditions:* Conditions refers to the protocols followed for each patient group. The number of conditions, and hence the number of patient groups, is determined by the number of variables generated by the study objectives. For example, a study designed to assess the efficacy of a new treatment method would likely have three conditions: a group receiving the study treatment, a group receiving the standard treatment, and a group receiving no treatment (the "control") group.
- *Controls:* Controls refers to aspects of the experimental design that help eliminate variables that might otherwise influence the experimental results. The controls defined here include randomization, blinding, prospective and retrospective data collection, and parameters (objective, subjective).
- *Randomization:* Randomly assigning patients to each condition or patient group increases the likelihood that the patients in each condition remain equal — within and among conditions — in every important way.
- *Blinding:* In blinding, researchers or patients (or sometimes both) do not know which condition or study group the patient has been assigned. This minimizes the possible effects that such knowledge can have on the results. In a *single-blind study,* the patients but not the researchers are uninformed about their condition status. In a *double-blind study,* neither the patients nor the researchers know about the patients' status during the trial. *Open-label* and *nonblind studies* make no attempts to conceal which treatment a patient receives.
- *Data collection:* In a *prospective* study, the events are measured as they occur; in a *retrospective* study, the events are measured after they occur; in this case, data usually are collected from medical records of previously treated patients.
- *Parameters:* Parameters are variables (such as efficacy or safety) that must be tested or measured to meet the study's objectives. An *objective parameter* allows little room for interpretation (for example, measuring the area of adhesions with a calibrated probe). A *subjective parameter* requires interpretation (such as quantifying the degree of pelvic pain). The reader must be sure that the parameters are appropriate (valid) for the type of conclusion made by the researchers.

Results

The results section describes the data that were recorded by the researchers. The data are commonly represented as the *mean* (the average of a group of numerical values), plus or minus the *standard deviation* (the numerical value that reflects the variation around the mean). The results of the statistical analysis also are presented, particularly for data that attain statistical significance. However, data that are not statistically significant may be clinically useful.

Results terminology

Statistical analysis refers to the mathematical manipulation of facts, or data, that allows researchers to organize their results. The analysis helps to determine whether the measured differences between two conditions were anything more than a chance occurrence and whether the results can be generalized from a small clinical trial to a larger population of patients.

Level of significance refers to the difference between the same bits of data in two study groups (such as treatment group versus control group, dosage group A versus dosage group B) expressed as the probability (P) value. If the P value is low enough to essentially rule out chance as a factor in the result ($P = < 0.05$ or $P = < 0.01$ are generally considered acceptable limits), then the result is considered statistically significant.

(continued)

How to read a clinical quantitative research paper *(continued)*

Confidence interval (CI) refers to the range of values that is likely to cover the true but unknown difference between treatment groups. If a study were repeated 100 times under the same conditions, a CI of 95% would be expected to include the true value 95 times. The CI is calculated from the estimate of the population value, the standard deviation from the sample, the sample size, and a factor related to the degree of confidence sought. A 95% CI is reported, which can be related to a P value of 0.05 (that is, any observed value within the CI would not be significant at the 0.05 level) and a 99% CI can be related to a P value of 0.01. Researchers may report the CI instead of or in addition to the significance level.

Clinical significance. When the observed results affect the clinical status of the patient, they are said to have clinical significance, even though the results may not have attained statistical significance.

Discussion

In the discussion (or summary) section, researchers describe their interpretation of the data, discuss the statistical and clinical significance of their results, and compare their results to those of related studies in the literature.

References

Authors should cite other research papers pertinent to their study. In the introduction, references serve as background material and can provide evidence for the need for the data sought in the presented study. In the methods section, references may support the researchers' choice of experimental design. References in the discussion section can help the reader interpret the results of the study.

Adapted from Supplement to Advances in Wound Care, 1001 Wound Care references, page 3, 1998.

Selected references

Allman, R.M., et al. "Pressure ulcers: Hospital complications and disease severity: Impact on hospital costs and length of stay," *Advances in Wound Care* 12(1):12-30, 1999.

Berquest, S., and Frantz, R.A. "Pressure ulcers in community-based older adults receiving home health care," *Advances in Wound Care* 12(7):339-351, 1999

Cali, T.J., and Bruce, M. "Pressure ulcer treatment: Explaining selected costs of therapeutic failure," *Advances in Wound Care* 12(S2):8-11, 1999.

Hoffman, D.R. "The federal effort to eliminate fraud and ensure quality care," *Advances in Wound Care* 10(5): 36-38, 1997.

Klingel, P. "Exploring the process of a skin care team," *Ostomy/Wound Management* 42(10):40-44, 1996.

Maklebust, J., and Magnan, M.A. "Risk factors associated with having a pressure ulcer: A secondary data analysis," *Advances in Wound Care* 7(6):25-42, 1994.

1001 Wound Care References: How to Read a Clinical Research Paper, Advances in Wound Care (suppl) pages 3-4, October 1998.

Sperling, R. "Suggestions for implementing the QI/OASIS Data Set," *Home Health Manager* 2(4):9-11, 1998.

Thomas, D.R., and Hess, C.T. "Evidence-Based Medicine," in: "Ask 'What works?'," *Resources in Wound Care*, page 2, 1998.

Xakellis, G.C. "Quality assurance program for pressure ulcers," *Clinics in Geriatric Medicine* 13:599-606, 1997.

Zulkowski, K. "MDS items not contained in the pressure ulcer RAP associated with pressure ulcer prevalence in newly institutionalized elders," *Ostomy/Wound Management* 45(1):24-33, 1999.

Chapter 13
Meeting future needs

The health care environment is in turmoil. In the search for the highest quality of care for the least cost, no one has yet found a model that is acceptable to patients, providers, and payers. Health care delivery systems are being downsized and restructured. Health care businesses are merging or purchasing one another. Reimbursement has changed from prospective payment to capitated payment for covered lives.

Many of these structural changes affect patients with pressure ulcers. This chapter reviews aspects of managed care, quality-of-life issues, legal and ethical issues, and governmental issues related to the future of pressure ulcer care.

Wound care under managed care

Originally, managed care was seen as a system that stressed continuity of care and a full range of services from prevention to complicated intervention in an inpatient setting. It was a system of organizing care, not just a mechanism of financing. It has become a method of cost containment. In Medicare and Medicaid, fixed negotiated rates have replaced charges. Changes in funding rules are the norm rather than the exception.

Agencies that deliver health care are trying to find innovative ways to stay cost-effective. Many are outsourcing services, such as physical therapy, dietary services, and materials management, or are entering strategic planning and corporate buying agreements to help contain or neutralize costs. Computerized systems track use of patient supplies for replenishment and utilization purposes.

The Balanced Budget Act of 1997 was intended to curtail Medicare spending by shifting from fee-for-service to prospective payments. The Act specifically affects patients and providers in the clinical setting. In acute care, diagnostic related groups (DRGs) are subject to new transfer rules. In the long-term care industry, prospective payments began in 1999. A prospective payment system for home health care is scheduled to take effect in October 2000. It's similar in concept to the current DRG system for acute care.

Prospective payment systems bundle all health care services instead of providing separate reimbursements for wound care. Therefore, facilities that provide wound management under managed care contracts must know their costs. They must be able to deliver wound management for the agreed-upon price through appropriate use of products and resources, which include surgical dressings, support surfaces, nutritional supplements, laboratory and diagnostic tests, nursing care, physical therapy, and other rehabilitative therapies. In long-term care, wound care will be reimbursed according to how sick the patient is. It is up to the provider to predict total costs for patient care. After calculating the cost, the agency must then monitor the actual cost of delivering the care. A postdischarge analysis can determine if resources could have been used more efficiently.

Wound care specialists need to develop and promote model pressure ulcer programs that their provider organizations can use to incorporate management of chronic wounds. In a sense, wound care has become a product line with competitive bidding for the best managed chronic wound care program. Standard reporting measures allow comparison of clinical outcomes, functional outcomes, patient satisfaction, and cost so that competing managed care plans can choose the most cost-effective wound management program. It will take a dedicated group of wound care specialists to design the most cost-effective pressure ulcer programs. Skilled clinicians from multiple disciplines are needed to embark on such an initiative.

New models of health care delivery

Market forces, health care legislation, and managed care have combined to change the delivery of health care services. As a managed care survival strategy, many health care providers are implementing new delivery models. The old model focused on care providers. The new models focus on the patient to improve continuity, quality, operational efficiency, and cost structure. Although patient-focused initiatives vary among facilities, the following common themes have emerged:

- grouping patients with similar resource needs
- decentralization or redeployment of ancillary services
- cross-training to produce multiskilled workers
- multidisciplinary team approach
- management restructuring and empowerment of employees
- clinical pathways (CareMaps)
- charting by exception (CBE).

Using multiskilled workers

In a common model, multiskilled workers — given such titles as "care partners" or "care associates" — are trained to perform tasks and carry responsibilities that once were assumed by health care professionals. They feed and bathe patients, monitor vital signs, change dressings, perform phlebotomies, and help patients ambulate, transfer, and do range-of-motion exercises. Some multiskilled workers also apply traction, casts, and continuous passive motion machines. Other duties vary, depending on the patient mix of the work setting. Certified wound care professionals are likely to find themselves in expanded roles of mentor and teacher of paraprofessionals who will put into practice the hands-on skills they have been taught.

The hoped-for increase in quality and quantity of time spent interacting with patients has not yet materialized. As multiskilled workers assume a larger share of patient care, it will be interesting to evaluate outcome data on satisfaction among patients, physicians, nurses, and other licensed and unlicensed health care personnel. To evaluate outcomes from newer delivery models, quality and cost data need to be collected before implementation; otherwise, valid comparisons of cost-effectiveness claims will be impossible.

Case management

Under managed care, the cost of pressure ulcers takes on new meaning. Patients who develop pressure ulcers may require intense care and longer hospital stays. Yet, under managed care contracts, health care providers receive no additional money for pressure ulcer care. For health care providers to afford delivery of needed care, they must be able to document the hidden costs of pressure ulcers. In addition, they must have consistent management protocols that emphasize primary care prevention to avoid unnecessary hospital care. Under managed care, every at-risk patient must have a comprehensive skin integrity and pressure ulcer risk assessment, and pressure ulcer prevention should be started before risk becomes reality.

As Medicare and Medicaid payments shrink, health care providers must establish control over the cost of providing care to patients with pressure ulcers. Case management of these patients is a way to support performance improvement efforts, meet internal and external documentation requirements, develop wound care pathways, improve patient and staff communication, streamline variance tracking, cut skyrocketing wound care costs, reduce length of stay, and boost agency revenues. The overall goal of case management is to provide a service delivery model that ensures cost-effective health care, offers alternatives to hospitalization, provides access to care, coordinates supportive services, and improves the patient's functional capacity.

A specialized wound care program with an accountable case manager can streamline care and maintain standards across settings. Specialized nurse case managers can develop staff and patient education programs for pressure ulcer management, allocate appropriate resources for care with patient and family input, and develop wound care pathways that can be superimposed on care pathways for other patient conditions or procedures.

Clinical pathways

Clinical pathways, or care maps, are multidisciplinary plans of care that give direction to the health care team. (See Chapter 8.) They can help providers give consistent, comprehensive, quality care for patients with pressure ulcers by describing the interventions that should be delivered to the patient each day. Patient outcomes are predefined, and progress toward these outcomes is documented. If expected patient outcomes are not achieved by the intervention of health care professionals, the plan of care must be reevaluated or the patient outcomes modified accordingly.

Reimbursement may be based on what is consistently documented in the medical record. In the acute care setting, documentation plays a significant role in case mix and DRG assignment, and external peer review organizations now review charts. Underestimating the importance of documentation in proper coding and DRG assignment can have disastrous consequences. Omissions in the medical record are costly for any health care provider. A model pressure ulcer pathway can help staff document required information efficiently.

Using telemedicine

The use of telecommunications technology to deliver medical services at a distance is called telemedicine. This technology, although controversial, is rapidly improving, and new and innovative uses are being tested throughout the country. Some argue that video visits lack the range of clinical assessment and treatment capability and personal touch of traditional therapeutic relationships. Others insist that they increase the patient's access to care for homebound patients, reduce resource consumption, and improve use of scarce health professionals. In one study, researchers used a telerehabilitation program to manage pressure ulcers in persons with spinal cord injuries. They explored the use of a still-image videophone to capture and send images for weekly wound assessments from the patients' homes to the clinic. The study found that pressure ulcers can be successfully managed via telemedicine. Participants and their families accepted and often preferred this method of care over traditional visits. Controlled studies are under way to determine validated outcomes and to determine cost-effectiveness and cost utility. It is believed that ongoing research in this area will provide new and better ways to help individuals and families reclaim their independence. Their involvement may be enhanced by the patient's ability to see the wound enlarged on a video monitor, making the pressure ulcer more real. It can also provide proof of healing progress for patients who become discouraged.

Quality-of-life issues

Quality of life has become a crisis in America. Human suffering, the financial costs of care, and legal and ethical problems created by life-or-death decisions are paramount to the issue. The tremendous improvement in life-sustaining techniques has created equally tremendous ethical challenges. As the population ages, health care administrators are increasingly concerned about the strain on physical and financial resources. Patients and families are concerned about their right to control their own health care. The courts are concerned about mental competency and the right to refuse life-sustaining treatments. Providers now have ethics committees that help patients and professionals reach decisions with peace of mind and some degree of certainty. Many states have advance directive guidelines that help patients document their wishes concerning the use of life-prolonging technology and delegate surrogates to make decisions in their behalf. An apparently overwhelming public consensus on individual rights seems to be changing society's attitude about what constitutes living and what constitutes dying. The public is demanding that more attention be paid to their needs and desires.

Ethical issues

Ethical and legal issues are becoming more prominent in the literature on pressure ulcers. The causes of pressure ulcers in "at-risk" patients have been known for years, but the overall incidence has not changed. The underlying question of why this problem persists has yet to be answered.

Ethics is the philosophical study of moral values and right decisions and actions. Health care is filled with choices regarding treatment, cost, and distribution of scarce resources. Ethical dilemmas occur when conflicting values support alternative choices for the same situation. According to one ethical principle, beneficence, a patient should derive benefit and experience no harm as a result of a choice. Decisions using this principle are made based on the greater good, or the lesser of two evils, and always in the best interest of the patient. This principle is often used by practitioners.

The utilitarian principle, on the other hand, states that resources should be given to those who would reap the most benefit or who are of greater value to society as a whole. Populations at risk for pressure ulcers, such as nursing home residents, elderly frail patients, and those who depend on others for basic care, may be considered less worthy recipients of scarce resources than other citizens. Individuals who are dependent and unable to contribute to society may have decisions made for them that are different from the decisions made for others. If an individual or a group is in a high-risk category, and a pressure ulcer is considered an inevitable characteristic of that patient population, then resources for prevention may be directed elsewhere.

What to do? Decisions about pressure ulcer management must consider factors such as the patient's general medical status, the condition of the ulcer, the potential for rehabilitation, and the patient's ability to comply with treatment recommendations. Treatment plans aim to improve the patient's condition or effect a cure. Health care providers and researchers historically have been concerned with treating disease and illness rather than fostering prevention and well-being. Because the perceived value of prevention efforts is low, societal and financial investment is lacking. The incipient trend toward valuing prevention efforts must be reinforced. Outcome research is needed to show the value of using resources to prevent pressure ulcers in high-risk individuals.

This is not to say that all high-risk patients should be treated unconditionally. The decision to treat conditions that place individuals at high risk for pressure ulcer development (immobility, incontinence, and malnutrition) is based in the goal set by the patient or the patient's advocate. A goal of comfort at the end of life is inconsistent with orders to turn every 2 hours to avoid pressure when such turning is painful for the patient. The ethical obligation is to provide care that is consistent with the patient's goal.

Legal issues

There has been a dramatic increase in pressure ulcer litigation over the past few years. Pressure ulcer injuries can lead to large financial compensation. Pressure ulcer litigation can occur from negligence or for fraud and abuse. Liability for negligence occurs when there is failure to provide necessary and appropriate care. The patient must show that there was a duty owed by the practitioner/agency and that this duty was breached. Then it must be shown that the probable cause of the pressure ulcer was the failure of the practitioner/agency to provide the necessary care to prevent the injury.

The federal False Claims Act states that documentation submitted to Medicare or Medicaid for payment must represent services that were actually rendered. Documentation that is untrue and is submitted for reimbursement is fraudulent. In addition, the provider is required to provide care that is necessary and appropriate. Providing and billing for services that will not benefit the patient, such as treatments known to be ineffective, are also fraudulent.

By implementing and following clinical practice guidelines, caregivers can reduce the likelihood of malpractice lawsuits. Guidelines and protocols are often cited as standards of care and therefore are considered expected practice. Violating guideline recommendations places the practitioner at risk. Conversely, following such guidelines in practice can be beneficial in litigation defense. It is the responsibility of each practitioner to keep up with changes in standards of practice. Caregivers can best protect themselves from litigation by carefully documenting objective findings, patient and ulcer assessments, risk factors, treatment provided, and outcomes obtained.

Nationwide cooperative efforts

In 1989, Congress established the Agency for Health Care Policy and Research (AHCPR) to improve the quality, appropriateness, and effectiveness of health care and to improve access to health care services. Social and economic factors giving rise to the AHCPR included delivery of inappropriate health care, lack of science-based health care, high health care costs, and consumer demands for greater participation in health care decision making.

Over the years, the AHCPR released numerous clinical practice guidelines for health-related conditions. Multidisciplinary panels of expert health care professionals and consumers designed the guidelines to help health care professionals and patients make better choices about treatment options. Much more scientific evidence is needed to support areas of the guidelines for which science is lacking, and many of the concepts in the guidelines need further testing. However, the agency's guidelines on prediction, prevention, and treatment of pressure ulcers still represent the soundest basis for comprehensive management of pressure ulcers and are the standard of care used by many accrediting and regulating bodies. Recent research on pressure ulcers has not revealed a need for changes to these clinical practices.

On December 6, 1999, Congress reauthorized the AHCPR and changed the name to the Agency for Healthcare Research and Quality (AHRQ). The new legislation validates the agency's core mission and its role as a science partner working with the public and private sector organizations to improve quality and safety of patient care.

AHRQ's stated theme is Closing the Gap. To make sure that knowledge gained from health care research is translated into measurable improvements, four such "gaps" need to be addressed, namely, those between:
■ current knowledge and current practices in health care
■ evidence now available and evidence needed to improve care in the future
■ questions confronting health care decision makers and available information
■ minority and predominant populations' access to health care services and the quality and outcomes of care.

The legislation included funding to support the AHRQ mission — to foster the use of evidence as the foundation for informed health care decision making by patients, clinicians, health care system leaders, purchasers, and policymakers.

National Pressure Ulcer Advisory Panel

The National Pressure Ulcer Advisory Panel (NPUAP) is a nonprofit multidisciplinary organization of health care professionals dedicated to the prevention of pressure ulcers. Their mission is to provide leadership, recommendations, guidance, and action toward pressure ulcer management. The panel acts as a steering committee for the country's efforts toward eradicating pressure ulcers. Through educational and legislative activities, the NPUAP stresses the responsibility of all health-related professionals in the management of pressure ulcers.

In 1987, the group was instrumental in amending the Omnibus Budget Reconciliation Act (OBRA) to strengthen language relating to quality of care in long-term settings. OBRA encouraged the Secretary of Health and Human Services to list pressure ulcers as a parameter for evaluating the quality of care delivered by long-term care facilities.

The National Academy of Sciences (NAS) invited NPUAP to participate in formulating the Health Care Objectives of the Nation for the year 2000. As part of the alliance of organizations involved in Healthy People 2000, one of the Panel's goals was to reduce the incidence of pressure ulcers by 50% by 2000, which was completed successfully. The NPUAP also introduced objectives pertaining to pressure ulcers in Healthy People 2000 and provided testimony at regional hearings sponsored by the U.S. Public Health Service. The NPUAP continues its alliance with the NAS and participated in formulating the Healthy People 2010 objectives for the nation. The NPUAP successfully sponsored an objective to reduce the proportion of nursing home residents with current diagnoses of pressure ulcers. The target is no more than 9 in 1,000 residents based on a baseline of 16 of 1,000 (1997 data). That is a 50% decrease in prevalence and improvement over baseline.

The NPUAP is also active in third-party reimbursement for prevention and treatment of pressure ulcers. Quality patient care and effective pressure ulcer interventions are difficult to provide when the required materials are not reimbursable. The NPUAP has been actively working with the Health Care Financing Administration on medical policy for durable medical equipment and supplies related to wound care. Meetings with the medical directors of the durable medical equipment regional carriers have been beneficial in reviewing and negotiating medical policy for surgical dressings and support surfaces.

In March 1989, the NPUAP sponsored the first National Consensus Development Conference in Washington, D.C., to focus on the pressure ulcer problem. The second and third national conferences sponsored by the NPUAP were formal multidisciplinary critiques of drafts of the AHRQ *Guideline on Prediction and Prevention of Pressure Ulcers* and *Guideline on Treatment of Pressure Ulcers*.

NPUAP national conferences are held biannually to address the most critical issues related to pressure ulcers. Recent NPUAP conferences have focused on avoidable versus unavoidable pressure ulcers and on the cost of care for pressure ulcers. The NPUAP has submitted a grant proposal to the AHRQ to examine the evidence base for pressure ulcer practices to produce outcomes, research, and benchmarking data to improve the standards of practice for wound care.

Summary

The dynamic state of the health care system challenges patients, clinicians, and providers. The crisis of care cuts across the boundaries of all health care professions. Patients in hospitals feel depersonalized and wonder if professionals really care about them. Caregivers seem to be rewarded for efficiency, technical skill, and measurable results while their concern and attentiveness go unnoticed by provider institutions.

The ethics of care and the sources from which caregivers draw inspiration must be restored to caregiving practices in the helping professions. In the future, as patient satisfaction becomes a marker of excellence, emphasis may swing from high technology to caring. As the health care system redefines itself, caring for and about patients must remain our overriding mission.

While continuously examining advances in pressure ulcer research, health care providers must remember that maintaining skin integrity remains a critical part of the complex management of ill, disabled, and elderly patients. Key challenges include:

■ education of the patient and family, focusing on early detection and intervention to decrease pressure ulcer risk factors

■ an aggressive patient/team approach to pressure ulcer management when skin integrity is already compromised

■ implementation of a coordinated team approach using the expertise of all related disciplines to manage the pressure ulcer problem.

Selected references

Barr, J.E. "Integrating disease management and wound care critical pathways in home care," *Home Healthcare Nurse* 17(10):651-663, 1999.

Beckrich, K., and Aronovitch, S.A. "Hospital acquired pressure ulcers: A comparison of costs in medical vs. surgical patients," *Nursing Economics* 17(5):263-271, 1999.

Bergstrom, N., et al. *Treatment of Pressure Ulcers.* Clinical Practice Guideline No. 15. AHCPR Publication No. 95-0652. Rockville, Md: Agency for Health Care Policy and Research, Public Health Service, U.S. Department of Health and Human Services, December 1994.

Fenner, S. "Developing and implementing a wound care program in long term care," *JWOCN* 26(5): 254-260, 1999.

Goebel, R.H., and Goebel, M.R. "Clinical practice guidelines for pressure ulcer prevention can prevent malpractice lawsuits in older patients," *JWOCN* 26(4):175-184, 1999.

Hoffman, D.R. "The federal effort to eliminate fraud and ensure quality care," *Advances in Wound Care* 10(5):36-38, 1997.

Josey, P., and Gustke, S. "How to merge telemedicine with traditional clinical practice," *Nursing Management* 30(4):33-36, 1999.

Knapp, M.T. "Nurses' basic guide to understanding the Medicare PPS," *Nursing Management* 30(5): 14-15, 1999.

McNichol, L., et al. "Notes from the regulatory and reimbursement subcommittee: Establishing reimbursement outpatient services," *JWOCN* 26(6): 22A-31A, 1999.

Motta, G.J. "Documentation and reimbursement by clinical setting," *Ostomy/Wound Management* 42(4): 18-23, 1996.

Motta, G.J. "Can SNFs under PPS afford to use support surfaces?," *Extended Care Product News* 61:5-6, 1999.

Murphy, R.N. "Legal and practical impact of clinical practice guidelines on nursing and medical practice," *Advances in Wound Care* 9(5):31-34, 1996.

National Pressure Ulcer Advisory Panel. "Proceedings of the Pressure Ulcer Conference: Controversy to Consensus: Assessment, Measurement and Outcomes," *Advances in Wound Care* 8(4): entire issue, 1995.

Panel for the Prediction and Prevention of Pressure Ulcers in Adults. *Pressure Ulcers in Adults: Prediction and Prevention.* Clinical Practice Guideline No. 3. AHCPR Publication No. 92-0047. Rockville, Md.: Agency for Health Care Policy and Research, Public Health Service, U.S. Department of Health and Human Services, May 1992.

Salcido, R. "Certification and competency in the year 2000 ... and beyond," *Advances in Wound Care* 12(1):8-9, 1999.

Soloway, D.N. "Civil claims relating to pressure ulcers: A claimant's lawyer's perspective," *Ostomy/Wound Management* 44(2):20-26, 1998.

Turnbull, I.G.B. "Understanding the balanced budget act of 1997," *Ostomy/Wound Management* 46(l): 40-47, 2000.

van Rijswijk, L.I. "Clinical practice guidelines: Moving into the 21st century," *Ostomy/Wound Management* 45(IA):47S-53S, 1999.

Vesmarovich, S., et al. "Use of telerehabilitation to manage pressure ulcers in persons with spinal cord injuries," *Advances in Wound Care* 12(5):264-269, 1999.

Winnington, P. "How to make the Internet work for you," *Skin and Aging* 6(11):38-43, 1998.

Appendices and Index

Appendix A: Norton scale

Physical Condition		Mental Condition		Activity		Mobility		Incontinent		Total Score
Good	4	Alert	4	Ambulatory	4	Full	4	Not	4	
Fair	3	Apathetic	3	Walks with help	3	Slightly limited	3	Occasionally	3	
Poor	2	Confused	2	Chairbound	2	Very limited	2	Usually/ Urine	2	
Very bad	1	Stupor	1	Bedbound	1	Immobile	1	Doubly	1	

Appendix B: Gosnell scale

I.D.: _____   Medical diagnosis: _____
Age: _____ Sex: _____   Primary: _____
Height: _____ Weight: _____   Secondary: _____
Date of admission: _____   Nursing diagnosis: _____
Date of discharge: _____   _____
_____

Instructions: Complete all categories within 24 hours of admission and every other day thereafter. Refer to the accompanying guidelines for specific rating details.

Date	Mental Status:	Continence:	Mobility:	Activity:	Nutrition:	Total Score
	1. Alert controlled	1. Fully	1. Full	1. Ambulatory	1. Good	
	2. Apathetic controlled	2. Usually limited	2. Slightly Assistance	2. Walks with	2. Fair	
	3. Confused controlled	3. Minimally limited	3. Very	3. Chairfast	3. Poor	
	4. Stuporous of control 5. Unconscious	4. Absence	4. Immobile	4. Bedfast		

Pressure Sore Risk Assessment Medication Profile

Medication	Dosage	*Frequency	Route	Date begun	Date discontinued

*If PRN, record pattern past 48 hours.

Guidelines for Numerical Rating of the Defined Categories

Rating	1	2	3	4	5
Mental status: An assessment of one's level of response to the environment	**Alert:** Oriented to time, place, and person (TPP); responsive to all stimuli, and understands explanations	**Apathetic:** Lethargic, forgetful, drowsy, passive and dull; sluggish, depressed; able to obey simple commands; possibly disoriented to time	**Confused:** Partial and/or intermittent disorientation to TPP; purposeless response to stimuli; restless, aggressive, irritable, anxious, and may require tranquilizers or sedatives	**Stuporous:** Total disorientation; does not respond to name, simple commands, or verbal stimuli	**Unconscious:** Nonresponsive to painful stimuli
Continence: The amount of bodily control of urination and defecation	**Fully controlled:** In total control of urine and feces	**Usually controlled:** Incontinent of urine, feces or both not more often than once q 48 hrs; **OR** has Foley catheter and is incontinent of feces	**Minimally controlled:** Incontinent of urine or feces at least once q 24 hrs	**Absence of control:** Consistently incontinent of both urine and feces	
Mobility: The amount and control of movement of one's body	**Full:** Able to control and move all extremities at will; may require use of a device but turns, lifts, pulls, balances, and attains sitting position at will	**Slightly limited:** Able to control and move all extremities but a degree of limitation is present; requires assistance of another person to turn, pull, balance, and/or attain a sitting position at will, but self-initiates movement or request for help to move	**Very limited:** Can assist another person who must initiate movement via turning, lifting, pulling, balancing, and/or attaining a sitting position (contractures, paralysis may be present)	**Immobile:** Does not assist self in any way to change position; unable to change position without assistance; completely dependent on others for movement	
Activity: The ability of an individual to ambulate	**Ambulatory:** Able to walk unassisted; rises from bed unassisted; with a device such as cane or walker is able to ambulate without help from another person	**Walks with help:** Able to ambulate with assistance of another person, braces, or crutches; may have stairs limitation	**Chairfast:** Ambulates only to a chair, requires assistance to do so, **OR** is confined to a wheelchair	**Bedfast:** Confined to bed 24 hours a day	
Nutrition: The process of food intake	Eats some food from each basic food category every day and the majority of each meal served **OR** is on tube feeding	Occasionally refuses a meal or frequently leaves at least half of a meal	Seldom eats a complete meal; eats only a few bites of food at a meal		

					Color	General skin appearance						
						Moisture	Tempera-ture	Texture				
					1. Pallor 2. Mottled 3. Pink 4. Ashen 5. Ruddy 6. Cyanotic 7. Jaundice 8. Other	1. Dry 2. Damp 3. Oily 4. Other	1. Cold 2. Cool 3. Warm 4. Hot	1. Smooth 2. Rough 3. Thin/ trans- parent 4. Scaly 5. Crusty 6. Other				
	Vital signs				24-hour fluid balance					Interventions		
Date	T	P	R	BP	Diet	Intake	Output			No	Yes	Describe

Vital signs: Take and record temperature, pulse, respiration, and blood pressure at every assessment rating.

Skin appearance: Describe observed skin characteristics: color, moisture, temperature, and texture.

Diet: Record the specific diet order.

24-hour fluid balance: Record the amount of fluid intake and output during the previous 24-hour period.

Interventions: List all devices, measures, and/or care activity being used for pressure sore prevention.

Medications: List name, dosage, frequency, and route for all prescribed medications. If a PRN order, list the pattern for the period since last assessment.

Comments: Use this space to add explanation or further detail regarding any of the previously recorded data or patient condition *or* describe anything that you believe to be of importance but not accounted for previously.

NOTE: For any item marked "other," please describe.
If you observe any signs of pressure on bony prominences or other body parts, describe in detail the location, color, temperature, moisture, texture, size, and any other pertinent items.

Appendix C: **Braden scale**

Patient's Name: _____

Sensory perception Ability to respond meaningfully to pressure-related discomfort	**1. Completely limited:** Unresponsive (does not moan, flinch, or grasp) to painful stimuli, due to diminished level of consciousness or sedation **OR** Limited ability to feel pain over most of body surface	**2. Very limited:** Responds only to painful stimuli; cannot communicate discomfort except by moaning or restlessness **OR** Has a sensory impairment which limits the ability to feel pain or discomfort over $1/2$ of body
Moisture Degree to which skin is exposed to moisture	**1. Constantly moist:** Skin kept moist almost constantly by perspiration, urine, other secretions; dampness detected every time patient is moved or turned	**2. Very moist:** Skin often (but not always) moist; linen must be changed at least once a shift
Activity Degree of physical activity	**1. Bedfast:** Confined to bed	**2. Chairfast:** Ability to walk severely limited or nonexistent; cannot bear own weight and/or must be assisted into chair or wheelchair
Mobility Ability to change and control body position	**1. Completely immobile:** Does not make even slight changes in body or extremity position without assistance	**2. Very limited:** Makes occasional slight changes in body or extremity position, but unable to make frequent or significant changes independently
Nutrition *Usual* food intake pattern	**1. Very poor:** Never eats a complete meal; rarely eats more than $1/3$ of any food offered; eats 2 servings or less of protein (meat or dairy products) per day; takes fluids poorl; does not take a liquid dietary supplement **OR** Is NPO and/or maintained on clear liquids or I.V.s for more than 5 days	**2. Probably inadequate:** Rarely eats a complete meal and generally eats only about $1/2$ of any food offered; protein intake includes only 3 servings of meat or dairy products per day; occasionally will take a dietary supplement **OR** Receives less than optimum amount of liquid diet or tube feeding
Friction and shear	**1. Problem:** Requires moderate to maximum assistance in moving; complete lifting without sliding against sheets is impossible; frequently slides down in bed or chair, requiring frequent repositioning with maximum assistance; spasticity, contractures, or agitation leads to almost constant friction	**2. Potential problem:** Moves feebly or requires minimum assistance; during a move, skin probably slides to some extent against sheets, chair restraints, or other devices; maintains relatively good position in chair or bed most of the time but occasionally slides down

Evaluator's Name:_____ Date of Assessment: _____

3. Slightly limited:
Responds to verbal commands, but cannot always communicate discomfort or need to be turned
OR
Has some sensory impairment limiting ability to feel pain or discomfort in 1 or 2 extremities

4. No impairment:
Responds to verbal commands; has no sensory deficit that would limit ability to feel or voice pain or discomfort

3. Occasionally moist:
Skin occasionally moist, requiring an extra linen change approximately once a day

4. Rarely moist:
Skin usually dry; linen only requires changing at routine intervals

3. Walks occasionally:
Walks occasionally during day, but for very short distances, with or without assistance; spends majority of each shift in bed or chair

4. Walks frequently:
Walks outside the room at least twice a day and inside room at least once every 2 hours during waking hours

3. Slightly limited:
Makes frequent though slight changes in body or extremity position independently

4. No limitations:
Makes major and frequent changes in position without assistance

3. Adequate:
Eats over half of most meals; eats a total of 4 servings of protein (meat, dairy products) each day; occasionally will refuse a meal, but will usually take a supplement if offered
OR
Is on a tube feeding or TPN regimen, probably meeting most nutritional needs

4. Excellent:
Eats most of every meal; never refuses a meal; usually eats a total of 4 or more servings of meat and dairy products; occasionally eats between meals; does not require supplementation

3. No apparent problem:
Moves in bed and in chair independently and has sufficient muscle strength to lift completely during move; maintains good position in bed or chair at all times

Total score

Appendix D: Bates-Jensen pressure sore status tool

General guidelines

Fill out the attached rating sheet to assess a pressure sore's status after reading the definitions and methods of assessment described below. Evaluate once a week and whenever a change occurs in the wound. Rate each item by selecting the response that best describes the wound and entering that score in the item score column for the appropriate date. When you have rated the pressure sore on all items, determine the total score by adding together the 13 item scores. The *higher* the total score, the more severe the pressure sore status. Plot total score on the Pressure Sore Status Continuum on the last page to determine progress.

Specific instructions

Item 1. **Size:** Use ruler to measure the longest and widest aspect of the wound surface in centimeters; multiply length x width.

Item 2. **Depth:** Choose the depth and thickness most appropriate to the wound, using these additional descriptions:
1 = tissues damaged but no break in skin surface
2 = superficial, abrasion, blister, or shallow crater. Even with, and/or elevated above, skin surface (such as hyperplasia)
3 = deep crater with or without undermining of adjacent tissue
4 = visualization of tissue layers not possible due to necrosis
5 = supporting structures include tendon and joint capsule

Item 3. **Edges:** Use this guide:

Indistinct, diffuse	=	unable to clearly distinguish wound outline
Attached	=	even or flush with wound base; *no* sides or walls present; flat
Not attached	=	sides or walls *are* present; floor or base of wound is deeper than edge
Rolled under, thickened	=	soft to firm and flexible to touch
Hyperkeratosis	=	callouslike tissue formation around wound and at edges
Fibrotic, scarred	=	hard, rigid to touch

Item 4. **Undermining:** Assess by inserting a cotton-tipped applicator under the wound edge; advance it as far as it will go without using undue force; raise the tip of the applicator so it may be seen or felt on the surface of the skin; mark the surface with a pen; measure the distance from the mark on the skin to the edge of the wound. Repeat these steps around the wound. Then use a transparent metric measuring guide with concentric circles divided into four (25%) pie-shaped quadrants to help determine percentage of wound involved.

Item 5. **Necrotic tissue type:** Pick the type of necrotic tissue that is *predominant* in the wound according to color, consistency, and adherence, using this guide:

White/gray nonviable tissue	=	may appear prior to wound opening; skin surface is white or gray
Nonadherent, yellow slough	=	thin, mucinous substance; scattered throughout wound bed; easily separated from wound tissue
Loosely adherent, yellow slough	=	thick, stringy clumps of debris; attached to wound tissue
Adherent, soft, black eschar	=	soggy tissue; strongly attached to tissue in center or base of wound
Firmly adherent, hard and black eschar	=	firm, crusty tissue; strongly attached to wound base *and* edges (like a hard scab)

Item 6. **Necrotic tissue amount:** Use a transparent metric measuring guide with concentric circles divided into four (25%) pie-shaped quadrants to help determine percentage of wound involved.

Item 7. **Exudate type:** Some dressings interact with wound drainage to produce a gel to trap liquid. Before assessing exudate type, gently cleanse wound with normal saline or water. Pick the exudate type that is *predominant* in the wound according to color and consistency, using this guide:

Bloody	=	thin, bright red
Serosanguineous	=	thin, watery, pale red to pink
Serous	=	thin, watery, clear
Purulent	=	thin or thick, opaque, tan to yellow
Foul purulent	=	thick, opaque, yellow to green with offensive odor

Item 8. **Exudate amount:** Use a transparent metric measuring guide with concentric circles divided into four (25%) pie-shaped quadrants to determine percentage of dressing involved with exudate. Use this guide:

None	=	wound tissues dry
Scant	=	wound tissues moist; no measurable exudate
Small	=	wound tissues wet; moisture evenly distributed in wound; drainage involves ≤25% dressing
Moderate	=	wound tissues saturated; drainage may or may not be evenly distributed in wound; drainage involves >25% to ≤75% dressing
Large	=	wound tissues bathed in fluid; drainage freely expressed; may or may not be evenly distributed in wound; drainage involves >75% of dressing

Item 9. **Skin color surrounding wound:** Assess tissues within 4 cm of wound edge. Dark-skinned persons show the colors "bright red" and "dark red" as a deepening of normal ethnic skin color or a purple hue. As healing occurs in such persons, the new skin is pink and may never darken.

Item 10. **Peripheral tissue edema:** Assess tissues within 4 cm of wound edge. Nonpitting edema appears as skin that is shiny and taut. Identify pitting edema by firmly pressing a finger down into the tissues and waiting for 5 seconds; on release of pressure, tissues fail to resume previous position and an indentation appears. *Crepitus* is accumulation of air or gas in tissues. Use a transparent metric measuring guide to determine how far edema extends beyond wound.

Item 11. **Peripheral tissue induration:** Assess tissues within 4 cm of wound edge. Induration is abnormal firmness of tissues with margins. Assess by gently pinching the tissues. Induration results in an inability to pinch the tissues. Use a transparent metric measuring guide with concentric circles divided into four (25%) pie-shaped quadrants to determine percentage of wound and area involved.

Item 12. **Granulation tissue:** Granulation tissue consists of small blood vessels and connective tissue that fills in full-thickness wounds. Tissue is healthy when bright, beefy red, shiny, and granular with a velvety appearance. Poor vascular supply appears as pale pink to dull, dusky red.

Item 13. **Epithelialization:** Epithelialization is the process of epidermal resurfacing and appears as pink or red skin. In partial-thickness wounds, it can occur throughout the wound bed as well as from the wound edges. In full-thickness wounds, it occurs from the edges only. Use a transparent metric measuring guide with concentric circles divided into four (25%) pie-shaped quadrants to help determine percentage of wound involved and to measure the distance the epithelial tissue extends into the wound.

Pressure sore status tool   Name: _____

Complete the rating sheet to assess pressure sore status. Evaluate each item by picking the response that best describes the wound and entering the score in the item score column for the appropriate date.

Location: Anatomic site. Circle, identify right (R) or left (L) and use "X" to mark site on body diagrams:

__Sacrum and coccyx   __Lateral ankle
__Trochanter   __Medial ankle
__Ischial tuberosity   __Heel
__Other site

Shape: Overall wound pattern; assess by observing perimeter and depth. Circle and *date* appropriate description:

__Irregular   __Linear or elongated
__Round or oval   __Bowl or boat
__Square or rectangle   __Butterfly
__Other shape

Item	Assessment	Date	Date	Date
		Score	Score	Score
1. Size	1 = Length x width <4 cm² 2 = Length x width 4 to 16 cm² 3 = Length x width 16.1 to 36 cm² 4 = Length x width 36.1 to 80 cm² 5 = Length x width >80 cm²			
2. Depth	1 = Nonblanchable erythema on intact skin 2 = Partial-thickness skin loss involving epidermis and/or dermis 3 = Full-thickness skin loss involving damage or necrosis of subcutaneous tissue; may extend down to but not through underlying fascia; and/or mixed partial- and full-thickness skin loss and/or tissue layers obscured by granulation tissue 4 = Obscured by necrosis 5 = Full-thickness skin loss with extensive destruction, tissue necrosis, or damage to muscle, bone, or supporting structure			
3. Edges	1 = Indistinct, diffuse, none clearly visible 2 = Distinct, outline clearly visible, attached, even with wound base 3 = Well-defined, not attached to wound base 4 = Well-defined, not attached to base, rolled under, thickened 5 = Well-defined, fibrotic, scarred or hyperkeratotic			
4. Undermining	1 = Undermining <2 cm in any area 2 = Undermining 2 to 4 cm involving <50% wound margins 3 = Undermining 2 to 4 cm involving >50% wound margins 4 = Undermining >4 cm in any area 5 = Tunneling and/or sinus tract formation			
5. Necrotic tissue type	1 = None visible 2 = White or gray nonviable tissue and/or nonadherent yellow slough 3 = Loosely adherent yellow slough 4 = Adherent, soft black eschar 5 = Firmly adherent, hard, black eschar			
6. Necrotic tissue amount	1 = None visible 2 = <25% of wound bed covered 3 = 25% to 50% of wound covered 4 = >50% and <75% of wound covered 5 = 75% to 100% of wound covered			
7. Exudate type	1 = None or bloody 2 = Serosanguineous: thin, watery, pale red or pink 3 = Serous: thin, watery, clear 4 = Purulent: thin or thick, opaque, tan or yellow 5 = Foul purulent: thick, opaque, yellow or green with odor			
8. Exudate amount	1 = None 2 = Scant 3 = Small 4 = Moderate 5 = Large			

Item	Assessment	Date	Date	Date
		Score	Score	Score
9. Skin color surrounding wound	1 = Pink or normal for ethnic group 2 = Bright red and/or blanches to touch 3 = White or gray pallor or hypopigmented 4 = Dark red or purple and/or nonblanchable 5 = Black or hyperpigmented			
10. Peripheral tissue edema	1 = Minimal swelling around wound 2 = Nonpitting edema extends <4 cm around wound 3 = Nonpitting edema extends ≥4 cm around wound 4 = Pitting edema extends <4 cm around wound 5 = Crepitus and/or pitting edema extends ≥4 cm			
11. Peripheral tissue induration	1 = Minimal firmness around wound 2 = Induration <2 cm around wound 3 = Induration 2 to 4 cm extending <50% around wound 4 = Induration 2 to 4 cm extending ≥50% around wound 5 = Induration >4 cm in any area			
12. Granulation tissue	1 = Skin intact or partial-thickness wound 2 = Bright, beefy red; 75% to 100% of wound filled and/or tissue overgrowth 3 = Bright, beefy red; <75% and >25% of wound filled 4 = Pink and/or dull, dusky red and/or fills ≤25% of wound 5 = No granulation tissue present			
13. Epithelialization	1 = 100% wound covered; surface intact 2 = 75% to <100% wound covered and/or epithelial tissue extends >0.5 cm into wound bed 3 = 50% to <75% wound covered and/or epithelial tissue extends to <0.5 cm into wound bed 4 = 25% to <50% wound covered 5 = <25% wound covered			
Total score				
Signature				

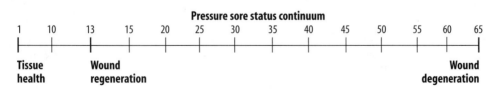

Pressure sore status continuum

1   10   13   15   20   25   30   35   40   45   50   55   60   65

Tissue health   **Wound regeneration**   **Wound degeneration**

Plot the total score on the Pressure Sore Status Continuum by putting an "X" on the line and the date beneath the line. Plot multiple scores with their dates on the same line to see at a glance if regeneration or degeneration of the wound is occurring.

Appendix E: **PUSH tool**

The Pressure Ulcer Scale for Healing (PUSH) is a simple, easy-to-use tool for evaluating healing.

Patient name_____   Patient I.D.# _____

User location _____   Date _____

Directions
Observe and measure the pressure ulcer. Categorize the ulcer with respect to surface area, exudate, and type of wound tissue. Record a subscore for each of the ulcer characteristics. Add the subscores to obtain the total score. A comparison of total scores measured over time provides an indication of the improvement or deterioration in pressure ulcer healing.

Length	0	1	2	3	4	5	Blank
	0 cm²	< 0.3 cm²	0.3 to 0.6 cm²	0.7 to 1.0 cm²	1.1 to 2.0 cm²	2.1 to 3.0 cm²	
× width		6	7	8	9	10	Subscore
		3.1 to 4.0 cm²	4.1 to 8.0 cm²	8.1 to 12.0 cm²	12.1 to 24.0 cm²	>24.0 cm²	
Exudate amount	0	1	2	3			Subscore
	None	Light	Moderate	Heavy			
Tissue type	0	1	2	3	4		Subscore
	Closed	Epithelial tissue	Granulation tissue	Slough	Necrotic tissue		
							Total score

Length × width
Measure the greatest length (head to toe) and the greatest width (side to side) using a centimeter ruler. Multiply these two measurements (length x width) to obtain an estimate of surface area in square centimeters (cm²). Do not guess! Always use a centimeter ruler and always use the same method each time the ulcer is measured.

Exudate amount
Estimate the amount of exudate (drainage) present after removal of the dressing and before applying any topical agent to the ulcer. Estimate the exudate as none, light, moderate, or heavy.

Tissue type
This refers to the types of tissue that are present in the wound (ulcer) bed. Score as a "4" if there is any necrotic tissue present. Score as a "3" if there is any amount of slough present and necrotic tissue is absent. Score as a "2" if the wound is clean and contains granulation tissue. A superficial wound that is reepithelializing is scored as a "1." When the wound is closed, score as a "0."

>**4-Necrotic tissue (eschar):** Black, brown, or tan tissue that adheres firmly to the wound bed or ulcer edges and may be either firmer or softer than surrounding tissue.
>**3-Slough:** Yellow or white tissue that adheres to the ulcer bed in strings or thick clumps or is mucinous.
>**2-Granulation tissue:** Pink or beefy red tissue with a shiny, moist, granular appearance.
>**1-Epithelial tissue:** For superficial ulcers, new pink or shiny tissue (skin) that grows in from the edges or as islands on the ulcer surface.
>**0-Closed/resurfaced:** The wound is completely covered with epithelium (new skin).

PUSH tool version 3.0, © 1998 National Pressure Ulcer Advisory Panel, Reston, Va.; used with permission.

Appendix F: Decision tree: Pressure ulcers

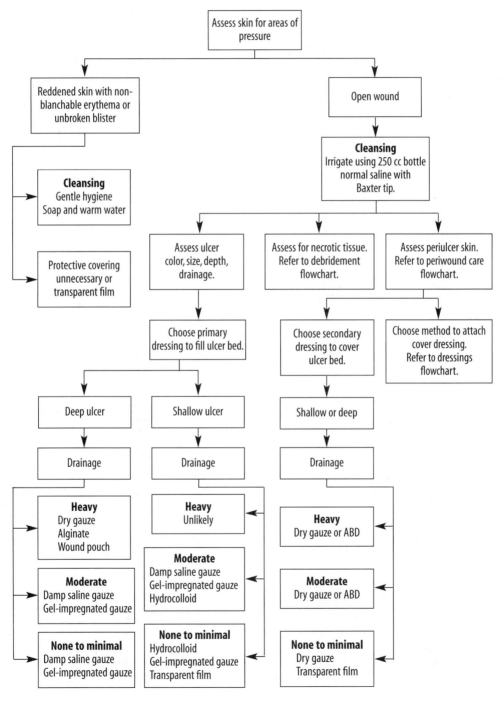

Appendix G: Decision tree: Leg ulcers

All leg ulcers should be assessed for etiology. Venous ulcers require external compression if there are no contraindications.

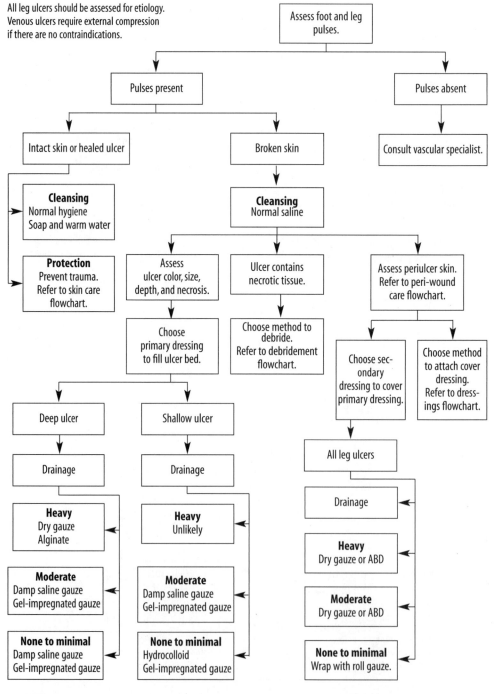

Assess foot and leg pulses.

Pulses present | Pulses absent

Intact skin or healed ulcer | Broken skin | Consult vascular specialist.

Cleansing
Normal hygiene
Soap and warm water

Cleansing
Normal saline

Protection
Prevent trauma.
Refer to skin care flowchart.

Assess ulcer color, size, depth, and necrosis.

Ulcer contains necrotic tissue.

Assess periulcer skin. Refer to peri-wound care flowchart.

Choose primary dressing to fill ulcer bed.

Choose method to debride.
Refer to debridement flowchart.

Choose secondary dressing to cover primary dressing.

Choose method to attach cover dressing. Refer to dressings flowchart.

Deep ulcer | Shallow ulcer

All leg ulcers

Drainage | Drainage

Drainage

Heavy
Dry gauze
Alginate

Heavy
Unlikely

Heavy
Dry gauze or ABD

Moderate
Damp saline gauze
Gel-impregnated gauze

Moderate
Damp saline gauze
Gel-impregnated gauze

Moderate
Dry gauze or ABD

None to minimal
Damp saline gauze
Gel-impregnated gauze

None to minimal
Hydrocolloid
Gel-impregnated gauze

None to minimal
Wrap with roll gauze.

Appendix H: **Decision tree: Surgical wounds**

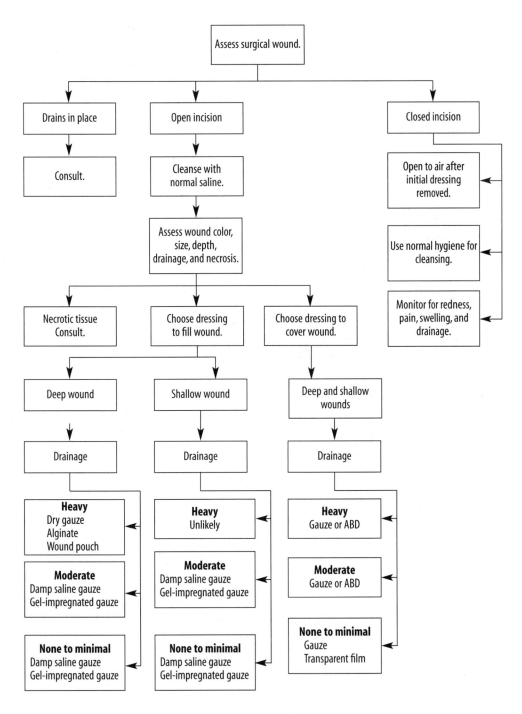

Appendix I: Decision tree: Peri-wound care

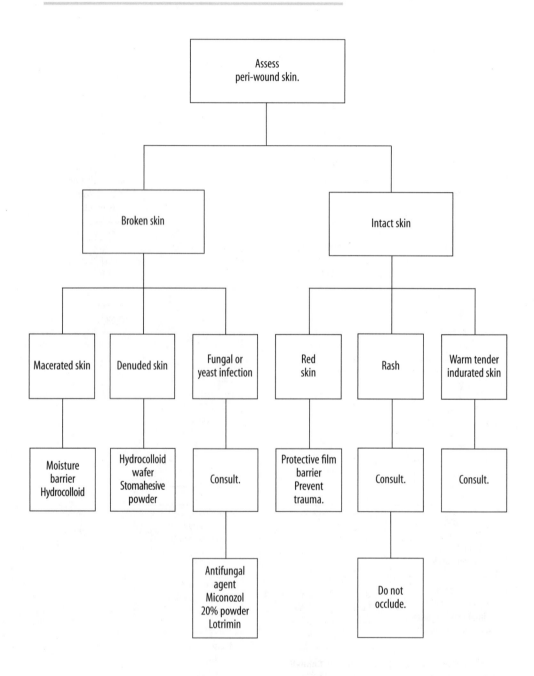

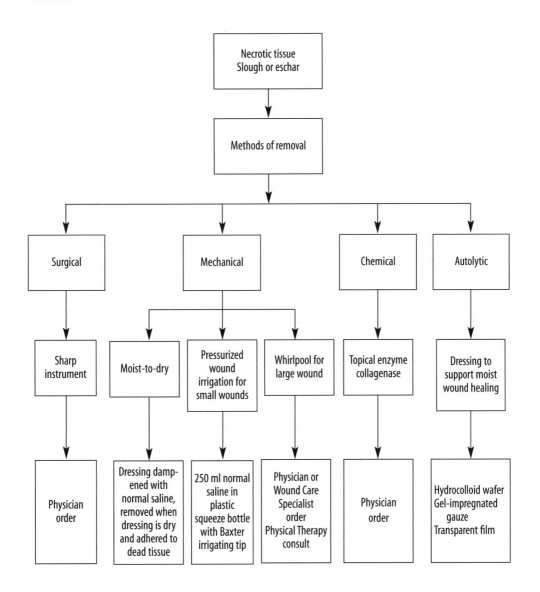

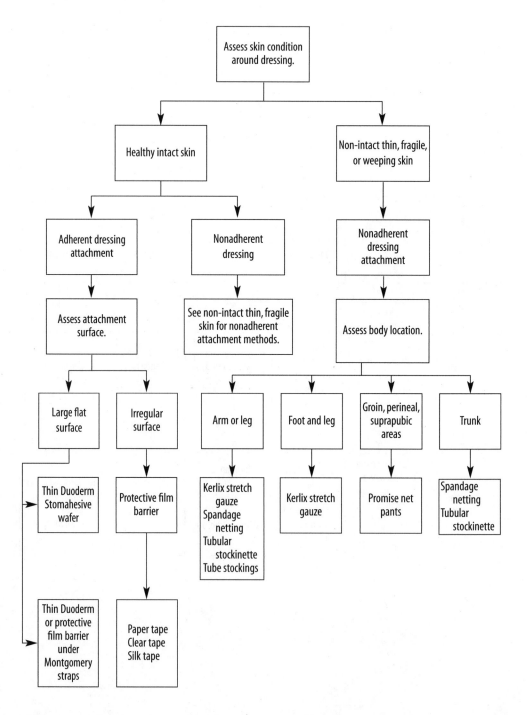

Appendix L: Decision tree: Pressure ulcer prevention

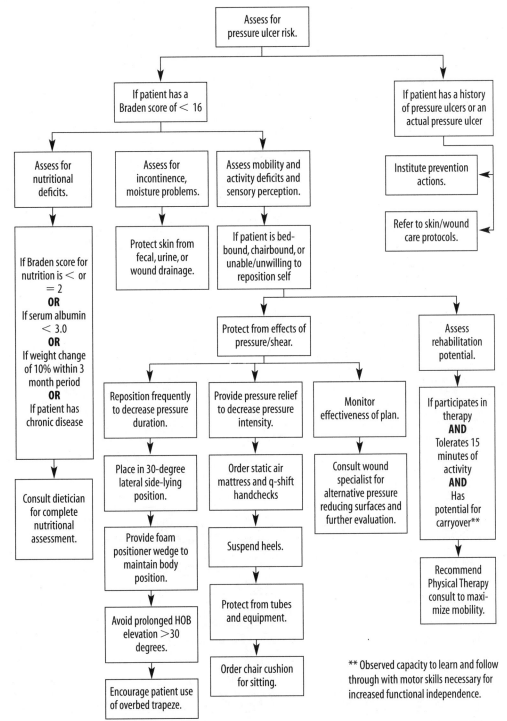

Assess for pressure ulcer risk.

If patient has a Braden score of < 16

If patient has a history of pressure ulcers or an actual pressure ulcer

Assess for nutritional deficits.

Assess for incontinence, moisture problems.

Assess mobility and activity deficits and sensory perception.

Institute prevention actions.

Refer to skin/wound care protocols.

If Braden score for nutrition is < or = 2 **OR** If serum albumin < 3.0 **OR** If weight change of 10% within 3 month period **OR** If patient has chronic disease

Protect skin from fecal, urine, or wound drainage.

If patient is bed-bound, chairbound, or unable/unwilling to reposition self

Protect from effects of pressure/shear.

Assess rehabilitation potential.

Consult dietician for complete nutritional assessment.

Reposition frequently to decrease pressure duration.

Provide pressure relief to decrease pressure intensity.

Monitor effectiveness of plan.

If participates in therapy **AND** Tolerates 15 minutes of activity **AND** Has potential for carryover**

Place in 30-degree lateral side-lying position.

Order static air mattress and q-shift handchecks

Consult wound specialist for alternative pressure reducing surfaces and further evaluation.

Provide foam positioner wedge to maintain body position.

Suspend heels.

Recommend Physical Therapy consult to maximize mobility.

Avoid prolonged HOB elevation >30 degrees.

Protect from tubes and equipment.

Encourage patient use of overbed trapeze.

Order chair cushion for sitting.

** Observed capacity to learn and follow through with motor skills necessary for increased functional independence.

275

Appendix M: Patient admission database

<table>
<tr><td rowspan="3">Wayne State University
Detroit Medical Center
Patient Admission Database</td><td>☐ DRH   ☒ HAR
☐ HTZ   ☐ HVS
☐ SIN   ☐ GRC</td><td>*Brown, Janella*
04592036
10-7-71
Feldspar, Jasper MD
Arrival date: *01/01/00*   Time: *1400*</td></tr>
</table>

Section I General information and orientation

Admit/Transfer from: ☒ Home   ☐ Observation   ☐ ECF   ☐ Another hospital:
☐ OR/PACU, Same Day   ☐ UCC/ED   ☐ Clinic   ☐ Other:

Information given by: ☒ Patient   ☒ Family Member   ☐ Patient unresponsive/no family present   ☐ Other:
Emergency contact/Relationship: *Ella Brown, Mother*   Daytime # *(313) 555-5678*   Evening #
Patient's Legal Guardian/Relationship: Daytime #:   Evening #:

Orientation to room/environment: ☒ ID/Allergy band   ☒ Call light   ☒ Smoking policy   ☒ Telephone   ☒ TV
☒ Visiting hours   ☒ Bed controls   ☒ Cellular phone policy   ☒ Patient rights

Disposition of property: ☒ Sent home   ☐ With patient   Height: *5'4"*   ☒ appr   Weight: *112 #*   ☐ appr *Actual*

Shaded area may be completed by the patient or family

Section II Reason for hospitalization?

PATIENT MEDICAL HISTORY (check all that apply)   ☐ No problems
Do you have or have you had: **Describe**

	Describe
☐ Neurological problems? for example: headaches, dizziness, fainting, or head injury	
☒ Numbness/tingling, paralysis, seizures, or tremors?	*Legs paralyzed since accident 4 years ago*
☐ Problems with your eyes? for example: glaucoma or cataract	
☐ Problems with your ears, nose, sinuses, or throat?	
☐ Heart disease, heart attack, high blood pressure, or stroke?	
☐ Chest pain, heart palpitations, or a pacemaker?	
☐ Circulation problems, heart valve problems, heart murmur, or blood clots?	
☐ Breathing or lung problems? for example: asthma, bronchitis, emphysema, or TB	
☐ Digestive, gastrointestinal, or abdominal problems?	
☒ Stomach pain, nausea/vomiting, heartburn, or ulcers?	*Sometime heartburn*
☐ Are you always hungry or always thirsty?	
☐ Diabetes or thyroid problems?	
☒ Unintended weight loss or gain of 10 pounds?	*Lost 30 pounds since accident.*
☐ Liver problems? for example: yellow jaundice, ascites, or cirrhosis	
☒ Bowel problems?	*I need help with bowel movements.*
☐ A change in bowel habit, constipation, diarrhea, or blood in stool?	
☐ Last bowel movement?_____	
☐ Ostomy? Type:	
☒ Bladder problems? for example: incontinence, dribbling, urgency, or frequency	*use catheter every 4 hours*
☐ Difficulty starting stream, burning, pain, or blood with urination?	
☐ Kidney problems or kidney stones?	
☐ Genital problems? ☐ Sexually transmitted disease?	
☐ Last menstrual period?_____ ☐ Painful/heavy periods?	
☐ Number of pregnancies_____ Number of live births_____ ☐ Pregnant now?	
☐ Joint, muscle, or bone problems? for example: arthritis or pain/swelling	
☒ Skin problems? for example: rash, sore, itching, bruise easily, or change in moles	*ulcers on buttocks*
☐ Emotional, mental, or psychiatric problems?	
☐ Blood problems, anemia, bleeding, or sickle cell anemia?	
☐ Cancer?	
☐ Recent fever or infection?	

Section III Family history   ☐ No problems

☐ Unknown   ☐ Lung disease   ☒ Hypertension   ☐ Liver disease   ☒ Stroke   ☒ Diabetes
☐ Asthma   ☐ Heart disease   ☐ Kidney disease   ☐ Alcohol abuse   ☐ Cancer   ☐ Other:

Section IV Allergy: Drug/Food/Other   ☒ None   If yes, please describe, including reaction

Section V Latex sensitivity assessment

Have you ever had swelling, itching, or hives on your lips or around your mouth after blowing up a balloon?   ☐ Yes   ☒ No
Have you ever had swelling, itching, or hives after a dental, vaginal, or rectal exam/procedure or after contact with a condom or diaphragm?   ☐ Yes   ☒ No
Have you ever had swelling, itching, hives, runny nose, eye irritation, wheezing, or asthma after contact with latex or rubber products?   ☐ Yes   ☒ No

Section VI Past surgeries, hospitalizations, accidents   ☐ None
If Yes, please describe, including dates, if known
  Appendix 1991
  Car accident 1996

Are you currently being treated for any chronic conditions?   ☐ None
If **Yes**, please describe, including treatments such as physical therapy
  Pressure sore

Do you drink alcohol or beer?	☐ Yes	☒ No	How often? _____	Most recent use? _____
Do you smoke or chew tobacco?	☐ Yes	☒ No	How much? _____	How many years? _____
Do you use marijuana?	☐ Yes	☒ No	How often? _____	Most recent use? _____
Do you use street drugs?	☐ Yes	☒ No	How often? _____	Most recent use? _____

Section VII Present medications   List all types of medicine taken, including home remedies, herbal treatments, store bought/off the shelf, nonprescription and prescription medications.

Name of medication	Amount/Dose	Frequency	Time last taken	Name of medication	Amount/Dose	Frequency	Time last taken
Vicodin	2 tabs	2-3 times/ day	1100				

Section VIII Diet/Nutrition
How is your appetite?   ☐ Excellent   ☐ Good   ☒ Fair   ☐ Poor
Are you on a special diet?   ☒ No   ☐ Yes, type: _____
Do you have problems chewing or swallowing?   ☒ No   ☐ Yes, describe: _____
Do you have loose/missing teeth?   ☒ No   ☐ Yes
If you have dentures, please check: ☐ Upper   ☐ Lower   ☐ Partial   Did you bring them with you?   ☐ Yes   ☐ No

Section IX Perceptual
Hearing   ☒ Normal   ☐ Impaired   ☐ R   ☐ L   ☐ Normal   **Eyesight**   ☐ Normal   ☐ Impaired
Hearing aid   ☐ Left Ear   ☐ Right Ear   ☒ Glasses   ☐ Contacts
What did you bring with you?   ☐ Hearing aid(s)   ☐ Glasses   ☐ Contacts   ☐ Prosthesis

Section X Personal values/Beliefs
Is it important for us to know your religious or cultural background?   ☐ Yes   ☒ No
Would you like assistance contacting someone from a religion or faith tradition?   ☐ Yes   ☒ No
Are there any religious or cultural practices you would like us to be aware of?   ☐ Yes   ☒ No

Section XI Home environment (Anticipated needs/Discharge plan)
☒ Single   ☐ Married   ☐ Separated   ☐ Divorced   ☐ Widowed   ☐ Occupation _____   Retired?   ☐ Yes   ☐ No
Number of dependents? *None*   Who lives at home with you? *Mother*
Are you concerned about the care of dependents or others while you are in the hospital?   ☐ Yes   ☒ No
Has anyone hurt you? Threatened to hurt you? Forced you to engage in unwanted sexual activity?   ☐ Yes   ☒ No

Section XII Activity/Self-care ability
Do you tire easily?   ☒ Yes   ☐ No
Do you need help with any of the following? (Check all that apply)   ☐ None
☐ Getting out of bed   ☐ Toileting   ☐ Medication administration   ☐ Laundry
☐ Walking *Can't walk*   ☐ Dressing   ☐ Cooking   ☐ Housework
☐ Bathing   ☐ Feeding   ☐ Shopping   ☒ Transportation
Who currently helps you at home?   ☐ No one   ☐ Family/Friend   ☐ Home Health Care   ☒ Other: *mother*
Name and phone number: *Ella Brown (313) 555-5678*

What medical equipment and/or supplies do you currently have at home?   ☐ None
☐ Walker   ☒ Wheelchair   ☒ Hospital bed   ☐ Oxygen   ☐ Suction machine
☐ Cane   ☐ Crutches   ☐ Commode   ☐ Respiratory/Breathing equipment   ☐ Ostomy supplies
☐ IV/Feeding pump   ☐ Other equipment or supplies: _____

What company supplies your equipment? _____ *W/F* _____

Remainder of patient admission database to be completed by a registered nurse

Section XIII Coping/Stress tolerance/Self-perception
Do you have any special concerns regarding this hospitalization or illness? [X] No   [ ] Yes, describe:

Have you recently experienced any big changes in your life? [X] No   [ ] Yes, describe:

How do you cope with stressful situations? Describe:

Would you like to talk to someone about your stress management? [X] No   [ ] Yes, describe:

What can we do as caregivers to help you with the health needs that brought you into the hospital? *Heal my sore*

Section XIV Sleep/Rest/Comfort
Do you feel rested after sleep? [ ] Yes   [X] No
[X] Difficulty sleeping, describe: *Awake several times during night*
[ ] Sleeping aids, describe:
Are you currently experiencing pain? [ ] No   [X] Yes, describe: *Dull, aching and throbbing*
            Type: [ ] Acute   [X] Chronic   Pain level ___5___ (VAS Scale 1-10)
How do you manage pain? *Vicodin*

Section XV Venous access device screen
Does the patient have a long-term venous access device? [X] No   [ ] Yes, type/location:
Is there adequate venous access for anticipated therapy? [ ] N/A   [X] Yes   [ ] No   [ ] Unknown

Section XVI Dialysis   [X] N/A   [ ] Physician: Dialysis center:
Type/Location/Age of Access: [ ] HD schedule:
         [ ] CAPD   [ ] CCP   PD exchange times: Liters/Exchange:

Section XVII Braden scale (score of ≤ 18 indicates risk for pressure ulcer development)   **Total:** *13*

Assess	1	2	3	4
Patient's ability to respond to pressure related discomfort	[X] Completely limited	[ ] Very limited	[ ] Slightly limited	[ ] No impairment
Degree to which the patient's skin is exposed to moisture	[ ] Completely moist	[ ] Very moist	[X] Occasionally moist	[ ] Rarely moist
Degree of physical activity the patient is capable of	[ ] Bedfast	[X] Chairfast	[ ] Walks occasionally	[ ] Walks frequently
Patient's ability to change and control body position	[ ] Completely immobile	[ ] Very limited	[X] Slightly limited	[ ] No limitation
Patient's usual food intake pattern	[ ] Very poor	[X] Probably inadequate	[ ] Adequate	[ ] Excellent
Friction/shear of the patient's skin when moving in bed	[ ] Problem	[X] Potential problem	[ ] No apparent problem	

Section XVIII Fall/Injury risk screen (Initiate interventions if ≥ 2 risk factors are present.)
[ ] No risk factors identified at time of admission   [ ] Current ETOH/drug abuse history
[ ] Medication affecting LOC, gait, elimination   [X] Sensory/motor deficit
[ ] General anesthesia within last 24 hours   [ ] General weakness, unsteady gait
[ ] Seizure activity within 1 week of admission   [ ] Restraint use
[ ] New onset/alteration in LOC, mobility, cognition, gait [ ] History of previous fall
[ ] Unable to follow safety instructions, confused, impaired mental status   [ ] Orthostatic hypotension

Section XIX Nutrition screen (Consult dietitian if any risk factors present.)
[ ] No risk factors identified at time of admission   [X] Diagnosis and/or diet implies risk
[ ] Has newly prescribed diet or has questions about current diet   [ ] Is on TPN or tube feedings
[X] Usual food intake pattern appears insufficient   [ ] Difficulty swallowing or chewing
[ ] Has risk of food/drug interaction (that is, MAOI or Coumadin)   [ ] NPO or clear liquid diet ≥ 5 days
[X] Has pressure ulcers and/or Total Braden Score ≤ 18   [X] Open or nonhealing wound
[ ] Has unplanned weight change ± 10# in last 3 months

Section XX Barriers to learning   [X] None
[ ] Vision   [ ] Hearing   [ ] Speech   [ ] Mobility   [ ] Learning disability
[ ] Anxious   [ ] Withdrawn   [ ] Uncooperative [ ] Motivation   [ ] Unable to follow instructions
[ ] Language   [ ] Read/write   [ ] Religious   [ ] Cultural   [ ] Age/Development
[ ] Other:

Section XXI Readiness to learn (Check all that apply.)
[X] Aware of diagnosis   [X] Accepts diagnosis   [X] Requests information   [X] Accepts information
[ ] Unaware of diagnosis   [ ] Denies diagnosis   [ ] Avoids information   [ ] Other:
How do you learn best?   [ ] Written   [X] Verbal [X] Demonstration   [ ] Other:

Section XXII

Care Management Specialist Screen
Consult if any risk factors present.

☐ No medical insurance ☐ No prescription coverage
☐ Military: ☐ CHAMPUS ☐ Veteran
☐ Two or more ED visits/hospitalizations in the past 3 months
☐ Discharged from hospital within 72 hours
☒ Currently receiving treatment for chronic illness or condition; specify: *Pressure ulcer*
☐ Barriers to treatment (Patient/Parent/Child) check all that apply: ☐ Language ☐ Cognitive ☐ Sensory ☐ Physical
☐ Transferred from another facility; type/name:
☒ Needs assistance with ADLS
☒ Current or past use of Home Health Care Agency; Agency Name: *Renaissance Home Care*
☐ May need special placement after discharge
☐ Nursing home ☐ Rehab ☐ Foster care ☐ Hospice
☐ Other:
☒ May need post acute services (check all that apply)
☐ PT/OT therapy ☒ Home care
☐ Respiratory care ☒ Medical equipment/supplies
☐ Other:

Referral to CMS ☒ *7 - 700* **Time:** *1400* **Initials:** *WBC*

Section XXIII

Clinical Social Worker Screen
Consult if any risk factors present.

☐ Patient unable to provide information, family unavailable
☐ Financial concerns (disability, income, vocational, insurance)
☐ Problems with obtaining medications/treatments
☐ Problems with adjustment to illness and/or treatment
☐ Assess for substance abuse history and need for treatment
☒ Assess need for self help, emotional support group
☐ Lives in a shelter or is homeless or displaced
☒ Evaluate home situation (specify in comments area)
☐ Patient/family advocacy, crisis intervention, conflict management
☐ Suspected physical emotional abuse, neglect, rape

☐ Identify J. Doe
☐ Locate family/caregiver
☐ Legal concerns/guardianship issues
☐ Failure to thrive
☐ Death/dying/loss/grieving issues
☐ Assess need for community resources
☐ Transportation needs
☐ Cares for dependents with special needs
☐ Psychiatric issues/emotional disorder
☐ Victim of crime

Referral to CMS ☒ *7-7-00* **Time:** *1400* **Initials:** *WBC*

Time	COMMENTS
1400	*Pt. Lives with mother since accident. Mother has been managing wound care for pressure ulcer.*
	Pt. Has been sleeping on a regular mattress and has a foam WC cushion.
	Pt. Will need home nursing and supplies including dressings, a mattress overlay, and a pressure reducing wheelchair
	cushion.

Time	Signature/Title	Initials	Time	Signature/Title	Initials
1400	*Willa Beth Cummings RN*	*WBC*			

Wayne State University
Detroit Medical Center
Patient Outcome Record
Tissue integrity, impaired: Pressure ulcer

☒ Nursing diagnosis   ☐ Collaborative problem

Brown, Janella
04592036
10-7-11
Feldspar, Jasper MD

Outcomes mutually set with patient/family on admission
☒ Yes   ☐ No If no,. state rationale _____

☐ Initiated by: Initial/date/time SW RN 1/7/00 1800 Outcome statement	1/7/00 Date	1/8/00 Date	1/9/00 Date	1/10/00 Date	1/11/00 Date	1/12/00 Date	1/13/00 Date
1. Ulcer bed moist	☐ Met ☒ Unmet	☒ Met ☐ Unmet	☒ Met ☐ Unmet	☒ Met ☐ Unmet	☒ Met ☐ Unmet	☒ Met ☐ Unmet	☒ Met ☐ Unmet
2. Ulcer bed beefy red color over entire surface	☐ Met ☒ Unmet	☐ Met ☒ Unmet	☐ Met ☒ Unmet	☐ Met ☒ Unmet	☐ Met ☒ Unmet	☐ Met ☒ Unmet	☒ Met ☐ Unmet
3. Evidence of new skin growth at borders of wound	☐ Met ☒ Unmet	☐ Met ☒ Unmet	☐ Met ☒ Unmet	☐ Met ☒ Unmet	☐ Met ☒ Unmet	☒ Met ☐ Unmet	☒ Met ☐ Unmet
4. Ulcer length, width, and depth decreased in size from baseline	☐ Met ☒ Unmet	☐ Met ☒ Unmet	☐ Met ☒ Unmet	☐ Met ☒ Unmet	☐ Met ☒ Unmet	☐ Met ☒ Unmet	☐ Met ☒ Unmet
5. Skin surrounding ulcer not indurated, inflamed, warm, or painful to touch	☐ Met ☒ Unmet	☐ Met ☒ Unmet	☐ Met ☒ Unmet	☒ Met ☐ Unmet	☒ Met ☐ Unmet	☒ Met ☐ Unmet	☒ Met ☐ Unmet
6. Skin surrounding ulcer not macerated (waterlogged)	☐ Met ☒ Unmet	☐ Met ☒ Unmet	☒ Met ☐ Unmet	☒ Met ☐ Unmet	☒ Met ☐ Unmet	☒ Met ☐ Unmet	☒ Met ☐ Unmet
7. Adequate caloric and protein intake	☐ Met ☒ Unmet	☐ Met ☒ Unmet	☒ Met ☐ Unmet	☒ Met ☐ Unmet	☒ Met ☐ Unmet	☒ Met ☐ Unmet	☒ Met ☐ Unmet

☐ **Outcomes met: Initials:** _____ **Date:** _____ **Time:** _____

☒ **Instructions given to ⟨patient⟩/⟨other:⟩** *and Mother* _____

☒ **Home care**

☐ **Community resources**

☐ **Other**

Teaching Interventions

1. Teach:
   a.) Signs and symptoms of a healing pressure ulcer.

   b.) Individualized wound treatment regime.

   c.) Prevention techniques
       -repositioning q 2 hours or less according to tissue tolerance and prevent friction
       -suspending heels off surface of bed
       -pressure relieving devices

   d.) Adequate nutritional needs to facilitate wound healing.

   e.) Hygiene practices to prevent infection and skin breakdown.

   f.) Medications (purpose, dosage, route, frequency, and side effects).

   g.) Signs and symptoms to report to a health care professional (e.g., wound infection, urinary tract infection, and inability to maintain adequate fluid intake).

   h.) When and where to receive follow-up care.

Optional teaching interventions

Initial	Signature/Title	Initial	Signature/Title	Initial	Signature/Title
SW	Susan Wiltose RN				
JB	Jim Bates				
RR	Raquel Robertson				

Appendix O: Patient education outcome record

Brown, Janella
04592036
10-7-71
Feldspar, Jasper, MD

Learner (Check all that apply)
- [x] Patient
- [ ] Family
- [x] Parent/~~Guardian~~
- [ ] Other

Wayne State University
Detroit Medical Center
Patient Education Outcome Record
Tissue integrity, impaired: Pressure ulcer

Teaching Method Codes (Check all that apply)
- [ ] Audio/Video
- [ ] Telephone
- [ ] Class
- [ ] Written/Handouts
- [x] Verbal
- [x] Other *Demo*

Outcome statement	Date 1/7/00	Date 1/8/00	Date 1/9/00	Date 1/10/00	Date 1/11/00	Date 1/12/00	Date 1/13/00
1. Verbalizes understanding regarding repositioning and pressure relief interventions	☐ Met ☒ Needs reinforcement ☐ Not initiated	☐ Met ☒ Needs reinforcement ☐ Not initiated	☐ Met ☒ Needs reinforcement ☐ Not initiated	☐ Met ☒ Needs reinforcement ☐ Not initiated	☐ Met ☒ Needs reinforcement ☐ Not initiated	☐ Met ☒ Needs reinforcement ☐ Not initiated	☐ Met ☒ Needs reinforcement ☐ Not initiated
2. Verbalizes understanding regarding adequate nutrition needs	☐ Met ☐ Needs reinforcement ☒ Not initiated	☐ Met ☒ Needs reinforcement ☐ Not initiated	☐ Met ☒ Needs reinforcement ☐ Not initiated	☐ Met ☒ Needs reinforcement ☐ Not initiated	☐ Met ☒ Needs reinforcement ☐ Not initiated	☐ Met ☒ Needs reinforcement ☐ Not initiated	☐ Met ☒ Needs reinforcement ☐ Not initiated
3. Verbalizes characteristics of healing	☐ Met ☐ Needs reinforcement ☒ Not initiated	☐ Met ☒ Needs reinforcement ☐ Not initiated	☐ Met ☒ Needs reinforcement ☐ Not initiated	☐ Met ☒ Needs reinforcement ☐ Not initiated	☐ Met ☒ Needs reinforcement ☐ Not initiated	☐ Met ☒ Needs reinforcement ☐ Not initiated	☐ Met ☒ Needs reinforcement ☐ Not initiated
4. Verbalizes and demonstrates proper technique to complete treatment regime	☐ Met ☐ Needs reinforcement ☒ Not initiated	☐ Met ☒ Needs reinforcement ☐ Not initiated	☒ Met ☐ Needs reinforcement ☐ Not initiated	☐ Met ☐ Needs reinforcement ☐ Not initiated	☐ Met ☐ Needs reinforcement ☐ Not initiated	☐ Met ☐ Needs reinforcement ☐ Not initiated	☐ Met ☐ Needs reinforcement ☐ Not initiated
	☐ Met ☐ Needs reinforcement ☐ Not initiated	☐ Met ☐ Needs reinforcement ☐ Not initiated	☐ Met ☐ Needs reinforcement ☐ Not initiated	☐ Met ☐ Needs reinforcement ☐ Not initiated	☐ Met ☐ Needs reinforcement ☐ Not initiated	☐ Met ☐ Needs reinforcement ☐ Not initiated	☐ Met ☐ Needs reinforcement ☐ Not initiated
	☐ Met ☐ Needs reinforcement ☐ Not initiated	☐ Met ☐ Needs reinforcement ☐ Not initiated	☐ Met ☐ Needs reinforcement ☐ Not initiated	☐ Met ☐ Needs reinforcement ☐ Not initiated	☐ Met ☐ Needs reinforcement ☐ Not initiated	☐ Met ☐ Needs reinforcement ☐ Not initiated	☐ Met ☐ Needs reinforcement ☐ Not initiated
	☐ Met ☐ Needs reinforcement ☐ Not initiated	☐ Met ☐ Needs reinforcement ☐ Not initiated	☐ Met ☐ Needs reinforcement ☐ Not initiated	☐ Met ☐ Needs reinforcement ☐ Not initiated	☐ Met ☐ Needs reinforcement ☐ Not initiated	☐ Met ☐ Needs reinforcement ☐ Not initiated	☐ Met ☐ Needs reinforcement ☐ Not initiated

Interventions

1. Assess tissue characteristics and treatment plan according to Skin and Wound Flowcharts. Provide moist environment to facilitate wound healing.

2. Cleanse ulcer bed using normal saline delivered under pressure, 4 centimeters (1 inch) from surface of ulcer.

3. Assess and document wound:
    a. Location
    b. Size in centimeters on initial assessment, weekly, or at each hydrocolloid dressing change.
    c. Wound bed color and drainage
    d. Surrounding tissue for induration, maceration, erythema, pain, and warmth.
    e. Pain during dressing changes or positioning.

4. Institute nursing interventions for prevention of further breakdown:
    a. Provide pressure reduction (SofCare, elevate heels, SofCare cushion).
    b. Suspend heels with pillows or vascular boots.
    c. Maintain head of bed elevation at the lowest degree consistent with medical condition to limit shear force on sacral area.
    d. Protect tissue from incontinence.
    e. Reposition q 2 hours or less based on tissue tolerance. Use foam wedge positioner.
    f. Alternate elevation of cardiac chair while sitting q 15 to 30 minutes

5. Consult dietitian for nutritional assessment.

6. Maintain/provide adequate caloric and protein intake to facilitate wound healing.

Date	Site	Stage (I thru IV, or Eschar/Slough)	Size (cm)	Dressing/Therapy
1/1/00	Sacrum	Slough	10 X 12 cm	Moist saline
1/1/00	Rt heel	I	2X 2 cm	Suspend heels
1/1/00	Left heel	I	2X 3 cm	Suspend heels

Optional interventions

☐ Pad mouth, face, and ears to protect from tubes/ties.

☒ Consult for complex skin or wound issues and/or specialty bed needs ☒ APN ☒ ET Nurse

Consult ☒ Discharge planner
       ☒ Social worker
       ☐ Pharmacist
       ☒ Dietician
       ☒ PT/OT (with physician order)

Appendix P: Acute care flow record

Wayne State University Detroit Medical Center **Acute Care Flow Record**	☐ DRH ☒ HAR ☐ HTZ ☐ HVS ☐ SIN ☐ GRC	Brown, Janella 04592036 10/7/11 Feldspar, Jasper MD	**Date:** 01/08/00

Section 1	0700-1859		1900-0659
Activity	0700-1500	1501-2300	2301-0659
Up ad lib			
Up in chair			
Bathroom privileges			
Bed rest	✓	✓	✓
Repositions self	✓	✓	✓
Turn/Reposition q 2 hours			
Range of motion			
Side rails up x ?	x 2	x 2	x 2
Commode			
Air mattress hand-checked	✓	✓	✓

Self-care / Assist	0700-1500	1501-2300	2301-0659
Feeds self	✓	✓	
Feeds self with assistance			
Complete feed			
Performs own ADL			
ADL with assist	✓	✓	
Complete care			

Section II Nutrition/Metabolic

Breakfast ☐ 0% ☑ <50% ☐ >50% ☐ All ☐ NPO
Diet type (optional)/comments: *Regular Ensure*
Lunch ☐ 0% ☑ <50% ☐ >50% ☐ All ☐ NPO
Diet type (optional)/comments: *Regular Ensure*
Dinner ☐ 0% ☐ <50% ☑ >50% ☐ All ☐ NPO
Diet type (optional)/comments: *Regular Ensure*
☐ Fluid restrictions

Section III Assistive devices/Special equipment
☐ Telemetry ☐ Crutches/cane ☐ Walker ☒ Wheelchair ☐ Commode
☐ I.V. pumps ☒ 1 ☐ 2 ☐ 3 ☐ 4 ☐ Feeding pump
☐ Adaptive device-type: ☐ Specialty chair-type:
☐ Traction-type/location: ☒ Specialty bed-type: *Acucair*
☐ Splint/brace-location: ☐ Air mattress ☐ Chair cushion
☒ Trapeze ☒ Compression Device
☐ Other: ☐ Anti-embolitic Stockings

Section IV Safety/Care interventions
Precautions | **Isolation**
☐ Patient Injury Prevention Plan ☐ Type:
☐ Restraints — See Restraint Flow Record ☐ Type:
☐ Other: ☐ Type:

Section V I.V. therapy

I.V. site-location/type Date placed	Dressing Δ Type/Time Initials	D/C time Initials	I.V. start Location/Type Time/Initials
Location Date placed Rt AR 1-7-00 Type *peripheral*			
Location Date placed Type			
Location Date placed Type			
Location Date placed Type			

I.V. site location codes

rt	Right	angio	Angiocath	SubQ	Subcutaneous
lt	Left	SL	Saline lock	Grsg	Groshong
h	Hand	hl	Heparin lock	Hkmn	Hickman
wr	Wrist	M/L	Midline	QC	Quinton
AR	Arm	PICC	Peripherally inserted central catheter	IVAD	Implanted vascular access device
antecub	Antecubital				
ft	Foot				
lg	Leg				
fem	Femoral	MC	Minicath		
abd	Abdomen	IC	Intracath		
SC	Subclavian	CL	Central line		
ej	External jugular				
ij	Internal jugular				

I.V. dressing codes
B = Band-Aid T = Transparent G = Gauze

Section VI Specimen collection (optional)

Type	Time	Initials
urine - C&S	0900	SW
C&S - Wound	1000	SW

Section VII Dressing change/Treatments (Time/initial in box)

Location/Type	0700-1500	1501-2300	2301-0659
Sacral wound			

Section VIII Patient activity off unit (optional)

Time	Signature/Title	Initials	Time	Signature/Title	Initials
1500	Susan Wiltose RN	SW			
2300	Jim Bates RN	JB			
0639	Raquel Robertson	RR			

0700-1859	1900-0659

Gastrointestinal core assessment
☐ *Findings WNL: Mucous membranes moist, pink, intact, abdomen non-tender, nondistended, bowel sounds positive all 4 quadrants*

Variance/Additional findings

☐ Nausea ☐ Vomiting
☐ Diarrhea ☒ Constipation

Bowel sounds	rt	lt
Upper	+	+
Lower	+	+

Bowel sound codes: +active ↓hypoactive ↑hyperactive (—)absent

Mucous membranes: ☐ Dry ☐ Pale ☐ Lesions _____
Abdomen ☐ Rigid ☐ Distended ☐ Tender, location _____
☐ Incontinent of stool ☐ Rectal pouch ☐ Ostomy-type _____

	Purpose		Status	Drainage
☐ NGT	☐ Feeding	☐ Drain		
☐ GT	☐ Feeding	☐ Drain		
☐ J tube	☐ Feeding	☐ Drain		
☐ SBFT	☐ Feeding	☐ Drain		
☐ Other:				

Comments: *Pt. has daily BM. No BM today. Manual extraction. Started on Metamucil.*

Genital/Urinary core assessment
☐ *Findings WNL: Voiding clear, yellow to amber urine, no flank pain*

Variance/Additional findings
☐ Anuric ☐ Oliguric <800 ml/day ☐ Polyuric >2500ml/day
☐ Burning with urination ☐ Pain with urination☐ Bladder distention
☐ Urine: ☐ Hematuria ☐ Foul odor ☐ Cloudy ☐ Urinary retention
  ☐ Incontinent ☐ Frequency ☐ Urgency ☐ Nocturia
☐ Genital edema ☐ Genital discharge-describe _____
☐ Indwelling catheter: Status_____ Drainage_____
☐ Condom catheter: Status_____ Drainage_____
☐ Suprapubic catheter: Status_____ Drainage_____
☐ Nephrostomy: Status_____ Drainage_____
☐ Ostomy-type _____

Comments: *Self cath q 4 hr.*

Other tubes and drains

☐ Dialysis access-type/location:

Other	Location	Status	Drainage
☐ Hemovac _____			
☐ Penrose _____			
☐ J-P _____			
☐ J-P _____			
☐ _____			
☐ _____			

Comments:

Gastrointestinal core assessment
☐ *Findings WNL: Mucous membranes moist, pink, intact, abdomen non-tender, nondistended, bowel sounds positive all 4 quadrants*

Variance/Additional findings ☒ No change from previous assessment

☐ Nausea ☐ Vomiting
☐ Diarrhea ☐ Constipation

Bowel sounds	rt	lt
Upper	+	+
Lower	+	+

Bowel sound codes: +active ↓hypoactive ↑hyperactive (—)absent

Mucous membranes: ☐ Dry ☐ Pale ☐ Lesions _____
Abdomen ☐ Rigid ☐ Distended ☐ Tender, location _____
☐ Incontinent of stool ☐ Rectal pouch ☐ Ostomy-type _____

	Purpose		Status	Drainage
☐ NGT	☐ Feeding	☐ Drain		
☐ GT	☐ Feeding	☐ Drain		
☐ J tube	☐ Feeding	☐ Drain		
☐ SBFT	☐ Feeding	☐ Drain		
☐ Other:				

Comments:

Genital/Urinary core assessment
☐ *Findings WNL: Voiding clear, yellow to amber urine, no flank pain*

Variance/Additional findings ☒ No change from previous assessment
☐ Anuric ☐ Oliguric <800 ml/day ☐ Polyuric >2500ml/day
☐ Burning with urination ☐ Pain with urination☐ Bladder distention
☐ Urine: ☐ Hematuria ☐ Foul odor ☐ Cloudy ☐ Urinary retention
  ☐ Incontinent ☐ Frequency ☐ Urgency ☐ Nocturia
☐ Genital edema ☐ Genital discharge-describe _____
☐ Indwelling catheter: Status_____ Drainage_____
☐ Condom catheter: Status_____ Drainage_____
☐ Suprapubic catheter: Status_____ Drainage_____
☐ Nephrostomy: Status_____ Drainage_____
☐ Ostomy-type _____

Comments:

Other tubes and drains

☐ Dialysis access-type/location: ☐ No change from previous assessment

Other	Location	Status	Drainage
☐ Hemovac _____			
☐ Penrose _____			
☐ J-P _____			
☐ J-P _____			
☐ _____			
☐ _____			

Comments:

Feeding tube/Drain status codes						Drainage/Character codes								
Pa	Patent	cont sxn	Continuous suction	Cl	Clamped	bu	Bulb	R	Red	GRN	Green	ser	Serous	cly	Cloudy
NP	Nonpatent	inter sxn	Intermittent suction	grty	Gravity			Y	Yellow	BRN	Brown	c-grd	Coffee ground	N	None
		dc	Discontinued	WS	Waterseal			B	Black	bldy	Bloody	p	Purulent	X	No stoma

*****Remainder of ACFR must be completed by a registered nurse.*****

0700-1859	1900-0659
I.V. site assessment	**I.V. site assessment**

I.V. site location & assessment			Cap/Tubing Δ			I.V. site location & assessment			Cap/Tubing Δ		
#1 *Rt AR*	☒ WNL	☐ Variance:		☐ Cap	☐ Tubing	#1 *Rt AR*	☒ WNL	☐ Variance:		☐ Cap	☐ Tubing
#2	☐ WNL	☐ Variance:		☐ Cap	☐ Tubing	#2	☐ WNL	☐ Variance:		☐ Cap	☐ Tubing
#3	☐ WNL	☐ Variance:		☐ Cap	☐ Tubing	#3	☐ WNL	☐ Variance:		☐ Cap	☐ Tubing
#4	☐ WNL	☐ Variance:		☐ Cap	☐ Tubing	#4	☐ WNL	☐ Variance:		☐ Cap	☐ Tubing

I.V. site assessment variance codes: **P** Pain **R** Redness **S** Swelling **I** Infiltrated

---

Neurological/Muscular core assessment
☐ *Findings WNL: Alert, oriented x3, moves all extremities*

Variance/Additional findings
☐ Altered LOC ☐ Disoriented/Confused ☒ AO3
Facial: ☐ Asymmetry ☒ Symmetry
Pupils: ☐ Unequal ☐ Non-reactive ☒ PERRLA
Chewing: ☐ Difficulty ☐ WNL Swallowing: ☐ Difficulty ☒ WNL
Gait: ☐ Unsteady ☐ Steady *NA*
☐ Sensory impairment ☒ Paralysis - describe: *Below waist*

Extremity	rt	lt	Motor strength:	[F] Fair
Upper	6	6	[nl] Normal	[P] Poor
Lower	0	0	[G] Good	[O] Absent

Comments: *Pt in MVA 4 yrs ago - paralyzed from waist down - able to transfer bed to chair with assistance.*

Neurological/Muscular core assessment
☐ *Findings WNL: Alert, oriented x3, moves all extremities*

Variance/Additional findings ☒ No change from previous assessment
☐ Altered LOC ☐ Disoriented/Confused ☐ AO3
Facial: ☐ Asymmetry ☐ Symmetry
Pupils: ☐ Unequal ☐ Non-reactive ☐ PERRLA
Chewing: ☐ Difficulty ☐ WNL Swallowing: ☐ Difficulty ☐ WNL
Gait: ☐ Unsteady ☐ Steady
☐ Sensory impairment ☐ Paralysis - describe:

Extremity	rt	lt	Motor strength:	[F] Fair
Upper			[nl] Normal	[P] Poor
Lower			[G] Good	[O] Absent

Comments:

Motor strength grading scale:
Normal = Full ROM against gravity with maximum resistance provided by examiner
Good = Full ROM against gravity with moderate resistance provided by examiner
Fair = Full ROM against gravity with minimum resistance, to full ROM with slight assistance from examiner
Poor = Full ROM with gravity eliminated to partial ROM with gravity eliminated
Absent = No visible or palpable muscle contraction, muscle is paralyzed

Breath sounds codes:	
clr clear	**co** congested
crkl crackles	**iw** inspiratory wheeze
rhon rhonchi	**ew** expiratory wheeze
ab absent	**dm** diminished

Respiratory core assessment
☒ *Findings WNL: respirations regular and unlabored, breath sounds clear, airway patent*

Variance/Additional findings
Respirations: ☐ Irregular ☐ Labored
☐ O$_2$ therapy _____
☐ Chest tube: Status_____ Drainage_____
☐ Cough: ☐ Nonproductive ☐ Productive
Sputum/secretions-color_____
☐ Thick ☐ Thin ☐ Frothy ☐ Mucoid
☐ Copious ☐ Moderate ☐ Scant ☐ None
☐ Suctioning required
Artificial airway ☐ OET ☐ NET ☐ Trach size/mode

Comments:

Breath sounds

Respiratory core assessment
☒ *Findings WNL: respirations regular and unlabored, breath sounds clear, airway patent*

Variance/Additional findings ☒ No change from previous assessment
Respirations: ☐ Irregular ☐ Labored
☐ O$_2$ therapy _____
☐ Chest tube: Status_____ Drainage_____
☐ Cough: ☐ Nonproductive ☐ Productive
Sputum/secretions-color_____
☐ Thick ☐ Thin ☐ Frothy ☐ Mucoid
☐ Copious ☐ Moderate ☐ Scant ☐ None
☐ Suctioning required
Artificial airway ☐ OET ☐ NET ☐ Trach size/mode

Comments:

Breath sounds

Cardiovascular core assessment
☐ *Findings WNL: Heart rate and rhythm regular*

Variance/Additional findings
☐ Irregular rate/rhythm
Abnormal heart sound: ☐ Murmur ☐ Extra sound ☐ None
Capillary refill: ☐ > 3 seconds ☐ < 3 seconds
Diminished/absent peripheral pulse: ☐ rt ☐ lt ☐ WNL
Calf tenderness: ☐ rt ☐ lt ☐ None
Edema: ☐ Anasarca ☐ None

Extremity	rt	lt	Edema scale:	0 - Absent (None)
Upper			1 - Mild (<0.6 cm)	3 - Severe (> 1.3 cm)
Lower	/	/	2 - Moderate (0.7-1.3 cm)	NP - (Nonpitting)

Comments: *Pt. spends most of time in WC - legs depend. Slight edema always present - Pt states.*

Cardiovascular core assessment
☐ *Findings WNL: Heart rate and rhythm regular*

Variance/Additional findings ☒ No change from previous assessment
☐ Irregular rate/rhythm
Abnormal heart sound: ☐ Murmur ☐ Extra sound ☐ None
Capillary refill: ☐ > 3 seconds ☐ < 3 seconds
Diminished/absent peripheral pulse: ☐ rt ☐ lt ☐ WNL
Calf tenderness: ☐ rt ☐ lt ☐ None
Edema: ☐ Anasarca ☐ None

Extremity	rt	lt	Edema scale:	0 - Absent (None)
Upper			1 - Mild (<0.6 cm)	3 - Severe (> 1.3 cm)
Lower			2 - Moderate (0.7-1.3 cm)	NP - (Nonpitting)

Comments:

0700-1859	1900-0659

Psychosocial core assessment
☒ *Findings WNL: Responds to care, willing to participate in care, makes decisions and suggestions about care*

Psychosocial core assessment
☒ *Findings WNL: Responds to care, willing to participate in care, makes decisions and suggestions about care*

Variance/additional findings	Variance/additional findings ☐ No change from previous assessment
☐ Altered neurostatus ☐ Other variance(s) Describe:	☐ Altered neurostatus ☐ Other variance(s) Describe:

Comments: | Comments:

Rest and comfort core assessment
☐ *Findings WNL: Pain free, reported VAS pain score <5, and/or satisfaction with current pain control*

Rest and comfort core assessment
☐ *Findings WNL: Pain free, reported VAS pain score <5, and/or satisfaction with current pain control*

Variance/Additional findings	Variance/Additional findings ☐ No change from previous assessment
☒ Reported VAS _7_ ☒ Sleep disturbance	☒ Reported VAS _5_ ☐ Sleep disturbance
☐ Behavior cues indicative of pain/ Other (describe in Comments)	☐ Behavior cues indicative of pain/ Other (describe in Comments)

Comments: *Reports pain and difficulty sleeping. Troubled with oral meds — minor relief. IV push MS given c̄ good results.*

Comments:

Braden scale   (score of ≤ 18 indicates risk for pressure ulcer development; initiate interventions)   **Total** _15_

Assess	1	2	3	4
Patient's ability to respond to pressure related discomfort	☐ Completely limited	☐ Very limited	☒ Slightly limited	☐ No impairment
Degree to which the patient's skin is exposed to moisture	☐ Completely moist	☐ Very moist	☒ Occasionally moist	☐ Rarely moist
Degree of physical activity the patient is capable of	☐ Bedfast	☒ Chair fast	☐ Walks occasionally	☐ Walks frequently
Patient's ability to change and control body position	☐ Completely immobile	☐ Very limited	☒ Slightly limited	☐ No limitation
Patient's usual food intake pattern	☐ Very poor	☒ Probably inadequate	☐ Adequate	☐ Excellent
Friction/shear of the patient's skin when moving in bed	☐ Problem	☒ Potential problem	☐ No apparent problem	

Integumentary core assessment
☐ *Findings WNL: Skin warm, dry, intact, turgor adequate; Braden total > 18*
(Describe wounds, incisions, lesions, and pressure, ulcers in next section)

Integumentary core assessment
☐ *Findings WNL: Skin warm, dry, intact, turgor adequate; Braden total > 18*
(Describe wounds, incisions, lesions, and pressure, ulcers in next section)

Variance/additional findings	Variance/additional findings ☒ No change from previous assessment
(Describe location of variations in Comments)	(Describe location of variations in Comments)
☐ Cool to touch ☐ Rash ☐ Excoriation	☐ Cool to touch ☐ Rash ☐ Excoriation
☐ Diaphoretic ☐ Ecchymosis ☒ Blistered	☐ Diaphoretic ☐ Ecchymosis ☐ Blistered
☐ Turgor sluggish ☐ Petechiae ☐ Denuded	☐ Turgor sluggish ☐ Petechiae ☐ Denuded
☒ Redness ☐ Itching ☐ Weeping	☐ Redness ☐ Itching ☐ Weeping

Comments: *Redness and blisters noted around sacral ulcer. Heels reddened bilaterally.*

Comments:

Assessment of wounds, surgical incisions, lesions, pressure ulcers	Assessment of wounds, surgical incisions, lesions, pressure ulcers

Description of wound Type/Location/Size/Appearance/ Drainage: Color, Character, Amount	Surrounding skin	Description of wound Type/Location/Size/Appearance/ Drainage: Color, Character, Amount	Surrounding skin
PU-Sacrum - 8 x 9 cm - open c̄ green-grey necrosis in base draining green liq, saturat. ABD	*Red blistered*	☐ No change from previous assessment *Drainage down ↓* *GRN but not saturated through ABD*	*R, Blst*
Heels - Bilateral Rt - 2 x 2 cm Lt - 3 x 3 cm	*R* *R*	☒ No change from previous assessment	
		☐ No change from previous assessment	

Drainage character codes						Skin character codes				
N None	Y Yellow	BRN Brown	ser Serous	c-grd Coffee ground		D&I Dry and Intact	blst Blistered	mst Moist		
R Red	B Black	GRN Green	bldy Bloody	P Purulent		Ex Excoriated	dn Denuded			

0700-1859	1900-0659
Assessment completed by: **Time** _____ **Initials** _____	Assessment completed by: **Time** _____ **Initials** _____

Appendix Q: Discharge instruction form

Harper Hospital
Detroit Medical Center
Discharge Instruction Form (please take this form to your doctor)

Follow-up care	Make an appointment to see
Date of adm: *1-1-00*	Dr. *Feldspar* Date/Time: *1 week* Phone #: *313-555-4569*
	Dr. _____ Date/Time: _____ Phone #: _____
Date of discharge: *1-21-00*	Dr. _____ Date/Time: _____ Phone #: _____

Physical activity

Resume usual activities: ☐ Yes ☒ No
Specific limitations: *Remain off ulcer at all times*

Diet

Type of diet: ☐ Regular ☒ Modified, specify *Ensure supp.*
Printed instructions given: ☐ Yes ☒ No
Instructions: *Take one 3x a day*

Medication

Special instructions: ☐ None

Vicodin ES	*Take one or 2 every 4-6 hours as needed*
Pepcid 20 mg	*Take one 2x day*
Cipro 750 mg	*Take one 2x day x 14 days*
Multivitamins	*Take one daily*
Vit C 1000 mg	*Take one daily*

Post-discharge plan

1) *Change dressing every 8 hours - use saline gauze in wound. Keep wound moist. Use protective barrier on skin around ulcer.*
2) *Monitor wound and skin as instructed.*

Physician Signature _*J. Feldspar MD*_ Date *1-21-00*

Special instructions

(i.e. equipment/ supplies /treatments)

Home care agency: *RENAISSANCE HOMECARE* Date of visit: *1-28-00*
Equipment supplier: *W&F Medical Supplies* Delivery date: *1-21-00*

I have been instructed and understand the above information.

Signature *Janella Brown* Date *1/21/00*
(patient or person receiving instructions)
Signature of Nurse *Raquel Robertson, RN* Date *1/21/00*

Appendix R: Continuing patient care form

Harper Hospital
Detroit Medical Center

Continuing Patient Care Form (Side 1)

Patient	Last name	First name	TO: Agency name and address
	Brown,	Janella	Renaissance

Address for care	City or Twp.	FROM: Hospital, Clinic, E.C.F. and address
4291 West	Detroit MI 48203	Harper Hospital
Phone 555-123-4561		

Patient's address, if not same as above	Phone	Referral date 1/21/00	Reported by:
N/a		Agency 1st Visit 1/21/00	Reported to:

Complete birth date	Sex	Marital status	Date
10/1/11	M /F	S M W D Sep	Hospital for drugs or services

Responsible relative or friend.		Medicare No.
Ella Brown		Medicaid No.

Relationship Mother	Phone 555-123-5618	Blue Cross No. XYZ 411 590 803 320 GP# 666444

Hospital Case No.	Room No.	Admission	Other Ins. (Give name)
480-55-4856	302W	Discharge 1/21/00	

II. Report by physician

Diagnoses: List primary first and date of onset
Infected sacral pressure ulcer

Prognosis	Good ☐	Fair ☒	Guarded ☐	Poor ☐
Patient informed of diagnosis		Yes ☒	No ☐	
Family informed of diagnosis		Yes ☒	No ☐	

Surgery performed (Type and date)
Bedside debridement

Brief medical history:
1996-MVA Paraplegia
Multiple UTIs — now on IS q4h
Sacral pressure ulcer

Complications
None

Rehabilitation or treatment goal:
Healed ulcer - Prevent further ulceration
Maximize function

Date and place of physician's next visit:
Home ☐   Office ☐   Clinic ☐   E.C.F. ☐

Medical orders and plan of treatment

Minimum number of hosp. days saved. ☐

Rehabilitation or treatment goal:

Diet (Specify)
Reg 1800 cal Ē Ensure supplements TID

Dressings or treatment (Specify)
Change dressing q8h-use saline gauze in wound. Keep wound moist. use protective barrier on skin around ulcer.

Catheter ☐ Size 16 Self-cath q4h **Frequency of change** _____ **Irrigation Solution** _____ **Amount** _____ **Frequency** _____

Enema (Specify)

Medications: Vicodin Es 1-2 q 4-6h prn pain   Multivitamins 1 daily   Pepcid 20 mg - 1 2X day
Cipro 750 mg BID x 14 days   Vitamin C 1000 mg daily

Specify therapeutic Exercise Program
Turn q 2 h while in bed. ↑upper body strength with upper body exercises. Schedule small shifts in body wt.

Activity allowance:
May be in chair no more than 20 minutes at a time

Patient Uses: Prostheses ☐   Brace ☐   Walker ☐   Wheelchair ☒   Cane ☐   Other ☐ vascular boots
Physical therapy ☒   Occupational therapy ☒   Social service ☐   Speech ☐   Evaluate need for home health aide ☒

Teaching patient or family RN   X
Teach pt. & mother to recognize infection, manage wound, develop schedule to relieve pressure.

I certify that the above patient is under my care and requires the above home health services because he is confined to his home. These professional services are to be provided on an intermittent basis and the established plan contained in the record will be reviewed by me at least every 2 months. These services are needed to treat all of the conditions for which the patient was treated during the related inpatient hospital or posthospital extended care facility approved stay.

Date	Physician's signature	Address	Phone	Signed by Resident
1/21/00	J. Feldspar, MD	3990 John Road, Detroit, MI 42201	555-123-4569	

Continuing patient care form (Side 2)

III. Hospital nurse's assessment: Reason for referral?

Activity limitations:
Ambulatory ☐
Ambulatory with assistance ☐
Confined to Bed ☒   Chair ☒
Chair for 20 mins

Activities of daily living
Independent ☐
Needs assistance ☒
Unable to do ☐

Vital signs with ranges & dates:
TPR *98-78-18*
BP *110/70*
WT *110*

Mental state:
Alert ☐   Depressed ☐
Apathetic ☐   Disoriented ☐
Confused ☐   Other ☐

Incontinence:

	None	Partial	Complete
Bowel	☒	☐	☐
Bladder	☒	☐	☐

X-Ray: Findings & dates
7/9/00 chest-neg

Disabilities and impairments:
Mentality ☐   Amputation ☐
Speech ☐   Paralysis ☒
Hearing ☐   Contractures ☐
Vision ☐   Decubitus ☒
Sensation ☐

In-hospital teaching:
Bowel training ___*const.*___
Bladder training ___*CISC*___
Colostomy care _____
Insulin administration _____
Modified diet Instruction ☐
Copy of diet to patient ☐
Copy of diet to agency ☐
Other ___*Dressings - sacral ulcer and*___
___*around G tube*___

Laboratory: Findings & dates:
Hb.   *10.3*   *7/9/00*
B.S. *100*   *7/9/00*
BUN *1.3*   *7/9/00*
Culture
Serology
Other significant findings:

Allergies
NKA

Special problems and other narrative:
Pt. Lives with mother. Pt is dependent on mother for housekeeping & cooking. Needs reinforcement for pressure ulcer prevention & education.

Diagram to show location, size, and extent of wound, stoma, burn, decubitus, graft, or other affected area.

10 cm
8 cm

Open, granulating base - 3 cm deep at center
Healed blister

1. Place moist N.S. gauze against open wound bed.
2. Cover with fluff gauze and ABD pad.
3. Place film dressing or hydrocolloid on intact skin next to wound.
4. Secure dressing with tape adhered to film or hydrocolloid. Avoid tape on skin.

Signature ___*Rachael Robertson*___   Title ___*RN*___

IV. Report of special hospital services: Dietitian, physical therapist, or social worker, etc.

Treatment plan for G tube:
Dietary - Ensure 1 can TID
*   - Reinforce balanced diet*   *JPW, RD*
*   - Vitamin C and Multi vit daily*

PT/OT-use of trapeze to minimize friction when moving in bed. Teach/reinforce safe transfer techniques.

Signature ___*Andy Winter*___   Title ___*RPT*___

Appendix S: Pressure ulcer home health care plan

PRESSURE ULCERS: PREVENTION AND CARE

CARE PLAN: To be filled in by the nurse or doctor and information explained to the caregiver, patient, or family.

1. Turning schedule — Use the "turn clock."
   Left hip to right hip - Mini shifts - move arms and legs - turn slightly - support back with pillows - keep off back

2. Times for dressing changes
   Sacral/tailbone area daily in a.m.

3. Wash hands.

4. Get supplies together.
   Normal saline   Collagenase ointment   Barrier film packet   Gel-impregnated gauze   Gauze squares   Outer dressing pad
   Paper tape

5. Remove old dressing and throw away in plastic trash bag.

6. Wash hands.

7. Wear "hospital gloves."

8. Clean or rinse ulcer with:
   Normal saline   use gauze squares to dry skin around ulcer

9. Rinse again with:
   Apply small amount of collagenase ointment to yellow areas on ulcer using gloved finger

10. Cover or fill with:
    use hydrogel gauze dressing to fill ulcer. Cover with large pad dressing

11. Tape or wrap dresing with:
    use Barrier film to wipe skin around ulcer. Allow Barrier film to dry. Apply paper tape.

12. Throw gloves away in plastic trash bag.

13. Wash hands.

14. Special supplies

15. Extra foods or vitamins
    vit C 500 mg 2 x day (Crush and pour into syringe barrel connected to feeding tube. Fill syringe with water and allow to run
    through. Give extra water to rinse syringe.)

M. Palmer, RN, ET	Sharon Major
Nurse' signature	Patient/family signature

Appendix T: Outcome and assessment information set

Medicare Home Health Care Quality Assurance and Improvement Demonstration
Outcome and Assessment Information Set (OASIS-B)

OASIS Items to Be Used at Specific Time Points

Start of Care (or Resumption of Care Following Inpatient Facility Stay): 1-69
Follow-Up: 1, 4, 9-11, 13, 16-26, 29-71
Discharge (not to inpatient facility): 1, 4, 9-11, 13, 16-26, 29-74, 78-79
Transfer to Inpatient Facility (with or without agency discharge): 1, 70-72, 75-79
Death at Home: 1, 79
Note: For items 51-67, please note special instructions at the beginning of the section.

CLINICAL RECORD ITEMS

a. (M0010) Agency ID: _269381HC_

b. (M0020) Patient ID Number: _SM962_

c. (M0030) Start of Care Date:
_05_ / _02_ / _2000_
month   day   year

d. (M0040) Patient's Last Name:
ELLIOT

e. (M0050) Patient State of Residence: _PA_

f. (M0060) Patient Zip Code:
_10981_

g. (M0063) Medicare Number: (including suffix if any)
_123456189A_
☐ NA- No Medicare

h. (M0066)7 Birth Date:
_01_ / _08_ / _1924_
month   day   year

I.(M0080) Discipline of Person Completing Assessment:
☒ X 1-RN   ☐ 2-LPN   ☐ 3-PT
☐ 4-SLP/ST   ☐ 5-OT   ☐ 6-MSW

j. (M0090) Date Assessment Information Recorded:
_05_ / _02_ / _2000_
month   day   year

Demographics and patient history

1. (M0100) This Assessment Is Currently Being Completed for the Following Reason:
☒ 1 - Start of care
☐ 2 - Resumption of care (after inpatient stay)
☐ 3 - Discharge from agency — not to an inpatient facility [Go to M0150]
☐ 4 - Transferred to an inpatient facility —discharged from agency [Go to M0830]
☐ 5 - Transferred to an inpatient facility — not discharged from agency [Go to M0830]
☐ 6 - Died at home [Go to M0906]
☐ 7 - Recertification reassessment (follow-up) [Go to M0150]
☐ 8 - Other follow-up [Go to M0150]

2. (M0130) Gender:
☒ 1 - Male   ☐ 2 - Female

3. (M0140) Race/Ethnicity (as identified by patient):
☒ 1 - White, non-Hispanic
☐ 2 - Black, African-American
☐ 3 - Hispanic
☐ 4 - Asian, Pacific Islander
☐ 5 - American Indian, Eskimo, Aleut
☐ 6 - Other
☐ UK - Unknown

4. (M0150) Current payment sources for home care: (Mark all that apply.)
☐ 0 - None: no charge for current services
☒ 1 - Medicare (traditional fee-for-service)
☐ 2 - Medicare (HMO/managed care)
☐ 3 - Medicaid (traditional fee-for-service)
☐ 4 - Medicaid (HMO/managed care)
☐ 5 - Workers' compensation
☐ 6 - Title programs (e.g., Title III, V, or XX)
☐ 7 - Other government (e.g., CHAMPUS, VA, etc.) _____
☐ 8 - Private insurance
☐ 9 - Private HMO/managed care
☐ 10 - Self-pay
☐ 11 - Other (specify)
☐ UK - Unknown

5. (M0160) Financial factors limiting the ability of the patient/family to meet basic health needs: (Mark all that apply.)
☐ 0 - None
☐ 1 - Unable to afford medicine or medical supplies
☐ 2 - Unable to afford medical expenses that are not covered by insurance/Medicare (e.g., copayments)
☐ 3 - Unable to afford rent/utility bills
☐ 4 - Unable to afford food
☒ 5 - Other (specify) _Has PACE_

6. (M0170) From which of the following inpatient facilities was the patient discharged during the past 14 days? (Mark all that apply.)
- ☐ 1 - Hospital
- ☐ 2 - Rehabilitation facility
- ☐ 3 - Nursing home
- ☐ 4 - Other (specify)
- ☒ NA - Patient was not discharged from an inpatient facility
    [If NA, go to M0200]

7. (M0180) Inpatient discharge date (most recent):

_____ / _____ / _____

month   day   year
- ☐ UK - Unknown

8. (M0190) Inpatient diagnoses and three-digit ICD code categories <u>for only those conditions treated during an inpatient facility stay within the last 14 days</u> (no surgical or V-codes):

Inpatient facility diagnosis	ICD
a. _____	(___)
b. _____	(___)

9. (M0200) Medical or treatment regimen change within past 14 days: Has this patient experienced a change in medical or treatment regimen (e.g., medication, treatment, or service change due to new or additional diagnosis, etc.) within the last 14 days?
- ☐ 0 - No [If no, go to M0220]
- ☒ 1 - Yes

10. (M0210) List the patient's medical diagnoses and three-digit ICD code categories for those conditions requiring changed medical or treatment regimen (no surgical or V-codes):

Changed medical regimen diagnosis	ICD
a. *Open wound @ ankle*	(*891*)
b. _____	(___)
c. _____	(___)
d. _____	(___)

11. (M0220) Conditions prior to medical or treatment regimen change or inpatient stay within past 14 days: If this patient experienced an inpatient facility discharge or change in medical or treatment regimen within the past 14 days, indicate any conditions that existed prior to the inpatient stay or change in medical or treatment regimen. (Mark all that apply.)
- ☐ 1 - Urinary incontinence
- ☐ 2 - Indwelling/suprapubic catheter
- ☐ 3 - Intractable pain
- ☐ 4 - Impaired decision making
- ☐ 5 - Disruptive or socially inappropriate behavior
- ☐ 6 - Memory loss to the extent that supervision required
- ☒ 7 - None of the above
- ☐ NA - No inpatient facility discharge and no change in medical or treatment regimen in past 14 days
- ☐ UK - Unknown

12. (M0230/M0240) Diagnoses and Severity Index: List each medical diagnosis or problem for which the patient is receiving home care and ICD code category (no surgical or V-codes), and rate them using the following severity index. (Choose one value that represents the most severe rating appropriate for each diagnosis.)

0 - Asymptomatic, no treatment needed at this time
1 - Symptoms well controlled with current therapy
2 - Symptoms controlled with difficulty, affecting daily functioning; patient needs ongoing monitoring
3 - Symptoms poorly controlled, patient needs further adjustment in treatment and dose monitoring
4 - Symptoms poorly controlled, history of rehospitalizations

Primary diagnosis	ICD	Severity rating					Date of onset
a. *Open wound @ ankle*	(*891*)	☐ 0	☐ 1	☒ 2	☐ 3	☐ 4	*04/28/00*
Other diagnosis	ICD						
b. *Type 2 diabetes*	(*250*)	☐ 0	☐ 1	☒ 2	☐ 3	☐ 4	*1984*
c. *PVD*	(*443*)	☐ 0	☐ 1	☐ 2	☒ 3	☐ 4	*1995*
d. _____	(___)	☐ 0	☐ 1	☐ 2	☐ 3	☐ 4	_____
e. _____	(___)	☐ 0	☐ 1	☐ 2	☐ 3	☐ 4	_____
f. _____	(___)	☐ 0	☐ 1	☐ 2	☐ 3	☐ 4	_____

Surgical procedure _____   Code _____   Date _____

13. (M0250) Therapies the patient receives at home: (Mark all that apply.)
- ☐ 1 - Intravenous or infusion therapy (excludes TPN)
- ☐ 2 - Enteral nutrition (nasogastric, gastrostomy, jejunostomy, or any other artificial entry into the alimentary canal)
- ☒ 4 - None of the above

14. (M0260) Overall prognosis: BEST description of patient's overall prognosis for recovery from this episode of illness
- ☐ 0 - Poor: little or no recovery is expected and/or further decline is imminent
- ☒ 1 - Good/Fair: partial to full recovery is expected
- ☐ UK - Unknown

15. (M0270) Rehabilitative prognosis: BEST description of patient's prognosis for functional status
- [×] 0 - Guarded: minimal improvement in functional status is expected; decline is possible
- [ ] 1 - Good: marked improvement in functional status is expected
- [ ] UK - Unknown

16. (M0280) Life expectancy: (Physician documentation is not required.)
- [×] 0 - Life expectancy is greater than 6 months
- [ ] 1 - Life expectancy is 6 months or fewer

17. (M0290) High risk factors characterizing this patient: (Mark all that apply.)
- [×] 1 - Heavy smoking
- [ ] 2 - Obesity
- [ ] 3 - Alcohol dependency
- [ ] 4 - Drug dependency
- [ ] 5 - None of the above
- [ ] UK - Unknown

Living arrangements

18. (M0300) Current residence:
- [×] 1 - Patient's owned or rented residence (house, apartment, or mobile home owned or rented by patient/couple/significant other)
- [ ] 2 - Family member's residence
- [ ] 3 - Boarding home or rented room
- [ ] 4 - Board and care or assisted living facility
- [ ] 5 - Other (specify)

19. (M0310) Structural barriers in the patient's environment limiting independent mobility: (Mark all that apply.)
- [ ] 0 - None
- [×] 1 - Stairs inside home that must be used by the patient (e.g., to get to toileting, sleeping, eating areas)
- [ ] 2 - Stairs inside the home that are used optionally (e.g., to get to laundry facilities)
- [×] 3 - Stairs leading from inside house to outside
- [ ] 4 - Narrow or obstructed doorways

20. (M0320) Safety hazards found in the patient's current place of residence: (Mark all that apply.)
- [ ] 0 - None
- [ ] 1 - Inadequate floor, roof, or windows
- [ ] 2 - Inadequate lighting
- [ ] 3 - Unsafe gas/electric appliance
- [ ] 4 - Inadequate heating
- [ ] 5 - Inadequate cooling
- [×] 6 - Lack of fire safety devices
- [ ] 7 - Unsafe floor coverings
- [ ] 8 - Inadequate stair railings
- [ ] 9 - Improperly stored hazardous materials
- [ ] 10 - Lead-based paint
- [ ] 11 - Other (specify)

21. (M0330) Sanitation hazards found in the patient's current place of residence: (Mark all that apply.)
- [×] 0 - None
- [ ] 1 - No running water
- [ ] 2 - Contaminated water
- [ ] 3 - No toileting facilities
- [ ] 4 - Outdoor toileting facilities only
- [ ] 5 - Inadequate sewage disposal
- [ ] 6 - Inadequate/improper food storage
- [ ] 7 - No food refrigeration
- [ ] 8 - No cooking facilities
- [ ] 9 - Insects/rodents present
- [ ] 10 - No scheduled trash pickup
- [ ] 11 - Cluttered/soiled living area
- [ ] 12 - Other (specify)

22. (M0340) Patient lives with: (Mark all that apply.)
- [ ] 1 - Lives alone
- [×] 2 - With spouse or significant other
- [ ] 3 - With other family member
- [ ] 4 - With a friend
- [ ] 5 - With paid help (other than home care agency staff)
- [ ] 6 - With other than above

Supportive assistance

23. (M0350) Assisting person(s) other than home care agency staff: (Mark all that apply.)
- [ ] 1 - Relatives, friends, or neighbors living outside the home
- [×] 2 - Person residing in the home (excluding paid help)
- [ ] 3 - Paid help
- [ ] 4 - None of the above (If none of the above, go to M0390)
- [ ] UK - Unknown (If unknown, go to M0390)

24. (M0360) Primary caregiver taking lead responsibility for providing or managing the patient's care, providing the most frequent assistance, etc. (other than home care agency staff):
- [×] 0 - No one person (If no one person, go to M0390)
- [ ] 1 - Spouse or significant other
- [ ] 2 - Daughter or son
- [ ] 3 - Other family member
- [ ] 4 - Friend or neighbor or community or church member
- [ ] 5 - Paid help
- [ ] UK - Unknown (If unknown, go to M0390)

25. (M0370) How often does the patient receive assistance from the primary caregiver?
- [×] 1 - Several times during day and night
- [ ] 2 - Several times during day
- [ ] 3 - Once daily
- [ ] 4 - Three or more times per week
- [ ] 5 - One to two times per week
- [ ] 6 - Less often than weekly
- [ ] UK - Unknown

26. (M0380) Type of primary caregiver assistance: (Mark all that apply.)
- [X] 1 - ADL assistance (bathing, dressing, toileting, bowel/bladder, eating/feeding)
- [X] 2 - IADL assistance (meds, meals, housekeeping, laundry, telephone, shopping, finances)
- [ ] 3 - Environmental support (housing, home maintenance)
- [X] 4 - Psychosocial support (socialization, companionship, recreation)
- [X] 5 - Advocates or facilitates patient's participation in appropriate medical care
- [ ] 6 - Financial agent, power of attorney, or conservator of finance
- [ ] 7 - Health care agent, conservator of person, or medical power of attorney
- [ ] UK - Unknown

Sensory status

27. (M0390) Vision with corrective lenses if the patient usually wears them:
- [X] 0 - Normal vision: sees adequately in most situations; can see medication labels, newsprint
- [ ] 1 - Partially impaired: cannot see medication labels or newsprint, but can see obstacles in path and the surrounding layout; can count fingers at arm's length
- [ ] 2 - Severely impaired: cannot locate objects without hearing or touching them or patient nonresponsive

28. (M0400) Hearing and ability to understand spoken language in patient's own language (with hearing aids if the patient usually uses them):
- [X] 0 - No observable impairment; able to hear and understand complex or detailed instructions and extended or abstract conversation
- [ ] 1 - With minimal difficulty, able to hear and understand most multi-step instructions and ordinary conversation; may need occasional repetition, extra time, or louder voice
- [ ] 2 - Has moderate difficulty hearing and understanding simple, one-step instructions and brief conversation; needs frequent prompting or assistance
- [ ] 3 - Has severe difficulty hearing and understanding simple greetings and short comments; requires multiple repetitions, restatements, demonstrations, additional time
- [ ] 4 - Unable to hear and understand familiar words or common expressions consistently or patient nonresponsive

29. (M0410) Speech and oral (verbal) expression of language (in patient's own language):
- [X] 0 - Expresses complex ideas, feelings, and needs clearly, completely, and easily in all situations with no observable impairment
- [ ] 1 - Minimal difficulty in expressing ideas and needs (may take extra time, makes occasional errors in word choice, grammar or speech intelligibility; needs minimal prompting or assistance)
- [ ] 2 - Expresses simple ideas or needs with moderate difficulty (needs prompting or assistance, errors in word choice, organization or speech intelligibility); speaks in phrases or short sentences
- [ ] 3 - Has severe difficulty expressing basic ideas or needs and requires maximal assistance or guessing by listener; speech limited to single words or short phrases
- [ ] 4 - Unable to express basic needs even with maximal prompting or assistance but is not comatose or unresponsive (e.g., speech is nonsensical or unintelligible)
- [ ] 5 - Patient nonresponsive or unable to speak

30. (M0420) Frequency of pain interfering with patient's activity or movement:
- [ ] 0 - Patient has no pain or pain does not interfere with activity or movement
- [ ] 1 - Less often than daily
- [X] 2 - Daily, but not constantly
- [ ] 3 - All of the time

31. (M0430) Intractable pain: Is the patient experiencing pain that is not easily relieved, occurs at least daily, and affects his sleep, appetite, physical or emotional energy, concentration, personal relationships, emotions, or ability or desire to perform physical activity?
- [X] 0 - No
- [ ] 1 - Yes

Integumentary status

32. (M0440) Does patient have a skin lesion or an open wound (excluding "ostomies")?
- [ ] 0 - No (If no, go to M0490)
- [X] 1 - Yes

33. (M0450) Does patient have a pressure ulcer?
- [X] 0 - No (If no, got to M0468)
- [ ] 1 - Yes

33a. (M0450) Current number of pressure ulcers at each stage: (Circle one response for each stage.)

Pressure ulcer stages
a) Stage 1: Nonblanchable erythema of intact skin; heralding of skin ulceration. In darker skin, warmth, edema, hardness, or discolored skin may be indicators. Number of pressure ulcers 0   1   2   3   4 or more
b) Stage 2: Partial thickness skin loss involving epidermis and/or dermis. The ulcer is superficial and presents clinically as an abrasion, blister, or shallow crater. Number of pressure ulcers 0   1   2   3   4 or more
c) Stage 3: Full-thickness skin loss involving damage or necrosis of subcutaneous tissue that may extend down to, but not through, underlying fascia. The ulcer presents clinically as a deep crater with or without undermining of adjacent tissue. Number of pressure ulcers 0   1   2   3   4 or more
d) Stage 4: Full-thickness skin loss with extensive destruction, tissue, necrosis, or damage to muscle, bone, or supporting structures (e.g., tendon, joint capsule, etc.) Number of pressure ulcers 0   1   2   3   4 or more
e) In addition to the above, is there at least one pressure ulcer that cannot be observed due to the presence of eschar or a nonremovable dressing, including casts? [X] 0 - No   [ ] 1 - Yes

33b. (M0460) Stage of most problematic (observable) pressure ulcer:
- [ ] 1 - Stage 1
- [ ] 2 - Stage 2
- [ ] 3 - Stage 3
- [ ] 4 - Stage 4
- [ ] NA - No observable pressure ulcer

33c. (M0464) Status of most problematic (observable) pressure ulcer:
- ☐ 1 - Fully granulating
- ☐ 2 - Early/partial granulation
- ☐ 3 - Not healing
- ☐ NA - No observable pressure ulcer

34. (M0468) Does this patient have a stasis ulcer?
- ☐ 0 - No (If no, go to M0482)
- ☒ 1 - Yes

34a. (M0470) Current number of observable stasis ulcer(s):
- ☐ 0 - Zero
- ☒ 1 - One
- ☐ 2 - Two
- ☐ 3 - Three
- ☐ 4 - Four or more

34b. (M0474) Does this patient have at least one stasis ulcer that cannot be observed due to the presence of a nonremovable dressing?
- ☒ 0 - No
- ☐ 1 - Yes

34c. (M0475) Status of most problematic (observable) stasis ulcer:
- ☐ 1 - Fully granulating
- ☒ 2 - Early/partial granulation
- ☐ 3 - Not healing
- ☐ NA - No observable stasis ulcer

35. (M0482) Does this patient have a surgical wound?
- ☒ 0 - No (If no, go to M0490)
- ☐ 1 - Yes

35a. (M0484) Current number of (observable) surgical wounds: (If a wound is partially closed but has more than one opening, consider each opening as a separate wound.)
- ☐ 0 - Zero
- ☐ 1 - One
- ☐ 2 - Two
- ☐ 3 - Three
- ☐ 4 - Four or more

35b. (M0486) Does this patient have at least one surgical wound that cannot be observed due to the presence of a nonremovable dressing?
- ☐ 0 - No
- ☐ 1 - Yes

35c. (M0488) Status of most problematic (observable) surgical wound:
- ☐ 1- Fully granulating
- ☐ 2 - Early/partial granulation
- ☐ 3 - Not healing
- ☐ NA - No observable surgical wound

Respiratory Status
36. (M0490) When is the patient dyspneic or noticeably short of breath?
- ☐ 0 - Never; patient is not short of breath
- ☒ 1 - When walking more than 20 feet, climbing stairs
- ☐ 2 - With moderate exertion (e.g., while dressing, using commode, or bedpan, walking distances less than 20 feet)
- ☐ 3 - With minimal exertion (e.g., while eating, talking, or performing other ADLs) or with agitation
- ☐ 4 - At rest (during day or night)

37. (M0500) Respiratory treatments utilized at home: (Mark all that apply.)
- ☐ 1 - Oxygen (intermittent or continuous)
- ☐ 2 - Ventilator (continually or at night)
- ☐ 3 - Continuous positive airway pressure
- ☒ 4 - None of the above

Elimination status
38. (M0510) Has this patient been treated for a urinary tract infection in the past 14 days?
- ☒ 0 - No
- ☐ 1 - Yes
- ☐ NA - Patient on prophylactic treatment
- ☐ UK - Unknown

39. (M0520) Urinary incontinence or urinary catheter presence:
- ☒ 0 - No incontinence or catheter (includes anuria or ostomy for urinary drainage) (If no, go to M0540)
- ☐ 1 - Patient is incontinent
- ☐ 2 - Patient requires a urinary catheter (i.e., external, indwelling, intermittent, suprapubic) (Go to M0540)

40. (M0530) When does urinary incontinence occur?
- ☐ 0 - Timed voiding defers incontinence
- ☐ 1 - During the night only
- ☐ 2 - During the day and night

41. (M0540) Bowel incontinence frequency:
- ☒ 0 - Very rarely or never has bowel incontinence
- ☐ 1 - Less than once weekly
- ☐ 2 - One to three times weekly
- ☐ 3 - Four to six times weekly
- ☐ 4 - On a daily basis
- ☐ 5 - More often than once daily
- ☐ NA - Patient has ostomy for bowel elimination
- ☐ UK - Unknown

42. (M0550) Ostomy for bowel elimination: Does this patient have an ostomy for bowel elimination that (within the last 14 days): a) was related to an inpatient facility stay, or b) necessitated a change in medical or treatment regimen?
- ☒ 0 - Patient does not have an ostomy for bowel elimination
- ☐ 1 - Patient's ostomy was not related to an inpatient stay and did not necessitate change in medical or treatment regimen
- ☐ 2 - Ostomy was related to an inpatient stay or did necessitate change in medical or treatment regimen

Neuro/Emotional/Behavior status
43. (M0560) Cognitive functioning: (patient's current level of alertness, orientation, comprehension, concentration, and immediate memory for simple commands)
- ☐ 0 - Alert/oriented, able to focus and shift attention, comprehends and recalls task directions independently
- ☒ 1 - Requires prompting (cuing, repetition, reminders) only under stressful or unfamiliar conditions
- ☐ 2 - Requires assistance and some direction in specific situations (e.g., on all tasks involving shifting of attention), or consistently requires low stimulus environment due to distractibility
- ☐ 3 - Requires considerable assistance in routine situations; is not alert and oriented or is unable to shift attention and recall directions more than half the time
- ☐ 4 - Totally dependent due to disturbances such as constant disorientation, coma, persistent vegetative state, or delirium

44. (M0570) When confused (reported or observed):
- [x] 0 - Never
- [ ] 1 - In new or complex situations only
- [ ] 2 - On awakening or at night only
- [ ] 3 - During the day and evening, but not constantly
- [ ] 4 - Constantly
- [ ] NA - Patient nonresponsive

45. (M0580) When anxious (reported or observed):
- [ ] 0 - None of the time
- [ ] 1 - Less often than daily
- [x] 2 - Daily, but not constantly
- [ ] 3 - All of the time
- [ ] NA - Patient nonresponsive

46. (M0590) Depressive feelings reported or observed in patient: (Mark all that apply.)
- [ ] 1 - Depressed mood (e.g., feeling sad, tearful)
- [ ] 2 - Sense of failure or self-reproach
- [x] 3 - Hopelessness
- [ ] 4 - Recurrent thoughts of death
- [ ] 5 - Thoughts of suicide
- [ ] 6 - None of the above feelings observed or reported

47. (M0600) Patient behaviors (reported or observed): (Mark all that apply.)
- [ ] 1 - Indecisiveness, lack of concentration
- [ ] 2 - Diminished interest in most activities
- [ ] 3 - Sleep disturbances
- [ ] 4 - Recent change in appetite or weight
- [ ] 5 - Agitation
- [ ] 6 - A suicide attempt
- [x] 7 - None of the above behaviors observed or reported

48. (M0610) Behaviors demonstrated at least once a week (reported or observed): (Mark all that apply.)
- [ ] 1 - Memory deficit: failure to recognize familiar persons/places, inability to recall events of past 24 hours, significant memory loss so that supervision is required
- [ ] 2 - Impaired decision-making: failure to perform usual ADLs or IADLs, inability to appropriately stop activities jeopardizes safety through actions
- [ ] 3 - Verbal disruption: yelling, threatening, excessive profanity, sexual references, etc.
- [ ] 4 - Physical aggression: aggressive or combative to self and others (e.g., hits self, throws objects, punches, performs dangerous maneuvers with wheelchair or other objects)
- [ ] 5 - Disruptive, infantile, or socially inappropriate behavior (excludes verbal actions)
- [ ] 6 - Delusional, hallucinatory, or paranoid behavior
- [x] 7 - None of the above behaviors demonstrated

49. (M0620) Frequency of behavior problems (reported or observed) (e.g., wandering episodes, self-abuse, verbal disruption, physical aggression, etc.):
- [x] 0 - Never
- [ ] 1 - Less than once a month
- [ ] 2 - Once a month
- [ ] 3 - Several times each month
- [ ] 4 - Several times a week
- [ ] 5 - At least daily

50. (M0630) Is this patient receiving psychiatric nursing services at home provided by a qualified psychiatric nurse?
- [x] 0 - No
- [ ] 1 - Yes

ADL/IADLs

For Questions 51 to 67, complete the "current" column for all patients. For these same items, complete the "prior" column at start of care or resumption of care; mark the level that corresponds to the patient's condition 14 days prior to the start of care.
In all cases, record what the patient is able to do.

51. (M0640) Grooming: Ability to tend to personal hygiene needs (i.e., washing face and hands, hair care, shaving or makeup, teeth or denture care, fingernail care):

Prior	Current	
[x]	[ ]	0 - Able to groom self unaided, with or without the use of assistive devices or adapted methods
[ ]	[ ]	1 - Grooming utensils must be placed within reach before able to complete grooming activities
[ ]	[x]	2 - Someone must assist the patient to groom self
[ ]	[ ]	3 - Depends entirely upon someone else for grooming needs
[ ]		UK - Unknown

52. (M0650) Ability to dress upper body (with or without dressing aids), including pullovers, undergarments, front-opening shirts and blouses, managing zippers, buttons, and snaps:

Prior	Current	
[x]	[ ]	0 - Able to get clothes out of closets and drawers, put them on, and remove them from the upper body without assistance
[ ]	[x]	1 - Able to dress upper body without assistance if clothing is laid out or handed to the patient
[ ]	[ ]	2 - Someone must help put on upper body clothing
[ ]	[ ]	3 - Depends entirely upon another person to dress the upper body
[ ]		UK - Unknown

53. (M0660) Ability to dress lower body (with or without dressing aids), including slacks, undergarments, socks or nylons, shoes:

Prior	Current	
[x]	[ ]	0 - Able to obtain, put on, and remove clothing and shoes without assistance
[ ]	[ ]	1 - Able to dress lower body without assistance if clothing and shoes are laid out or handed to patient
[ ]	[x]	2 - Someone must help put on undergarments, slacks, socks or nylons, and shoes
[ ]	[ ]	3 - Depends entirely upon another person to dress lower body
[ ]		UK - Unknown

54. (M0670) Bathing: Ability to wash entire body; excludes grooming (washing face and hands only):

Prior	Current	
☐	☐	0 - Able to bathe self in shower or tub independently
☒	☐	1 - With the use of devices, able to bathe self in shower or tub independently
☐	☐	2 - Able to bathe in shower or tub with the assistance of another person: (a) for intermittent supervision or encouragement or reminders OR (b) to get in and out of the shower or tub OR (c) for washing difficult-to-reach areas
☐	☒	3 - Participates in bathing self in shower or tub, but requires presence of another person throughout the bath for assistance or supervision
☐	☐	4 - Unable to use the shower or tub and is bathed in bed or bedside chair
☐	☐	5 - Unable to effectively participate in bathing and is totally bathed by another person
☐		UK - Unknown

55. (M0680) Toileting: Ability to get to and from the toilet or bedside commode:

Prior	Current	
☒	☒	0 - Able to get to and from the toilet independently with or without a device
☐	☐	1 - When reminded, assisted, or supervised by another person, able to get to and from the toilet
☐	☐	2 - Unable to get to and from the toilet but is able to use a bedside commode (with or without assistance)
☐	☐	3 - Unable to get to and from the toilet or bedside commode but is able to use a bedpan/urinal independently
☐	☐	4 - Totally dependent in toileting
☐		UK - Unknown

56. (M0690) Transferring: Ability to move from bed to chair, on and off toilet or commode, into and out of tub or shower, and ability to turn and position self in bed if patient is bedfast:

Prior	Current	
☐	☐	0 - Able to transfer independently
☒	☒	1 - Transfers with minimal human assistance or with use of an assistive device
☐	☐	2 - Unable to transfer self but able to bear weight and pivot during the transfer process
☐	☐	3 - Unable to transfer self and unable to bear weight or pivot when transferred by another person
☐	☐	4 - Bedfast, unable to transfer but able to turn and position self in bed
☐	☐	5 - Bedfast, unable to transfer and unable to turn and position self
☐		UK - Unknown

57. (M0700) Ambulation/Locomotion: Ability to walk safely, once in a standing position, or use a wheelchair, once in a seated position, on a variety of surfaces:

Prior	Current	
☒	☐	0 - Able to walk independently on even and uneven surfaces and climb stairs with or without railings (i.e., needs no human assistance or assistive device)
☐	☒	1 - Requires use of a device (e.g., cane, walker) to walk alone or requires human supervision or assistance to negotiate stairs or steps or uneven surfaces
☐	☐	2 - Able to walk only with the supervision of assistance of another person at all times
☐	☐	3 - Chairfast, unable to ambulate but able to wheel self independently
☐	☐	4 - Chairfast, unable to ambulate and unable to wheel self
☐	☐	5 - Bedfast, unable to ambulate or be up in a chair
☐		UK - Unknown

58. (M0710) Feeding or eating: Ability to feed self meals and snacks: (Note: This refers only to the process of eating, chewing, and swallowing, not preparing the food to be eaten.)

Prior	Current	
☒	☒	0 - Able to feed self independently
☐	☐	1 - Able to feed self independently but requires: (a) meal set-up OR (b) intermittent assistance or supervision from another person; OR (c) a liquid, pureed, or ground meat diet
☐	☐	2 - Unable to feed self and must be assisted or supervised throughout the meal/snack
☐	☐	3 - Able to take in nutrients orally and receives supplemental nutrients through a nasogastric tube or gastrostomy
☐	☐	4 - Unable to take in nutrients orally and is fed nutrients through a nasogastric tube or gastrostomy
☐	☐	5 - Unable to take in nutrients orally or by tube feeding
☐		UK - Unknown

59. (M0720) Planning and preparing light meals (e.g., cereal, sandwich) or reheat delivered meals:

Prior	Current	
☒	☐	0 - (a) Able to independently plan and prepare all light meals for self or reheat delivered meals; OR (b) Is physically, cognitively, and mentally able to prepare light meals on a regular basis but has not routinely performed light meal preparation in the past (i.e., prior to this home care admission)
☐	☒	1 - Unable to prepare light meals on a regular basis due to physical, cognitive, or mental limitations
☐	☐	2 - Unable to prepare any light meals or reheat any delivered meals
☐		UK - Unknown

60. (M0730) Transportation: physical and mental ability to safely use a car, taxi, or public transportation (bus, train, subway):

Prior	Current	
☐	☐	0 - Able to independently drive a regular or adapted car, OR uses a regular or handicap-accessible public bus
☒	☒	1 - Able to ride in a car only when driven by another person; OR able to use a bus or handicap van only when assisted or accompanied by another per-son
☐	☐	2 - Unable to ride in a car, taxi, bus, or van, and requires transportation by ambulance
☐		UK - Unknown

61. (M0740) Laundry: Ability to do own laundry—to carry laundry to and from washing machine, to use washer and dryer, to wash small items by hand:

Prior	Current	
☐	☐	0 - (a) Able to take care of all laundry tasks independently; OR (b) Physically, cognitively, and mentally able to do laundry and access facilities, but has not routinely performed laundry tasks in the past (i.e., prior to this home care admission)
☒	☐	1 - Able to do only light laundry, such as minor hand wash or light washer loads; due to physical, cognitive, or mental limitations, needs assistance with heavy laundry such as carrying large loads of laundry
☐	☒	2 - Unable to do any laundry due to physical limitation or needs continual supervision and assistance due to cognitive or mental limitation
☐		UK - Unknown

62. (M0750) Housekeeping: Ability to safely and effectively perform light housekeeping and heavier cleaning tasks:

Prior	Current	
☐	☐	0 - (a) Able to independently perform all housekeeping tasks; OR (b) Physically, cognitively, and mentally able to perform all housekeeping tasks but has not routinely participated in housekeeping tasks in the past (i.e., prior to this home care admission)
☐	☐	1 - Able to perform only light housekeeping (e.g., dusting, wiping kitchen counters) tasks independently
☐	☐	2 - Able to perform housekeeping tasks with intermittent assistance or supervision from another person
☐	☐	3 - Unable to consistently perform any housekeeping tasks unless assisted by another person throughout the proces
☒	☒	4 - Unable to effectively participate in any housekeeping tasks
☐		UK - Unknown

63. (M0760) Shopping: Ability to plan for, select, and purchase items in a store and to carry them home or arrange delivery:

Prior	Current	
☐	☐	0 - (a) Able to plan for shopping needs and independently perform shopping tasks, including carrying packages; OR (b) Physically, cognitively, and mentally able to take care of shopping, but has not done shopping in the past (i.e., prior to this home care admission)
☐	☐	1 - Able to go shopping, but needs some assistance: (a) By self is able to do only light shopping and carry small packages, but needs someone to do occasional major shopping; OR (b) Unable to go shopping alone, but can go with someone to assist
☒	☒	2 - Unable to go shopping, but is able to identify items needed, place orders, and arrange home delivery
☐	☐	3 - Needs someone to do all shopping and errands
☐		UK - Unknown

64. (M0770) Ability to use telephone: Ability to answer the phone, dial numbers, and effectively use the telephone to communicate:

Prior	Current	
☒	☒	0 - Able to dial numbers and answer calls appropriately and as desired
☐	☐	1 - Able to use a specially adapted telephone (i.e., large numbers on the dial, teletype phone for the deaf) and call essential numbers
☐	☐	2 - Able to answer the telephone and carry on a normal conversation but has difficulty placing calls
☐	☐	3 - Able to answer the telephone only some of the time or is able to carry on only a limited conversation
☐	☐	4 - Unable to answer the telephone at all but can listen if assisted with equipment
☐	☐	5 - Totally unable to use the telephone
☐	☐	NA - Patient does not have a telephone
☐	☐	UK - Unknown

Medications

65. (M0780) Management of oral medications: Patient's ability to prepare and take all prescribed oral medications reliably and safely, including administration of the correct dosage at the appropriate times/intervals; excludes injectable and IV medications: (Note: This refers to ability, not compliance or willingness.)

Prior	Current	
☒	☒	0 - Able to independently take the correct oral medication(s) and proper dosage(s) at the correct times
☐	☐	1 - Able to take medication(s) at the correct time if: (a) individual dosages are prepared in advance by another person; OR (b) given daily reminders; OR someone develops a drug diary or chart
☐	☐	2 - Unable to take medication unless administered by someone else
☐	☐	NA - No oral medications prescribed
☐	☐	UK - Unknown

66. (M0790) Management of inhalant/mist medications: Patient's ability to prepare and take all prescribed inhalants/mist medications (nebulizers, metered dose devices) reliably and safely, including administration of the correct dosage at the appropriate times/intervals; excludes all other forms of medication (oral tablets, injectable and I.V. medications):

Prior	Current	
☐	☐	0 - Able to independently take the correct medication and proper dosage at the correct times
☐	☐	1 - Able to take medication at the correct times if: (a) individual dosages are prepared in advance by another person; OR (b) given daily reminders.
☐	☐	2 - Unable to take medication unless administered by someone else
☒	☒	NA - No inhalants/mist medications prescribed
☐		UK - Unknown

67. (M0800) Management of injectable medications: Patient's ability to prepare and take all prescribed injectable medications reliably and safely, including administration of correct dosages at appropriate times/intervals; excludes I.V. medications:

Prior	Current	
☒	☒	0 - Able to independently take the correct medication and proper dosage at the correct times
☐	☐	1 - Able to take injectable medication at the correct times if: (a) individual syringes are prepared in advance by another person, OR (b) given daily reminders
☐	☐	2 - Unable to take injectable medications unless administered by someone else
☐	☐	NA - No injectable medications prescribed
☐	☐	UK - Unknown

Equipment management

68. (M0810) Patient management of equipment (includes only oxygen, I.V./infusion therapy, enteral/parenteral nutrition equipment or supplies): Patient's ability to set up, monitor and change equipment reliably and safely, to add appropriate fluids or medication, and to clean/store/dispose of equipment or supplies using proper technique: (Note: This refers to ability, not compliance or willingness.)

☐ 0 - Patient manages all tasks related to equipment completely independently.
☐ 1 - If someone else sets up equipment (i.e., fills portable oxygen tank, provides patient with prepared solutions), patient is able to manage all other aspects of equipment.
☐ 2 - Patient requires considerable assistance from another person to manage equipment, but completes portions of the task independently.
☐ 3 - Patient is only able to monitor equipment (e.g., liter flow, fluid in bag) and must call someone else to manage the equipment.
☐ 4 - Patient is completely dependent on someone else to manage all equipment.
☒ NA - No equipment of this type used in care (If NA, go to M0830).

69. (M0820) Caregiver management of equipment (includes only oxygen, I.V./infusion equipment, enteral/parenteral nutrition, ventilator therapy equipment or supplies): Caregiver's ability to set up, monitor, and change equipment reliably and safely, to add appropriate fluids or medication, and to clean/store/dispose of equipment or supplies using proper technique: (Note: This refers to ability, not compliance or willingness.)

☐ 0 - Caregiver manages all tasks related to equipment completely independently.
☐ 1 - If someone else sets up equipment, caregiver is able to manage all other aspects.
☐ 2 - Caregiver requires considerable assistance from another person to manage equipment, but independently completes significant portions of task.
☐ 3 - Caregiver is only able to complete small portions of task (e.g., administer nebulizer treatment, clean/store/dispose of equipment or supplies).
☐ 4 - Caregiver is completely dependent on someone else to manage all equipment.
☐ NA - No caregiver
☐ UK - Unknown

Emergent care

70. (M0830) Emergent care: Since the last time OASIS data were collected, has the patient utilized any of the following services for emergent care (other than home care agency services)? (Mark all that apply.)

☒ 0 - No emergent care services (If no emergent care and patient discharged, go to M0855)
☐ 1 - Hospital emergency room (includes 23-hour holding)
☐ 2 - Doctor's office emergency visit/house call
☐ 3 - Outpatient department/clinic emergency (includes urgicenter sites)
☐ UK - Unknown

71. (M0840) Emergent care reason: For what reason(s) did the patient/family seek emergent care? (Mark all that apply.)

☐ 1 - Improper medication administration, medication adverse effects, toxicity, anaphylaxis
☐ 2 - Nausea, dehydration, malnutrition, constipation, impaction
☐ 3 - Injury caused by fall or accident at home
☐ 4 - Respiratory problems (e.g., shortness of breath, tracheobronchial obstruction, respiratory infection)
☐ 5 - Wound infection, deteriorating wound status, new lesion/ulcer
☐ 6 - Cardiac problems (e.g., fluid overload, exacerbation of heart failure, chest pain)
☐ 7 - Hypoglycemia/hyperglycemia, diabetes out of control
☐ 8 - GI bleeding, obstruction
☐ 9 - Other than above reasons
☐ UK - Reason unknown

Data items collected at inpatient facility admissions or agency discharge only

72. (M0855) To which inpatient facility has the patient been admitted?
- ☐ 1 - Hospital (Go to M0890)
- ☐ 2 - Rehabilitation facility (Go to M0903)
- ☐ 3 - Nursing home (Go to M0900)
- ☐ 4 - Hospice (Go to M0903)
- ☐ NA - No inpatient facility admission

73. (M0870) Discharge disposition: Where is the patient after discharge from your agency? (Choose only one answer.)
- ☐ 1 - Patient remained in the community (not in hospital, nursing home, or rehab facility)
- ☐ 2 - Patient transferred to a noninstitutional hospice (Go to M0903)
- ☐ 3 - Unknown because patient moved to a geographic location not served by this agency (Go to M0903)
- ☐ UK - Other Unknown (Go to M0903)

74. (M0880) After discharge, does the patient receive health, personal, or support services or assistance? (Mark all that apply.)
- ☐ 1 - No assistance or services received
- ☐ 2 - Yes, assistance or services provided by family or friends
- ☐ 3 - Yes, assistance or services provided by other community resources (e.g., Meals-on-Wheels, home health services, homemaker assistance, transportation assistance, assisted living, board and care) (Go to M0903)

75. (M0890) If the patient was admitted to an acute care hospital, for what reason was he/she admitted?
- ☐ 1 - Hospitalization for emergent (unscheduled) care
- ☐ 2 - Hospitalization for urgent (scheduled within 24 hours of admission) care
- ☐ 3 - Hospitalization for elective (scheduled more than 24 hours before admission) care
- ☐ UK - Unknown

76. (M0895) Reason for hospitalization: (Mark all that apply.)
- ☐ 1 - Improper medication administration, medication side effects, toxicity, anaphylaxis
- ☐ 2 - Injury caused by fall or accident at home
- ☐ 3 - Respiratory problems (shortness of breath, infection, obstruction)
- ☐ 4 - Wound or tube site infection, deteriorating wound status, new lesion/ulcer
- ☐ 5 - Hypoglycemia/hyperglycemia, diabetes out of control
- ☐ 6 - GI bleeding, obstruction
- ☐ 7 - Exacerbation of heart failure, fluid overload, heart failure
- ☐ 8 - Myocardial infarction, stroke
- ☐ 9 - Chemotherapy
- ☐ 10 - Scheduled surgical procedure
- ☐ 11 - Urinary tract infection
- ☐ 12 - I.V. catheter-related infection
- ☐ 13 - Deep vein thrombosis, pulmonary embolus
- ☐ 14 - Uncontrolled pain
- ☐ 15 - Psychotic episode
- ☐ 16 - Other than above reasons (Go to M0903)

77. (M0900) For what reason(s) was the patient admitted to a nursing home? (Mark all that apply.)
- ☐ 1 - Therapy services
- ☐ 2 - Respite care
- ☐ 3 - Hospice care
- ☐ 4 - Permanent placement
- ☐ 5 - Unsafe for care at home
- ☐ 6 - Other
- ☐ UK - Unknown

78. (M0903) Date of last (most recent) home visit:

<u>05</u> / <u>02</u> / <u>2000</u>

month day year

79. (M0906) Discharge/transfer/death date: Enter the date of the discharge, transfer, or death (at home) of the patient.

_____ / _____ / _____

month day year

- ☐ UK - Unknown

Appendix U: **Product categories**

Generic categories of wound care products are helpful in fostering standardization of language and understanding of product capabilities. The information included here is intended to assist with this understanding by defining the categories and offering general characteristics of the products within the categories. However, all products in these categories do not perform identically; it's the responsibility of the individual clinician to understand indications, contraindications, and labeled usage for each product.

Dressings

Alginates

Alginates, derived from brown seaweed, are composed of soft, nonwoven fibers shaped as ropes (twisted fibers) or pads (fibrous mats). Alginates are absorbent and conform to the shape of a wound. When packed into a wound, an alginate generally interacts with wound exudate to form a gel that maintains a moist healing environment. There must be enough exudate in the wound to convert the dry alginate fibers into a gel. General characteristics of dressings in this category: absorb up to 20 times their weight, form a gel within the wound, facilitate autolytic debridement, fill in dead space, often require a secondary dressing, and are easy to apply and remove.

Biosynthetics

Biosynthetics originally were developed as temporary coverage for burn wounds. Their use has since been extended to short- or long-term use on a variety of skin-loss wounds, including skin tears and donor sites. A biosynthetic dressing may be a gel or a semiocclusive sheet and may require freezing. Biosynthetics foster healing by reepithelialization.

Collagen

Collagen is a fibrous, insoluble protein produced by fibroblasts. Its fibers are found in connective tissues, including skin, bone, ligaments, and cartilage. During wound healing, collagen dressings may encourage the deposition and organization of newly formed collagen fibers and granulation tissue in the wound bed. Collagen dressings also may stimulate new tissue development and wound debridement. Collagen dressings are manufactured in sheets and pads and as particles and gels. General characteristics of dressings in this category: absorb exudate, maintain a moist wound-healing environment, may be used in combination with topical agents, conform to a wound surface, are nonadherent, require a secondary dressing, and are easy to apply and remove.

Composites

Composite dressings are a combination of two or more physically distinct products manufactured as a single dressing that provides multiple functions. To be classified as a composite, a dressing must include the following features: a bacterial barrier, an absorptive layer (other than an alginate, foam, hydrocolloid, or hydrogel), a semiadherent or nonadherent property for covering the wound, and an adhesive border. General characteristics of dressings in this category: may facilitate autolytic debridement, allow for exchange of moisture vapor, mold well, and are easy to apply and remove.

Contact layers

Contact layers are dressings that are manufactured with a single layer of a woven (polymer) net that does not adhere to the wound bed. These dressings allow wound exudate to pass through to a secondary dressing. Contact layers can protect the wound base from trauma during dressing changes and also can be used to introduce topical medications and wound fillers into the wound. The medication or filler is applied first to the contact layer, and then the contact layer is applied to the wound bed. Contact layer dressings require secondary dressings.

Foams

Foam dressings are nonlinting and absorbent. They vary in thickness and have a nonadherent layer that provides nontraumatic removal. Some foam dressings have an adhesive border and may have a film coating as an additional barrier to bacteria. Foams create a moist environment and provide thermal insulation to the wound. They are manufactured as pads, sheets, and cavity dressings. General characteristics of dressings in this category: are nonadherent, may repel contaminants, are easy to apply and remove, absorb light to heavy amounts of exudate, and may be used under compression. Foams may require a secondary dressing, tape, wrap, or net to anchor them in place.

Gauze

Gauze dressings may be cotton or synthetic and may be impregnated, nonadherent, woven, or nonwoven. General characteristics of dressings in this category: are moderately absorptive, cost-effective, and easily available; can be combined with topical agents or other types of dressings; can be packed loosely into tunneling wounds; and can be "fluffed" for maximum absorption capacity.

Hydrocolloids

Hydrocolloids are occlusive or semiocclusive dressings composed of materials such as gelatin, pectin, and carboxymethylcellulose. The composition of the layer that comes into contact with the wound varies considerably among dressings in this category. Hydrocolloids generally provide a moist healing environment that allows clean wounds to granulate and necrotic wounds to debride autolytically. Hydrocolloids are manufactured in a variety of shapes, sizes, adhesive properties, and forms, including wafers, pastes, and powders. General characteristics of dressings in this category: are impermeable to bacteria and other contaminants, are permeable to moisture vapor but not water, facilitate autolytic debridement, are self-adhesive, mold well, provide light to moderate absorption, minimize skin trauma and disruption of healing by being left in place for 3 to 5 days.

Hydrofibers

A hydrofiber is a sterile nonwoven pad or ribbon composed of sodium carboxymethylcellulose fibers. Conformable and absorbent, the hydrofiber interacts with wound exudate to form a gel, maintaining a moist wound environment for healing, debridement, and easy dressing removal. There must be enough exudate in the wound to convert the hydrofiber into a gel. Hydrofibers require a secondary dressing.

Hydrogels

Hydrogels are water- or glycerin-based amorphous gels, impregnated gauzes, or sheet dressings. Because of their high water content, hydrogels do not absorb large amounts of exudate. Hydrogels may help maintain a moist wound environment, promote granulation and epithelialization, and facilitate autolytic debridement. General characteristics of dressings in this category: are soothing, reduce pain, rehydrate the wound bed, facilitate autolytic debridement, fill in dead space, provide minimal to moderate absorption, and are easy to apply and remove.

Specialty absorptives

Specialty absorptive dressings are manufactured as a unitized multilayer product that provides either a semiadherent quality, nonadherent layer, or highly absorptive layers of fibers, such as absorbent cellulose, cotton, or rayon. These dressings may or may not have an adhesive border. General characteristics of dressings in this category: are nonadherent, absorbent, easy to apply and remove; can be used as secondary dressings over most primary dressings; and may have an adhesive border, making additional tape unnecessary.

Transparent films

Transparent films are adhesive, semipermeable polyurethane membrane dressings that vary in thickness and size. They are waterproof and impermeable to bacteria and contaminants, yet they permit water vapor to cross the barrier at various rates depending on porosity. These dressings do not absorb drainage and are changed when fluid accumulates beneath them. They generally maintain a moist environment, promoting formation of granulation tissue and autolysis of necrotic tissue. General characteristics of dressings in this category: retain moisture, are impermeable to bacteria and other contaminants, facilitate autolytic debridement, allow wound observation, and do not require secondary dressings.

Wound fillers

Wound fillers are manufactured in a variety of forms, including pastes, granules, powders, beads, and gels. They generally provide a moist wound healing environment, absorb exudate, and help debride the wound bed by softening necrotic tissue. General characteristics of dressings in this category: may be absorbent, promote autolytic debridement, are easy to apply and remove, may be used in combination with other products, require a secondary dressing, and fill dead space.

Prescription products

Dermal skin replacements

Dermal skin replacements are indicated for temporary wound coverage and maintenance of a viable wound bed while awaiting the availability of autologous tissue. These products are associated with reduced wound contraction and inflammation and provide an organized dermis or dermal analog upon which thin autologous skin grafts may be placed.

Enzymatic debriding agents

Enzymatic agents debride the wound by digesting necrotic tissue. Different types of enzymatic agents include proteolytic enzymes, fibrinolytic enzymes, collagenase, and papain. The enzymatic action of such agents may be affected by the presence of salts, heavy metals, and antimicrobials. Hard eschar should be scored or crosshatched to allow the enzymes to be effective.

Growth factors

Growth factors are proteins that occur naturally in the human body. They cause cellular growth and cell migration and may regulate the wound-healing process. Researchers have identified several families of growth factors: epidermal growth factor, platelet-derived growth factor, insulin-like growth factors, transforming growth factors and related polypeptides, and fibroblast growth factor. Each of these families of growth factors has different cellular activities with selected cells. For example, platelet-derived growth factors, such as becaplermin, are chemotactic for fibroblasts but not for monocytes. Use of a growth factor is an adjunct to standard wound practices, such as debridement, pressure relief, and infection control.

Pain management medications

Wound-related pain should be a primary assessment for patients with wounds. Wound pain can be managed with pharmacologics, positioning, appropriate dressing selection, and application and removal techniques.

Adjunctive therapies and products

Antimicrobial/antifungal/ antibiotic dressings

Topical antimicrobial, antifungal, and antibiotic products are available as ointments, impregnated into gauzes or other types of dressings, and as sprays or powders. Some antibacterial dressings may help decrease wound odor, although they also may emit a chemical odor of their own.

Deodorizers

High bacterial levels, infection, and tissue necrosis in a wound may cause problems with odor. Social isolation or depression are significant side effects of wound odor. Debriding and cleansing the wound are the first steps to reducing odor, along with more frequent dressing changes. Synthetic dressings that include a layer of charcoal also help decrease odor and are available as absorptive wafers and nonabsorptive pads. Air fresheners or odor eliminators may be used as adjuncts with the other methods discussed above.

Electrical stimulation

Electrical stimulation is the application of electrical impulses to treat musculoskeletal pain, muscle dysfunction, and soft tissue trauma by causing physiologic changes at the tissue and cellular level. Electrical stimulation delivers electrical current into wound tissues by the capacitive technique of placing two electrodes in direct contact with the periwound skin or through a moist dressing on the wound. The electrical current has positive or negative polarity depending on the therapeutic benefit desired, such as increased blood perfusion and cutaneous Po_2, increased migration of repair cells into the wound, autolysis, edema management, and bacteriostasis.

Irrigation devices

There are a variety of mechanical means of delivering a cleansing solution to the wound bed. Examples are a 35-ml syringe plus 19-gauge needle, a 35-ml syringe plus 19-gauge angiocatheter, a soft plastic bottle of cleanser/normal saline plus screw cap with irrigating tip, or a pulsed lavage device with various attachments for lavage pressure and vacuum aspiration of the irrigant and/or wound slough.

Normothermic and temperature therapy

Normothermic and temperature wound therapy warm the wound and periwound area, dilating cutaneous blood vessels, which allows for increased capillary blood perfusion and increased tissue oxygen saturation. Normothermic wound therapy does not make contact with the wound but adheres to the periwound skin and surrounds the wound. It transmits radiant infrared heat to the wound through 100% relative humidity.

Oxygen therapy, hyperbaric

Hyperbaric oxygen therapy is the administration of 100% oxygen inspired at a pressure greater than 2.0 to 6.0 atmospheres absolute. Hyperbaric oxygen therapy increases tissue oxygenation and fosters wound healing by supporting white blood cell phagocytic activity. Systemically elevated oxygen levels are translated to the tissues, allowing for stimulation of fibroblastic activity necessary for collagen formation. Thus new epithelial tissue is fostered. Hyperbaric oxygen therapy also may have an antimicrobial effect and may inhibit toxin production of both aerobes and anaerobes.

Tapes

Tapes are used to keep a dressing system (wound care products, pouches, tubes, and drains) in place. Tapes are available in various materials, widths, adhesive properties, and hypoallergenic qualities.

Wound pouching systems

Wound pouching systems are appropriate for wounds that drain more than 50 to 100 ml of fluid per 8 hours or that are draining fluid that is especially damaging to skin, such as pancreatic enzymes.

Tissue load management products

Adjunctive products

Adjunctive products for tissue load management include devices designed specifically for use on the lower limb, special support surface covers and cushions, pads designed especially for use on stretchers and tables, inflation pumps, and patient repositioning schedules.

Mattress overlays

Mattress overlays are designed to be placed on top of a standard hospital or home mattress. Mattress overlays may be static or dynamic and are constructed of foam, air, gel, water, beads, or a combination of materials.

Mattress replacements

Mattress replacements are designed to be placed directly on a hospital or home bed frame in lieu of the standard mattress. Mattress replacements may be static or dynamic and are constructed of foam, air, gel, water, beads, or a combination of materials.

Seating surfaces and back/neck support

Seating devices are available as foam, gel, or water cushions, pads, and chairs. They may be dynamic or static, with a variety of features such as ischial/coccygeal pockets and waterproof materials. Neck and back cushions and supports also are included in this category.

Total bed replacements

Total bed replacements, also termed "specialty beds," may be electric or semi-electric and are designed to replace both mattress and frame. Total bed replacements are available as low-air-loss and air-fluidized devices and may come with a variety of adjuvant features such as kinetic, pulsation, percussion, and vibration features.

Selected references

Bergstrom, N., et al. Treatment of pressure ulcers. Clinical Practice Guideline, No. 15. AHCPR Publication No. 95-0652. Rockville, Md.: Agency for Health Care Policy and Research, December 1994.

Gogia, P.P., editor. *Clinical wound management.* Thorofare, N.J.: SLACK Incorporated, 1995.

Hess, C.T. *Nurse's clinical guide: Wound care,* 3rd ed. Springhouse, Pa.: Springhouse Corporation, 2000.

Krasner, D., and Kane D., editors. *Chronic wound care: A clinical source book for healthcare professionals,* 2nd ed. Wayne, Pa.: Health Management Publications, 1997.

Maklebust. J., and Sieggreen, M. *Pressure ulcers: Guidelines for prevention and nursing management,* 2nd ed. Springhouse, Pa.: Springhouse Corporation, 1996.

McCulloch, J.M., Kloth, L.C., and Feedar, J.A., editors. *Wound healing: Alternatives in management,* 2nd ed. Philadelphia, Pa.: F.A. Davis, 1995.

Mulder, G.D., Fairchild, P.A., and Jeter, K.F., editors. *Clinicians' pocket guide to chronic wound repair,* 4th ed. Springhouse, Pa.: Springhouse Corporation, 1999.

Panel for the Prediction and Prevention of Pressure Ulcers in Adults. Pressure ulcers in adults: Prediction and prevention. Clinical Practice Guideline, No. 3. AHCPR Publication No. 920047. Rockville, Md.: Agency for Health Care Policy and Research, May 1992.

Appendix V: Glossary

Abrasion: A wearing away of the skin through some mechanical process, such as friction or trauma.

Abscess: A circumscribed collection of pus that forms in tissue as a result of acute or chronic localized infection. It is associated with tissue destruction and, frequently, swelling.

Alginate: A nonwoven, highly absorptive dressing manufactured from seaweed.

Blanchable erythema (reactive hyperemia):
A reddened area of the skin that temporarily turns white or pale when pressure is applied with a fingertip. Blanchable erythema over a pressure site is usually due to a normal reactive hyperemic response.

Bottoming out: Flattening of the support surface by the body, determined by the caregiver placing an outstretched hand (palm up) under the mattress overlay, below the part of the body at risk for ulcer formation. If the caregiver can feel less than 1 inch of support surface between the patient and the hand, the patient has "bottomed out."

Cellulitis: Inflammation of cellular or connective tissue, usually accompanied by local warmth, pain, swelling, and possibly fever. Inflammation may be diminished or absent in immunosuppressed individuals.

Chemical debridement: Topical application of biologic enzymes, such as Santyl (Collagenase or Accuzyme), to break down devitalized wound tissue.

Collagen: A main supportive protein of skin, tendon, bone, cartilage, and connective tissue.

Colonization: Presence of organisms on or in tissues in which no host-pathogen reaction subsequently occurs.

Contamination: Presence in or on tissues of bacteria, other microorganisms, or foreign material. The term usually refers to bacterial contamination. Wounds with bacterial counts of 10 or fewer organisms per gram of tissue are generally considered contaminated; those with higher counts are generally considered infected.

Continuously moist saline dressing: A dressing technique in which gauze moistened with normal saline solution is applied to the wound and remoistened frequently enough to prevent it from drying. The goal is to maintain a continuously moist wound environment.

Cytotoxic agents: Compounds that destroy both diseased and healthy cells. Examples of cytotoxic agents used to clean wounds include betadine, Dakin's solution, hydrogen peroxide, and some skin and wound care cleansers.

Dead space: An area of tissue loss leaving a cavity or tract. This area is lightly packed to avoid superficial closure before the wound fills in from the base.

Debridement, autolytic: A form of debridement in which self-digestion of eschar occurs.

Debris: Remains of broken-down or damaged cells or tissue or old dressing materials.

Denudation: Loss of superficial skin layers.

Dermis: The layer of skin lying beneath the epidermis. It is highly vascular, tough connective tissue, containing nerves, lymphatics, sebaceous glands, and hair follicles.

Desiccation: Loss of tissue moisture or drying out of the wound bed.

Differentiation: In wound healing, remodeling of collagen from a gel-like consistency to a mature scar. This maturation imparts mechanical strength to the tissue.

Drainage: Fluid produced by the wound, which may contain serum, cellular debris, bacteria, leukocytes, pus, or blood.

Enzyme: A protein that acts as a catalyst to induce chemical changes in other substances.

Epidermis: The outermost layer of skin, which is thin and avascular.

Epithelialization: Regeneration of epidermis across the wound surface.

Erythema: An inflammatory redness of the skin due to engorged capillaries.

Eschar: Nonviable (dead) wound tissue characterized by a leathery, black crust. It often covers an underlying necrotic process.

Excoriation: Abrasions or scratches on the skin.

Exudate: Any fluid that has been extruded from a tissue or its capillaries, usually due to injury or inflammation. It is characteristically high in protein and white blood cells.

Fascia: A band of white fibrous tissue that lies deep in relation to the skin and forms a supportive sheath for muscles and various organs of the body.

Fibrin: The insoluble protein formed from fibrinogen by the proteolytic action of thrombin; essential in blood clotting.

Fistula: An abnormal passage or communication, usually between an internal organ and the surface of the body, or from one internal organ to another.

Foam: A spongelike polymer dressing that may or may not be adherent; it may be impregnated or coated with other materials and has some absorptive properties.

Friction: Act of rubbing two surfaces against one another. It may lead to physiologic wearing away of tissue.

Gauze: A woven cotton or synthetic fabric dressing that is absorptive and permeable to water, water vapor, and oxygen. It may be impregnated with petrolatum, antiseptics, or other agents.

Granulation: Formation in wounds of soft, pink, fleshy projections during the healing process in a wound not healing by first intention, consisting of new capillaries surrounded by fibrous collagen. The tissue appears reddened from the rich blood supply.

Hydrocolloid: An adhesive, moldable wafer dressing (such as Duoderm) made of carbohydrate with a nonpermeable waterproof backing. It has some absorptive properties.

Hydrogel: A water-based nonadherent dressing (such as Transigel) having some absorptive properties.

Hydrophilic: The ability to readily absorb moisture.

Indicator: A well-defined objective and measurable variable used to monitor the quality, appropriateness, or both of an important aspect of care.

Induration: Tissue firmness that may occur around a wound margin. Occurs following reactive hyperemia or chronic venous congestion.

Infection: Pathogenic contamination that is reacted against but cannot be controlled by the body's immune system.

Inflammation: A localized protective response elicited by injury or destruction of tissue. It is characterized by heat, redness, swelling, pain, and loss of function.

Ischemia: A deficiency of blood and oxygen in a body part.

Maceration: Softening of a tissue by soaking until the connective tissue fibers are so weakened that the tissue components can be teased apart.

Mechanical debridement: Removal of foreign material and devitalized or contaminated tissue from a wound by physical force rather than by chemical (enzymatic) or natural (autolytic) forces. Examples are wet-to-dry dressings, wound irrigation, and whirlpool debridement.

Necrosis: Localized tissue death caused by disease or injury.

Necrotic tissue: Dead or avascular tissue.

Neovascularization: The outgrowth of new capillaries from existing capillaries.

Nonblanching erythema: Red or purple areas of the skin that persist when fingertip pressure is applied and released. Nonblanchable erythema over a pressure site is a sign of a Stage I pressure ulcer.

Pathogen: Any microorganism capable of producing disease.

Phagocytosis: The engulfing of microorganisms, other cells, and foreign particles by phagocytes.

Pressure: A unit of force that is applied vertically or perpendicular to a surface.

Pressure gradient: The difference in pressure between two points. The transmission of pressure from one tissue to another, as from the skin to the subcutaneous tissues, causes an increase in pressure to those tissues that are deeper.

Primary dressing: A dressing placed directly on the wound bed.

Pus: A thick, yellowish fluid composed of viable and necrotic polymorphonuclear lymphocytes with necrotic tissue debris partially liquefied by enzymes liberated from dead leukocytes and other tissue breakdown products.

Reactive hyperemia: An increased amount of blood in a body part following stoppage and subsequent restoration of the blood supply.

Sharp debridement: Removal of foreign material or devitalized (dead) tissue by a sharp instrument such as a scalpel. Laser debridement is also considered a type of sharp debridement.

Shear: A unit of force that is applied horizontally or parallel to a surface.

Sinus tract: A blind pouch; a cavity or channel that permits the drainage of wound contents.

Skin sealant: A clear liquid that creates a film barrier to seal and protect the skin from trauma.

Slough:
Nonviable tissue is loosely attached and characterized by string-like, moist, necrotic debris; yellow, green, or gray in color.

Tissue biopsy: Use of a sharp instrument to obtain a sample of skin, muscle, or bone for diagnostic purposes.

Transparent film: Clear, adherent nonabsorptive dressing (such as Tegaderm) that is permeable to oxygen and water vapor.

Undermining: A tunneling effect or pocket occurring under the pressure ulcer edges or margins. This is caused by the cone-shaped pressure gradient transmitted from the body surface toward the bone.

Vascular boot: A boot made from foam and designed to elevate the heel from the bed, thereby relieving pressure while the patient is in a supine position.

Wet-to-dry dressing: A debridement technique in which gauze moistened with normal saline is applied to the wound and removed once the gauze becomes dry and adheres to the wound bed. The goal is to debride the wound as the dressing is removed.

Wound irrigation: Pressurized cleansing of the wound by flushing with fluid (such as 250 ml sterile normal saline) with a nozzle tip.

Appendix W: Internet Resources

Agency for Healthcare Research and Quality
www.ahrq.gov

American Academy of Physical Medicine & Rehabilitation
www.aapmr.org

American Academy of Wound Management
members.aol.com/woundnet

American Association of Diabetes Educators
www.diabetesnet.com/aade.html

American Diabetes Association
www.diabetes.org

American Federation of Home Health Agencies
www.his.com/afhha/usa.html

American Health Care Association
www.ahca.org

American Occupational Therapy Association
www.aota.org

American Pain Society
www.ampainsoc.org

American Physical Therapy Association
www.apta.org

American Podiatric Medical Association
www.apma.org

American Society of Consultant Pharmacists
www.ascp.com

American Society of Plastic and Reconstructive Surgeons
www.plasticsurgery.com

American Spinal Injury Association
www.asia-spinalinjury.org

Association of Rehabilitation Nurses
www.rehabnurse.org/index.htm

Health Care Financing Administration
www.hcfa.gov

Medicare
www.medicare.gov

National Association for Home Care
www.nahc.org

National Institute of Health
www.nih.gov

National Pressure Ulcer Advisory Panel
www.npuap.org

Rehabilitation Engineering Society of North America
www.resna.org

Wound Healing Society
www.woundheal.org

Wound, Ostomy & Continence Nurses Society
www.wocn.org

Wound Source Product Book
www.woundsource.com

Index

i refers to an illustration; t refers to a table

i refers to an illustration; t refers to a table

i refers to an illustration; t refers to a table

Hydrofiber dressings, 304
Hydrogel dressings, 104, 304. *See also* Dressings.
  policies and procedures for, 161-162
Hydrogen dressings, 100t-101t. *See also* Dress-
  ings.
Hyperbaric oxygen, 108-109
Hypodermis, 7, 7i
Hypopigmentation
  postinflammatory changes in, 9
  in vitiligo, 9
Hypoxia, wound healing and, 33-34

IJ

Immobility, assessment of, 42
Incidence, 13-14. *See also* Prevalence.
  calculation of, 229-230
Incontinence, 26
  assessment of, 47, 48t
  skin care for, 83-86
Indentation load deformation, 71
Infection. *See* Wound infection.
Information sources, 16
Insurance, 187, 189, 195, 198-199, 247-248
Internet resources, 313-314
Irrigation, 95-97, 97t, 217
  devices for, 306
  policies and procedures for, 153-154
Ischemia, pressure and, 19-23

K

Keloids, 10
Keratinocytes, 3

L

Lactate, wound healing and, 33-34
Langerhan's cells, 3
Langer's lines, 32
Latex gloves, value analysis of, 238t-240t, 238-
  240
Learning. *See* Clinician education; Patient edu-
  cation.
Leg ulcers, decision tree for, 270t
Legal issues, 252-253
Linen savers, 86
Liquid copolymer film barriers, 86
Long-term care, 195-196
Lotions, 82
Low–air-loss beds, 72, 74-77, 75t-77t, 78i-80i.
  See also Beds.
  policies and procedures for, 172

M

Maceration, 26

Macrophages, in wound healing, 30
Malnutrition. *See also* Nutrition.
  assessment for, 42-47, 43t-46t, 216t
  risk factors for, 216t
  signs of, 43t, 44t, 216t
  wound healing and, 34-36, 90-91
Managed care, 247-250
Mattresses, 72, 89-90
  selection of, 74-77, 75t-77t, 78i-79i
  value analysis of, 235-238
Mattress overlays, 71-72, 73i, 89-90, 308
  policies and procedures for, 174-176
  selection of, 74-77, 75t-77t, 78i-79i
  value analysis of, 235-238
Mattress replacements, 308
Mechanical debridement, 94, 99
Medical record data sheet, 226-227, 227i
Medicare, 189, 195, 198-199, 247-248
Melanocytes, 4-5, 9
Melanosomes, 4-5, 9
Mental status assessment, 42
Minerals
  deficiencies of, 42-47, 43t-46t, 44t. *See also*
    Malnutrition.
  wound healing and, 35-36, 36, 90-92, 91t, 92t
Minimum Data Set, 195
Mobility, assessment of, 42
Moist-to-dry dressings, 94, 99. *See also* Dress-
  ings.
  policies and procedures for, 157-158
Moisture, 25-26
Moisturizers, 82-83
Multidisciplinary team, 188-189
Multiskilled workers, 249
Myofibroblasts, 32

N

National Pressure Ulcer Advisory Panel, 234,
  253-254
Neck supports, 308
Necrosis, care map for, 136-139
Negative pressure, 110
Negligence, 252-253
Nonblanchable erythema, 51
No-reflow phenomenon, 19-23
Normal saline, recipe for, 217t
Normothermic and temperature therapy, 307
Norton Scale, 49, 258t
NPUAP. *See* National Pressure Ulcer Advisory
  Panel.
Nursing care, goals of, 17
Nursing homes, 195-196

i refers to an illustration; t refers to a table

i refers to an illustration; t refers to a table

i refers to an illustration; t refers to a table

---

i refers to an illustration; t refers to a table